PSYCHOTHERAPY
for the TREATMENT *of*
SUBSTANCE ABUSE

PSYCHOTHERAPY
for the TREATMENT *of*
SUBSTANCE ABUSE

Edited by
Marc Galanter, M.D.
Herbert D. Kleber, M.D.

Assistant Editors
Helen Dermatis, Ph.D.
Caitlin McMahon

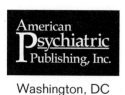

American **Psychiatric** Publishing, Inc.

Washington, DC
London, England

Tables and figures reproduced in this book, unless otherwise noted, are reprinted from *The American Psychiatric Publishing Textbook of Substance Abuse Treatment,* 4th Edition, edited by Marc Galanter and Herbert D. Kleber. Washington, DC, American Psychiatric Publishing, 2008. Copyright © 2008 American Psychiatric Publishing, Inc. Used with permission. *Network Therapy for Alcohol and Drug Abuse* (DVD) copyright ©1995 Marc Galanter, M.D. Used with permission.

Manufactured in the United States of America on acid-free paper
14   13   12   11   10   5   4   3   2   1
First Edition

Typeset in Adobe's New Baskerville and Folio.

American Psychiatric Publishing, Inc.
1000 Wilson Boulevard
Arlington, VA 22209-3901
www.appi.org

Library of Congress Cataloging-in-Publication Data
Psychotherapy for the treatment of substance abuse / edited by Marc Galanter, Herbert D. Kleber ; assistant editors, Helen Dermatis, Caitlin McMahon. — 1st ed.
    p. ; cm.
Includes bibliographical references and index.
  ISBN 978-1-58562-390-7 (alk. paper)
  1. Substance abuse—Treatment. 2. Psychotherapy. I. Galanter, Marc.
  [DNLM: 1. Substance-Related Disorders—therapy. 2. Psychotherapy—methods.
WM 270 P9755 2011]
  RC564.P865 2011
  362.29–dc22

                                                                          2010021471

British Library Cataloguing in Publication Data
A CIP record is available from the British Library.

If you would like to buy between 25 and 99 copies of this or any other APPI title, you are eligible for a 20% discount; please contact APPI Customer Service at appi@psych.org or 800-368-5777. If you wish to buy 100 or more copies of the same title, please e-mail us at bulksales@psych.org for a price quote.

Contents

Shelly F. Greenfield, M.D., M.P.H.
Grace Hennessy, M.D.

Robert L. DuPont, M.D.
Carl M. Selavka, Ph.D.

Nady el-Guebaly, M.D., D.Psych., D.P.H.

David R. Gastfriend, M.D.
David Mee-Lee, M.D.

Carlo C. DiClemente, Ph.D., A.B.P.P.
Miranda Garay Kofeldt, M.A.
Leigh Gemmell, Ph.D.

Contributors

David W. Brook, M.D.

Professor of Psychiatry, New York University School of Medicine, New York, New York

Kathleen M. Carroll, Ph.D.

Professor of Psychiatry, Division of Substance Abuse, Yale University School of Medicine, West Haven, Connecticut

Helen Dermatis, Ph.D. (assistant editor)

Research Scientist, Nathan Kline Institute for Psychiatric Research, Orangeburg, New York

Carlo C. DiClemente, Ph.D., A.B.P.P.

Professor of Psychology, University of Maryland, Baltimore County, Baltimore, Maryland

Robert L. DuPont, M.D.

President, Institute for Behavior and Health, Inc., Rockville, Maryland

Nady el-Guebaly, M.D., D.Psych., D.P.H.

Professor and Head, Division of Addiction Psychiatry, Department of Psychiatry, University of Calgary, and Consultant, Addictions Program and Centre, Alberta Health Services, Calgary, Alberta, Canada

Richard J. Frances, M.D.

Director of Professional and Public Education, Silver Hill Hospital, New Canaan, Connecticut; Clinical Professor of Psychiatry, New York University, New York, New York; Adjunct Professor of Psychiatry, University of Medicine and Dentistry of New Jersey, Newark, New Jersey

Marc Galanter, M.D. (editor)

Professor of Psychiatry and Director, Division of Alcoholism and Drug Abuse, New York University School of Medicine, New York, New York; Research Scientist, Nathan Kline Institute for Psychiatric Research, Orangeburg, New York

David R. Gastfriend, M.D.
Vice President for Scientific Communications, Alkermes, Inc., Waltham, Massachusetts

Leigh Gemmell, Ph.D.
Health Services Research and Development Postdoctoral Fellow, Center for Health Equity Research and Promotion, VA Pittsburgh Healthcare System, Pittsburgh, Pennsylvania

Shelly F. Greenfield, M.D., M.P.H.
Associate Professor of Psychiatry, Harvard Medical School, Boston, Massachusetts; Chief Academic Officer, McLean Hospital, and Director, Clinical and Health Services Research and Education, Alcohol and Drug Abuse Treatment Program, McLean Hospital, Belmont, Massachusetts

Grace Hennessy, M.D.
Director, Substance Abuse Recovery Program, VA New York Harbor Healthcare System, New York, New York

Stephen T. Higgins, Ph.D.
Professor, Departments of Psychiatry and Psychology, and Director, Center for Substance Abuse Research and Treatment, University of Vermont, Burlington, Vermont

Herbert D. Kleber, M.D. (editor)
Professor of Psychiatry, Columbia University College of Physicians & Surgeons, and Director, Division on Substance Abuse, New York State Psychiatric Institute, New York, New York

Miranda Garay Kofeldt, M.A.
Psychology Department, University of Maryland, Baltimore County, Baltimore, Maryland

Eric Leventhal, L.C.S.W.
Psychotherapist, Park West Associates, and Senior Psychiatric/Clinical Social Worker, Bellevue Hospital, New York, New York

Hallie A. Lightdale, M.D.
Assistant Professor of Clinical Psychiatry, Georgetown University School of Medicine, and Psychiatrist, Georgetown University Student Counseling and Psychiatric Services, Washington, D.C.

Avram H. Mack, M.D.

Assistant Professor of Clinical Psychiatry, Georgetown University School of Medicine, Washington, D.C.

Caitlin McMahon (assistant editor)

Research Associate, Division of Alcoholism and Drug Abuse, Department of Psychiatry, New York University School of Medicine, New York, New York

David Mee-Lee, M.D.

Chief Editor, American Society of Addiction Medicine Patient Placement Criteria, Second Edition–Revised; Senior Vice President, The Change Companies, Davis, California

Edgar P. Nace, M.D.

Clinical Professor of Psychiatry, University of Texas Southwestern Medical School, and Medical Director, Turtle Creek Manor, Dallas, Texas

Timothy J. O'Farrell, Ph.D.

Professor of Psychology, Families and Addiction Program, VA Boston Healthcare System, Brockton, Massachusetts; Department of Psychiatry, Harvard Medical School, Boston, Massachusetts

Richard K. Ries, M.D.

Professor and Director of Addictions Division, Department of Psychiatry and Behavioral Sciences, University of Washington School of Medicine, Seattle, Washington

Carl M. Selavka, Ph.D.

Forensic Analytical Chemist, Northeastern Bioscience Associates, Charlton, Massachusetts

Kenneth Silverman, Ph.D.

Professor, Department of Psychiatry and Behavioral Sciences, Johns Hopkins University School of Medicine, and Director, Center for Learning and Health, Johns Hopkins Bayview Medical Center, Baltimore, Maryland

J. Scott Tonigan, Ph.D.

Associate Research Professor, Department of Psychology, University of New Mexico, Albuquerque, New Mexico

Yukiko Washio, Ph.D.
Postdoctoral Fellow, Department of Psychiatry, University of Vermont, Burlington, Vermont

Laurence M. Westreich, M.D.
Clinical Associate Professor, Division of Alcoholism and Drug Abuse, Department of Psychiatry, New York University School of Medicine, New York, New York

Penelope P. Ziegler, M.D.
Medical Director, Virginia Health Practitioners Intervention Program, Richmond, Virginia

Disclosure of Interests

The following contributors to this book have indicated financial interest in or other affiliation with a commercial supporter, manufacturer of commercial products, provider of commercial services, nongovernmental organization, and/or government agency, as listed below. Grants directly supporting work on chapter preparation for this book are listed in footnotes to the individual chapters.

Robert L. DuPont, M.D. — *Grants/Research Support:* Bensinger DuPont & Associates, Washington/Baltimore High Intensity Drug Trafficking Area. *Other:* President, Institute for Behavior and Health, Inc. (nonprofit organization devoted to reducing the use of illegal drugs) and DuPont Associates, P.A. (private practice of psychiatry); Executive Vice President, Bensinger DuPont & Associates (contractual relationships to fund independent advisory committees with Ortho-McNeil Janssen Scientific Affairs, L.L.C., and Novartis Consumer Health, Inc.)

David R. Gastfriend, M.D. — *Employment:* Full-time employee, Alkermes, Inc.; Principal, RecoverySearch, Inc.

Herbert D. Kleber, M.D. — *Consultant:* Alkermes, Inc., Abbott Laboratories, Grünenthal, Johnson & Johnson, Purdue Pharma, Neuromed. *Scientific Advisory Board:* Grünenthal, U.S. World Med. *Speakers' Bureau:* Abbott, Johnson & Johnson.

David Mee-Lee, M.D. — *Royalties:* Level of Care Index and Dimensional Assessment for Patient Placement Engagement and Recovery (assessment instruments), ASAM 101 (home study course), Applying ASAM Placement Criteria (DVD and manual, Hazelden Foundation Clinical Innovators Series).

Richard K. Ries, M.D. — *Grants/Research Support:* National Institutes of Health, Substance Abuse & Mental Health Services Administration/Center for Substance Abuse Treatment. *Consultant/Advisor:* King County and Skagit County, Washington; occasional forensic consultation. *Speakers' Bureau:* AstraZeneca, Bristol-Myers Squibb, Janssen, Eli Lilly, Pfizer, Suboxone. *Other:* Editor, Mid-America Addiction Technology Transfer Center, University of Missouri–Kansas City.

Carl M. Selavka, Ph.D. — *Consulting Scientist:* National Laboratory Certification Program, U.S. Department of Health and Human Services; Trimega Laboratories, Inc. *Other:* Civilian manager, Production Services Division, U.S. Air Force Drug Testing Laboratory, San Antonio, Texas.

The following contributors have indicated that they had no competing interests during the year preceding manuscript submittal:

David W. Brook, M.D., Kathleen Carroll, Ph.D., Carlo DiClemente, Ph.D., Nady M. el-Guebaly, M.D., Marc Galanter, M.D., Leigh Gemmell, Ph.D., Shelly F. Greenfield, M.D., Grace Hennessy, M.D., Stephen T. Higgins, Ph.D., Miranda Garay Kofeldt, M.A., Eric Leventhal, L.C.S.W., Edgar P. Nace, M.D., Timothy J. O'Farrell, Ph.D., Kenneth Silverman, Ph.D., J. Scott Tonigan, Ph.D., Yukiko Washio, Ph.D., Laurence M. Westreich, M.D., Penelope P. Ziegler, M.D.

Introduction

Although over 20% of Americans may have a substance use problem at some time in their lives, only one in 10 of them is receiving treatment at any given time, partly because of a shortage of treatment providers. This shortage is compounded by the fact that many of the clinicians providing treatment have inadequate training in the various psychotherapy and behavioral interventions that have been shown to be effective in substance use disorders. This book attempts to remedy the training gap. The editors of this volume, Drs. Galanter and Kleber, are also the editors of *The American Psychiatric Publishing Textbook of Substance Abuse Treatment*, now in its fourth edition (2008), and the contents of this book have been adapted from that comprehensive textbook.

Although a number of effective medications exist for opioid-related disorders and to a lesser extent for alcohol-related ones, most individuals with those disorders either do not want or do not receive these medications. The situation is even more pronounced for individuals with disorders related to stimulants, sedatives, or marijuana, for which effective medications are lacking. The most common interventions for all of these disorders are psychotherapy and behavioral approaches. Even when medications are available, such interventions may be necessary to keep patients taking their medications and to help them cope with problems in their lives that were present prior to the substance use disorders or that occurred as a consequence of them.

The authors of the various chapters in this book are among the leading authorities on the particular interventions they address. The chapters include relevant case studies and are designed for both experienced clinicians and those new to the field. The book begins with Greenfield and Hennessy's chapter, "Assessment of the Patient," which combines key didactic points with the compassion and insights of two experienced therapists. In increasingly diverse societies in which addiction is an equal opportunity disease, the material that el-Guebaly presents in Chapter 3, "Cross-Cultural Aspects of Addiction Therapy," is of practical importance. The American Society of Addiction Medicine has developed patient placement criteria that are in widespread use by both clinicians and insurance companies; in Chapter 4, Gastfriend and Mee-Lee, who worked on these criteria, describe the reasons behind them.

Motivational enhancement, discussed by DiClemente and colleagues in Chapter 5; cognitive-behavioral therapies, addressed by Carroll in Chapter 7; and contingency management, covered by Higgins and colleagues in Chapter 8, likely represent the three most studied behavioral interventions for substance use disorders; however, these are not the most widely used interventions. We hope the materials presented in these chapters will give clinicians more confidence to try them. In contrast, psychodynamic psychotherapy, discussed by Lightdale and colleagues in Chapter 9, is probably more frequently used because of clinician familiarity but has been the focus of fewer empirical studies than the other three interventions. Its principles, however, can improve insights in and practice of the other modalities.

A self-help fellowship is probably the most commonly used approach in substance abuse interventions and certainly the most frequent referral from the criminal justice system. In the discussion of 12-step facilitation in Chapter 12, Ries and colleagues lay out how to improve the chance of a successful referral to Alcoholics Anonymous (AA), as well as how to use AA precepts in other settings. In Chapter 14, "The History of Alcoholics Anonymous and the Experiences of Patients," Nace presents case histories that can be of use both to clinicians and to patients reluctant to go to AA. In Chapter 10, Galanter and Dermatis discuss network therapy, a multimodal approach to rehabilitation that uses family members and friends to try to achieve prompt abstinence and to involve the willing patient in ongoing relapse prevention activities. The option is presented in a positive manner, and the network members try to be constructive and helpful. In contrast, the intervention approach, discussed by Westreich and Leventhal in Chapter 6, is at times used in situations where the abuser is not interested in halting use or entering therapy.

Other commonly used therapeutic modalities are described in Chapter 11 on group therapy, by Brook, and Chapter 13 on family therapy, by O'Farrell. Group therapy has been shown to be both clinically effective and cost-effective. Family therapy has become more widely available and accepted in the past two decades, though it is not as widespread as group therapy.

Given the addictive nature of abused substances and the stigma attached to the disorders, it is not surprising that self-reports of use often are not reliable either in initial diagnoses or in ongoing therapy. Therefore, Chapter 2, "Testing to Identify Recent Drug Use," by DuPont and Selavka, is of importance.

Overall, we believe this book can be of practical use to a variety of practitioners in the field.

Reference

Galanter M, Kleber HD (eds): The American Psychiatric Publishing Textbook of Substance Abuse Treatment, 4th Edition. Washington, DC, American Psychiatric Publishing, 2008

Use of the DVD on Network Therapy

In network therapy, family members and/or close friends meet together with the therapist and patient at intervals in parallel to the patient's individual therapy. One problem in conveying the nature of a psychotherapeutic treatment such as this in a written document is the difficulty of capturing the actual experience in therapy sessions. In preparing this volume, we were aware of the value of capturing this experience, and we decided to employ recorded segments of actual sessions. This text is therefore accompanied by a DVD that is associated specifically with Chapter 10, "Network Therapy," but is also relevant to other chapters. The video included here was prepared for the American Psychiatric Association to provide an illustration of how network therapy is carried out in practice.

Sessions conducted over the course of treatment were recorded and later transcribed. Identifying information was then removed from the transcript or altered so as to obscure the patient's identity and immediate circumstances. Those segments that best illustrated the nature of the treatment were then reproduced by actors and included in this DVD, along with a discussion between Dr. Galanter and Daniel Keller, Ph.D., following each segment.

Network therapy was a reasonable choice for this undertaking because it shows pragmatic use of a variety of modalities that are reflected in the various chapters of this book. Thus, the DVD deals with the following issues that are characteristic of addictive disorders:

1. Denial and shame are typically impediments to presentation of a comprehensive and valid history. Inclusion of collateral informants introduces information into the sessions that the patient might not reveal or might not be aware of.
2. The distress encountered by patients with addictions may drive them to succumb to the principal symptom the therapist wishes to address, namely, substance use. These patients then may avoid the treatment

setting during a relapse. A patient's fidelity to closely held network members may be helpful in retaining the patient in treatment.

3. Triggers to substance abuse abound in patients' daily lives and may operate outside the patient's awareness. People close to the patient can help to sort these out.

4. Relapse is possible at any time during the treatment, and even long after treatment has been terminated. Having a network of people helps the patient obtain needed help if a relapse occurs.

Evolving Issues in Network Therapy

Until the era in which specific treatments were developed for addictions, clinicians, by and large, had no format specifically tailored for approaching patients with addictions in the office setting. Practitioners would often do no more than tell a patient to return to treatment after achieving abstinence, or to attend AA. Counseling and psychodynamic approaches were found to be of limited impact in resolving addictive disorders.

By the 1970s, new treatments were being devised by clinicians and addiction specialists. Under a federal teaching grant for medical training in addictive disorders, an approach emerged that made use of the various new methods. Network therapy was further developed over the course of the late 1970s and the 1980s as a pragmatically grounded approach for treatment, using a variety of techniques developed by others. Many of those techniques are detailed in this book in the forms that have evolved over the ensuing decades. It is therefore useful for the reader to consider the following issues with regard to certain aspects of network therapy as they pertain to the techniques described in different chapters throughout the book.

Assessment

In network therapy, the assessment phase ideally includes participation of at least one potential network member, such as a spouse. This phase also includes discussion with the patient as to which parties would be appropriate for inclusion in a network.

Patient Placement Criteria

The network therapy approach deals primarily with patients who are substance dependent and who typically require augmentation beyond individual therapy alone to ensure their stability and progress. In this way, network therapy may provide an alternative to residential care.

Motivational Enhancement

Motivational enhancement is provided by supportive network members as well as the clinician. The network sessions are regarded as opportunities for enhancing the patient's motivation for recovery-oriented activity.

Intervention

Classical intervention techniques involve the implied threat of withdrawal of contact and support. In contrast, the network technique employs supportive and engaging social pressure from network members.

Cognitive-Behavioral Therapy

Cognitive-behavioral therapy is a key element of network therapy. Important goals in network therapy are understanding triggers for substance use and anticipating related behavioral change to avert relapse.

Psychodynamic Psychotherapy

Psychodynamic psychotherapy can be used in individual sessions concomitant with the network sessions. An understanding of the patient's dynamics is of great value in framing effective sessions held with network members.

Group Therapy

Network therapy, although it involves a group of people, differs from group therapy in that the patient alone is the focus of attention. Discussion therefore revolves specifically around support of the patient's abstinence and movement toward recovery; other members are not expected to be revealing of their personal issues.

Twelve-Step Facilitation

Twelve-step facilitation can be used to promote involvement of the patient in a 12-step program in both individual and network sessions.

1 | Assessment of the Patient

Shelly F. Greenfield, M.D., M.P.H.
Grace Hennessy, M.D.

Clinicians encounter patients with substance use disorders in all clinical settings. In 2005, federal and state government health care spending in the United States associated with alcohol, tobacco, and drug abuse was estimated to be more than $207.2 billion (National Center on Addiction and Substance Abuse 2009). Based on estimates, there were nearly 113 million emergency room admissions in 2006, and approximately 1.7 million of those were associated with drug use or misuse (Substance Abuse and Mental Health Services Administration 2008). Up to 40% of medical inpatient admissions are related to the complications of alcohol dependence (Horgan 1993), and on any given day, more than 900,000 individuals receive alcohol or drug treatment in specialized treatment programs, with most of these receiving treatment as outpatients (Horgan et al. 2001). In 2004, there were nearly 1.9 million admissions to publicly funded substance abuse treatment programs (Substance Abuse and Mental Health Services Administration 2006). Despite the prevalence of these disorders in both general and treatment-seeking populations, substance use disorders are often undetected and undiagnosed in a variety of clinical settings (Cummings and Cummings 2000; Deitz et al. 1994), and fewer than one-third of physicians in the United States carefully screen for addiction (National Center on Addiction and Substance Abuse 2000). A thorough and accurate substance use history should therefore be a part of any medical or psychiatric interview.

Work on this chapter was supported in part by Grant K24 DA019855 from the National Institute on Drug Abuse (Greenfield). The authors gratefully acknowledge assistance in preparing the manuscript from Rebecca Popuch, B.A.

A number of factors influence the accurate identification, assessment, and diagnosis of substance use disorders among patients presenting for treatment. These include the clinical setting; the style of interviewing; the attitude of the clinician; and patient characteristics, such as the patient's motivation and stage of readiness to change, the presence of another co-occurring medical or psychiatric disorder, and the stage of use or abuse of the substance (e.g., current intoxication, current withdrawal, early abstinence, sustained abstinence, recent relapse).

Successful treatment of substance use disorders depends on a careful, accurate assessment and diagnosis. The goals of assessment of patients with substance use disorders are 1) to identify the presence of substance abuse or dependence, as well as identify signs and symptoms of harmful or hazardous substance use, so that prevention and early intervention might take place; 2) to make an accurate diagnosis and relate this to any other co-occurring medical or psychiatric disorder; 3) to formulate and help to initiate appropriate interventions and treatment; and 4) to enhance the patient's motivation for change. In this chapter, we review principles of eliciting the history of substance abuse, key elements of the patient history, formulation of an accurate diagnosis, the use of biological tests and interviews with significant others, the use of screening instruments and structured interviews, and the enhancement of motivation through the interview.

Eliciting the Substance Abuse History

The interview and elicitation of the substance abuse history are essential to making an accurate diagnosis. The interview setting, the clinician's style of interviewing, and patient factors can influence the accuracy of the history.

Setting

Accurate assessment is facilitated by interview settings that provide privacy and patient confidentiality and permit adequate time to ask key questions, follow up on positive patient responses, and give feedback to the patient. Patients' concerns about confidentiality need to be addressed (Senay 1997). Patients may worry about whether their history will be transmitted to parents, spouses, employers, licensing boards, the courts, or other parties.

The laws governing patient confidentiality—especially with respect to substance abuse by minors—may vary according to state or federal jurisdiction or with respect to the class of drug involved (e.g., narcotic treatment supported by federal funds has strict safeguards for confidentiality). It is important for the clinician to be aware of these particular laws and to communicate them to the patient (Senay 1997). In particular, the U.S. Department of Health and Human Services (1996) issued the Standards for Privacy of Individually Identifiable Health Information as part of the provisions of the Health Insurance Portability and Accountability Act. This privacy rule requires that programs 1) notify patients that federal law and regulations protect the confidentiality of alcohol and drug abuse patient records and 2) give patients a written summary of the regulations' requirements (Substance Abuse and Mental Health Services Administration 2004). A statement that gives the patient accurate information regarding confidentiality can be critical in the patient's willingness to provide a valid self-report. Similarly, privacy in the interview setting can also allow the patient to feel comfortable providing an accurate history. Research studies have shown that patients give valid self-reports when honest self-reporting is encouraged (Weiss et al. 1998) and when they perceive few negative consequences.

The time allotted should be sufficient to accomplish the essential tasks of the interview. For example, the patient should be given several minutes to freely describe his or her problem. The clinician can then move toward a more active style of gathering the history through specific questions. After completion of the history taking, the clinician should take time to provide the patient with a summary of what he or she has heard from the patient, provide feedback about possible diagnoses and treatment options or recommendations, and address the patient's specific questions.

Interviewing Style

The clinician's attitude and style of history taking can facilitate a thorough and accurate assessment. One key to the accurate assessment of individuals with substance use disorders is to be mindful of the great heterogeneity among these patients. Patients with substance use disorders may be of any ethnic background, socioeconomic circumstance, age, gender, marital or partner status, and level of employment. The epidemiology of substance use disorders reveals that there is no "typical" person with substance abuse or dependence (Robins and Regier 1991). The first possible mistake a clinician can make in an assessment is not asking the appropriate questions to elicit the substance use history because the patient does not fit a particular profile that the clinician has in mind. A substance use history should therefore be obtained from all patients presenting for treatment.

Patients with substance use disorders often report that they do not discuss their substance use openly with physicians because of their feelings of shame, discomfort, fear, distrust, and hopelessness (Center for Substance Abuse Treatment 2004; Weiss et al. 2000b). They often exhibit certain typical defenses, including denial, minimization, rationalization, projection, and externalization (Schottenfeld and Pantalon 1999). The clinician needs to recognize these defenses and realize that they can present obstacles to obtaining an accurate history. A number of interview strategies and approaches can help to circumvent these obstacles. It is often useful to begin the interview by asking an open-ended question, such as "How can I help you?" or "What brought you here to see me today?" Allowing the patient to begin in this way can help the clinician understand how the patient defines the problem, and this can set the direction for the rest of the interview. At the start of the interview, the clinician can give the patient several minutes to further describe his or her understanding of the nature of the problem, before moving into a more active and detailed mode of history taking. This technique also allows the clinician to get to know the patient more fully before obtaining a detailed substance abuse history. For example, asking the patient about other areas of his or her life history that might be less threatening, including work, family, or relationships, helps develop rapport with the patient and can help the patient feel more at ease.

Patients with substance use disorders may vary in their insight into the nature of the problem, their readiness to change, their feelings of shame, or their own explanations for what has caused their problem. For this reason, as in most psychiatric interviewing, asking questions in a simple and straightforward manner and maintaining a nonjudgmental stance are most helpful. The clinician can help reduce a patient's shame by carefully phrasing specific questions. For example, the clinician can ask, "How has cocaine caused you problems?" rather than "How has your use of cocaine been a problem?" Instead of asking "Why did you drink alcohol then?" the clinician might ask "How were you feeling before you drank?" or "Do you think there were any specific circumstances or triggers to drinking at that time?" Another approach to diminishing shame can be to phrase questions in a less person-specific manner, such as "Some people with alcohol problems experience blackouts (or other negative consequence or behavior). I am wondering if you have ever had that experience." This technique can be used to convey to the patient a range of experiences that others with similar problems have had and can show that the clinician is knowledgeable about these experiences and is able to hear what the patient might have to say, thereby serving to reduce shame. To avoid using labels, clinicians can ask patients to describe their pattern of use without labeling it. For example, if the patient says, "I just drink socially but I am not an alcoholic," the clinician can explain, "It would be most helpful for me to be able to understand the pattern of your drinking, so if we look at this past week (month, etc.), tell me about your drinking."

As in all clinical interactions, asking questions in an honest, respectful, and matter-of-fact manner is likely to be most effective (Center for Substance Abuse Treatment 2004). Attributes of clinicians that have been shown to be effective in establishing a therapeutic alliance with patients presenting with addiction problems include respect, nonpossessive warmth, friendliness, genuineness, empathy, a supportive style, reflective listening, and a patient-centered approach (Center for Substance Abuse Treatment 2004; Miller and Rollnick 2002). Finally, the clinician's interviewing style should reflect cultural sensitivity, knowledge, and empathy (Westermeyer et al. 2004a). In practically all settings, clinicians will provide care for patients with diverse backgrounds, and such culturally competent assessment is necessary when interviewing patients to assess their substance use history. Clinicians' attitudes toward their own substance use or nonuse, as well as toward their own cultural identity, can affect their attitudes toward patients' substance use, as well as toward patients' cultural and ethnic identities (Westermeyer et al. 2004a).

Patient Characteristics

The interview can also be influenced by a number of patient characteristics that can affect the clinical presentation of a substance use disorder. Bearing in mind this matrix of patient characteristics can help the clinician adjust the interview to most effectively facilitate an accurate history. These patient characteristics include the following:

- Age, gender, partner or marital status, legal and employment status, and culture and ethnicity
- Degree of insight into and explanation for the nature of his or her problem
- Medical or psychiatric comorbidity
- Stage in the course of the illness (e.g., recovery, recent relapse, first treatment)
- Current phase of use (e.g., intoxicated, withdrawing, interepisode)
- Stage of readiness for change and motivation

A number of patient characteristics can influence the approach to the interview. For example, an interview with an adolescent who is dependent on marijuana is likely to require a different interview style than an interview with an elderly widow who has developed a drinking problem in the several years following her husband's death. Women may be more likely than men to explain their presenting problem as mood or anxiety related and may view their drinking or substance use as a consequence of these difficulties and not as the primary problem (Greenfield and

O'Leary 2002; Greenfield et al. 2007). Cultural norms may differ regarding the quantity or frequency of use of a substance and may affect the social acceptability and the patient's description of his or her use (Westermeyer 1997). A growing literature emphasizes an ethnoculturally competent substance abuse assessment that takes into account the patient's views of the effects ethnicity or cultural background may have on his or her substance abuse history or treatment (Straussner 2001). A clinician's lack of knowledge about the ways of life of others' cultures (e.g., social roles, life-cycle rituals, family and social organization, literature, art) or ethnic bias (e.g., bias toward a distinctive subgroup that exists within a culture) can lead to inappropriate diagnosis and treatment (Westermeyer et al. 2006). Clinically relevant areas of inquiry for cultural influences on substance use include normative versus deviant substance use, ceremonial versus secular substance use, and assessment of the patient's social network (Westermeyer et al. 2006). A patient's marital or partner status and employment status may also influence his or her presentation; individuals may present themselves for evaluation at the urging or demand of significant others or because of work or legal complications resulting from their substance use.

The clinical presentation may also vary depending on whether the patient presents for treatment early in the course of the illness or at a more advanced phase. For example, a patient who has intermittent binge alcohol use may present for treatment after a recent legal charge of driving while intoxicated. Although the patient's alcohol use may not yet qualify for a diagnosis of an alcohol use disorder, this interview may allow for identification of an alcohol problem early in its evolution and may provide an opportunity for early intervention. This interview will likely differ in scope and focus, for example, from that of a patient with a 15-year history of alcohol dependence who is presenting for a second admission for detoxification.

The current phase of a patient's drug use will also influence the clinical presentation and interview. Patients may present in different clinical settings in a state of intoxication, withdrawal, remission, slip, relapse, or maintenance. The clinician is unlikely to elicit a valid history from a patient who is acutely intoxicated (Babor et al. 1987). An interview during intoxication may be confined to the ascertainment of acute medical conditions in need of intervention (e.g., respiratory depression, pancreatitis, gastrointestinal bleeding). The complete history is best deferred to a time when the patient is no longer intoxicated.

When the clinician is interviewing substance-using patients who are requesting detoxification or exhibiting signs and symptoms of acute withdrawal (American Psychiatric Association 2006), the most important goals of the assessment are to ascertain the medical need for detoxification and to prevent withdrawal complications. Because untreated withdrawal from alcohol or sedative-hypnotics (e.g., benzodiazepines and barbiturates) can result in seizures, delirium tremens, and death, the clinician must first assess the patient for signs and symptoms of withdrawal. The presence of such signs and symptoms, such as tachycardia, diaphoresis, increased hand tremors, anxiety, psychomotor agitation, nausea or vomiting, and transient perceptual disturbances (American Psychiatric Association 2000), indicates a need for inpatient detoxification. Signs and symptoms of opioid withdrawal include dysphoric mood, muscle aches, nausea or vomiting, lacrimation or rhinorrhea, yawning, fever, insomnia, pupillary dilation, piloerection (gooseflesh), and diaphoresis (American Psychiatric Association 2000, 2006; Center for Substance Abuse Treatment 2004). Although opioid withdrawal is not associated with severe medical complications, inpatient detoxification may be necessary to ameliorate withdrawal symptoms that if left untreated, could result in ongoing opioid use. With the passing of the Drug Addiction Treatment Act of 2000, outpatient detoxification and treatment with buprenorphine or buprenorphine-naloxone may also be an option, and this can be assessed in the interview as well (Center for Substance Abuse Treatment 2004). The clinician can assess the patient's interest in buprenorphine treatment and the patient's appropriateness for such treatment by inquiring about the patient's understanding of the risks and benefits, ability to adhere to the treatment plan and follow safety procedures, and medical and psychiatric conditions, including pregnancy, among other factors (Center for Substance Abuse Treatment 2004). Generally, withdrawal syndromes associated with the use of marijuana and stimulants such as cocaine do not require inpatient detoxification (American Psychiatric Association 2006). Nicotine withdrawal is also managed on an outpatient basis (American Psychiatric Association 2006).

A patient may also present in full, sustained remission from a substance use disorder but may report symptoms of another medical or psychiatric illness or a new onset of urges and cravings. It is important in this instance for the clinician 1) to find out the supports the patient has used to maintain abstinence and recovery; 2) to examine how any other illness, whether it is chronic or of new onset, may be affecting the patient's ongoing recovery; and 3) to ascertain what types of treatments or interventions may help support the patient's ongoing recovery. Similarly, the interview with a patient who presents with a recent slip or relapse to substance use may be directed toward understanding the triggers to the recent drug use and identifying strategies that will help circumscribe the relapse and help the patient get back on the recovery track.

The patient's current stage of motivation for change will also affect the interview (Prochaska et al. 1992). The interview with a patient who is precontemplative (i.e., does not want to change his or her addictive behavior) will usually require more probing to elicit the history. Interview strategies that focus on establishing a pattern of use and that then elicit advantages and disadvantages of such use may be helpful. To establish a pattern of use, the clinician might say to the patient, "It would be helpful for me to understand the pattern of your alcohol (cocaine, marijuana, etc.) use. As you know, people's use of alcohol (cocaine, marijuana, etc.) varies greatly, and it would help me to understand the usual pattern for you." The clinician might then proceed to use a calendar method of ascertaining days of use in the past week, month, 3 months, 6 months, and year (Sobell et al. 1992). For the more recent time periods, the clinician can ask for patterns of use (type of substance, quantity, frequency, time of day, etc.) for each day of the past week or month. For the more distant time periods, it is helpful to anchor the questions in seasonal events or events important to the patient. For example, the clinician might ask whether the patient's substance use was the same during the previous winter holidays as it is currently. Alternatively, the clinician might ask the patient to compare the past week's or month's use of a substance to previous 6-month time intervals, such as by saying, "Would you say the current pattern of use that you just described is the same pattern you have had for the last 6 months? What about the previous 6 months? Was there ever a period when you were using more heavily? When was that?"

A similar style of interviewing can be used to obtain the patient's lifetime substance abuse history. The clinician can ask about patterns of use during successive developmental periods, such as, "Tell me about your first use. Your use in high school? College? Your 20s? After you were married?" until the clinician is satisfied that he or she has understood the course of use throughout the patient's life span.

After identifying these use patterns, the patient might be encouraged to identify any ways in which he or she perceives that the substance has caused negative consequences for him or her. This interview will likely differ from interviews with patients who have had a brief recent relapse after a sustained period of recovery. Elicitation of the latter patients' earlier history is likely to be more straightforward and to require less probing. Such patients are likely to provide an overview of their previous substance use problem and of what helped them in their recovery. These interviews may be more likely to focus on the nature of the recent relapse, the particular triggers to substance use, any consequences of the relapse, and plans to help the patient return to abstinence and recovery.

As in all psychiatric interviews, the clinician's empathic stance is helpful. An empathic capacity to feel the patient's experience but at the same time to maintain objectivity is critical (Frances and Franklin 1989). Patients often feel great relief when they are asked questions about their condition, because these questions reveal that the clinician is knowledgeable about the condition, can understand what the experience of the condition might be like, and may be able to offer the patient relief through some form of treatment. Therefore, the clinician should reserve time at the end of the interview to summarize for the patient what the clinician has heard about the patient's history, the way in which the clinician formulates this, any diagnostic implications that the clinician is considering, and any possible treatment options and recommendations. The clinician may begin this part of the interview by saying, "I would like to save some time to give you feedback about what we have discussed and to let you know some of my thoughts. Before I do this, is there anything else that is important that we have not had a chance to discuss or that you think I haven't asked you?" After the patient has had a chance to add any further information, the clinician can then present what he or she has heard. It is often useful to first let the patient know of any particular risk factors or vulnerabilities that he or she may have. For example, the clinician might say, "It sounds to me as if you have had a number of risk factors. You have told me that both of your parents had alcohol problems, and we know that this is likely to have made you more vulnerable to the substance. Second, you have told me that you have struggled with a mood disorder, and we know that often patients with other psychiatric disorders such as mood disorders are more vulnerable to developing problems with drugs and alcohol." The clinician might then proceed to summarize the history the patient has given and to relate the key elements of the history to specific diagnostic criteria. This should then lead to a formulation of the diagnosis and the treatment implications.

Diagnosing Substance Use Disorders

To elicit key elements of the history that allow the clinician to formulate the diagnosis and to relate these elements back to the patient in a straightforward manner, the clinician should have in mind the diagnostic criteria and use the interview to elicit history that will help establish a differential diagnosis and exclude or include the likely diagnosis for the particular patient. Psychiatric disorders attributable to substances of abuse can generally be divided into disorders produced by the substance's pharmacological effects—such as intoxication, withdrawal, and substance-induced disorders—and disorders related to the pattern or negative consequences of such use (Woody and Cacciola 1997). In DSM-IV and DSM-IV-TR (American Psychiatric Association 1994, 2000), both categories of these disorders are covered in the section "Substance-Related Disorders," which consists of two subsections, "Substance Use Disorders" and "Substance-Induced Disorders." The substance use disorders include both substance dependence and substance abuse.

Substance Use Disorders

According to DSM-IV-TR, a diagnosis of *substance dependence* is made when a patient has had a maladaptive pattern of substance use leading to clinically significant impairment or distress, as manifested by at least three of seven symptoms or behaviors occurring within the same 12-month period. The DSM-IV-TR criteria for substance dependence are listed in Table 1–1. In DSM-IV-TR, it is specified that the substance dependence diagnosis can be further characterized as being "with physiological dependence" if the substance dependence diagnosis is accompanied by evidence of tolerance or withdrawal or as being "without physiological dependence" when there is no evidence of either tolerance or withdrawal.

A diagnosis of *substance abuse* is made when the individual has never before met criteria for dependence and exhibits a maladaptive pattern of substance use leading to significant impairment or distress as manifested by one or more behaviors that have occurred within a 12-month period. The DSM-IV-TR criteria for substance abuse are provided in Table 1–2. Importantly, the criteria for substance abuse or dependence are the same regardless of substance of abuse. The presence of the behaviors and symptoms listed in Table 1–2 within the 12 months before the interview constitutes a current diagnosis, and their presence in any 12-month period earlier in the individual's life is consistent with a past diagnosis.

DSM-IV-TR also provides for a number of course specifiers. *Early full remission* is specified if no criteria for dependence or abuse have been met for at least 1 month but for less than 12 months. *Early partial remission* is specified if for at least 1 month but less than 12 months, one or more criteria for dependence or abuse (but less than the full criteria for dependence) have been met intermittently or continuously. *Sustained full remission* is specified when none of the criteria have been present for 12 months or longer. *Sustained partial remission* is used when the full criteria for dependence have not been met for a period of 12 months or longer but one or more criteria for dependence or abuse have been present. The specifier *on agonist therapy* is used if the individual is taking a prescribed agonist, partial agonist, or agonist/antagonist medication and no criteria for dependence or abuse have been met for that class of

TABLE 1–1.   **DSM-IV-TR criteria for substance dependence**

A maladaptive pattern of substance use, leading to clinically significant impairment or distress, as manifested by three (or more) of the following, occurring at any time in the same 12-month period:

(1) tolerance, as defined by either of the following:
    (a) a need for markedly increased amounts of the substance to achieve intoxication or desired effect
    (b) markedly diminished effect with continued use of the same amount of the substance

(2) withdrawal, as manifested by either of the following:
    (a) the characteristic withdrawal syndrome for the substance (refer to Criteria A and B of the criteria sets for withdrawal from the specific substances)
    (b) the same (or a closely related) substance is taken to relieve or avoid withdrawal symptoms

(3) the substance is often taken in larger amounts or over a longer period than was intended

(4) there is a persistent desire or unsuccessful efforts to cut down or control substance use

(5) a great deal of time is spent in activities necessary to obtain the substance (e.g., visiting multiple doctors or driving long distances), use the substance (e.g., chain-smoking), or recover from its effects

(6) important social, occupational, or recreational activities are given up or reduced because of substance use

(7) the substance use is continued despite knowledge of having a persistent or recurrent physical or psychological problem that is likely to have been caused or exacerbated by the substance (e.g., current cocaine use despite recognition of cocaine-induced depression, or continued drinking despite recognition that an ulcer was made worse by alcohol consumption)

Specify if:
    With physiological dependence: evidence of tolerance or withdrawal (i.e., either Item 1 or 2 is present)
    Without physiological dependence: no evidence of tolerance or withdrawal (i.e., neither Item 1 nor 2 is present)

Course specifiers:
    Early full remission
    Early partial remission
    Sustained full remission
    Sustained partial remission
    On agonist therapy
    In a controlled environment

TABLE 1–2. **DSM-IV-TR criteria for substance abuse**

A. A maladaptive pattern of substance use leading to clinically significant impairment or distress, as manifested by one (or more) of the following, occurring within a 12-month period:

   (1) recurrent substance use resulting in a failure to fulfill major role obligations at work, school, or home (e.g., repeated absences or poor work performance related to substance use; substance-related absences, suspensions, or expulsions from school; neglect of children or household)

   (2) recurrent substance use in situations in which it is physically hazardous (e.g., driving an automobile or operating a machine when impaired by substance use)

   (3) recurrent substance-related legal problems (e.g., arrests for substance-related disorderly conduct)

   (4) continued substance use despite having persistent or recurrent social or interpersonal problems caused or exacerbated by the effects of the substance (e.g., arguments with spouse about consequences of intoxication, physical fights)

B. The symptoms have never met the criteria for substance dependence for this class of substance.

Source. Reprinted from the *Diagnostic and Statistical Manual of Mental Disorders*, 4th Edition, Text Revision. Washington, DC, American Psychiatric Association, 2000, p. 199. Copyright 2000, American Psychiatric Association. Used with permission.

medication for at least 1 month. The specifier *in a controlled environment* is similarly used when the individual has been in full remission for a month or more and the individual is in an environment with restricted access to substances. Such an environment could be a locked hospital unit, a supervised residential setting, or a substance-free prison.

   In addition to individuals who meet criteria for substance abuse or dependence, a significant number of individuals use substances in a way that is harmful or hazardous even though their use does not meet criteria for abuse or dependence or for another substance-related disorder. With respect to alcohol, the World Health Organization defines *hazardous drinkers* as those whose pattern of drinking poses a high risk of future damage to physical or mental health (Babor et al. 2001; Bohn et al. 1995). It defines *harmful drinking* as a pattern of alcohol use that is already resulting in problems (Babor et al. 2001; Bohn et al. 1995). In addition to application of these definitions of *harmful* and *hazardous alcohol use*, in the 10th Revision of the *International Statistical Classification of Diseases and Related Health Problems* (ICD-10), *harmful substance use* is defined as "a pattern of substance use that is causing damage to health. The damage may be physical…or mental" (World Health Organization 1992/2007). This category of harmful use is the closest that ICD-10 comes to the DSM-IV-TR diagnosis of substance abuse. However, the DSM-IV-TR diagnosis of substance abuse focuses on social consequences of behavior, whereas the ICD-10 definition of harmful use focuses on psychological or physical harm. Importantly, the ICD-10 category of harmful use has greater utility cross-culturally, because the social acceptability of substance use may vary greatly from country to country (Woody and Cacciola 1997).

Although the DSM-IV-TR diagnoses of substance use disorders are in wide use in the United States, the concepts of hazardous or harmful substance use defined by the World Health Organization are especially useful to consider when the patient describes the overuse or misuse of substances and the pattern of use, though it does not meet criteria for a DSM-IV-TR definition of substance use disorder, nevertheless increases vulnerability to developing a substance use disorder or is currently creating some difficulties. Such an ascertainment allows the clinician the opportunity to provide education and recommendations that may constitute early intervention for an individual when problem use already exists or that may constitute prevention in the case of someone whose use places him or her at risk. Certainly, an assessment of a patient's risk factors for developing a substance use disorder (e.g., family history of substance use disorder, personal history of problems with the substance, presence of another psychiatric disorder) may lead the clinician to advise reduction or cessation of a particular substance even if abuse or dependence is not yet present. In the case of patients with new-onset psychiatric illness, such as bipolar disorder or schizophrenia, the risk of developing a substance use disorder is great. Moreover, intervention that leads to cessation of any substance use is a good example of prevention (Brems et al. 2002; Greenfield and Shore 1995).

Substance-Induced Disorders

Disorders produced by the direct pharmacological effects of a substance are referred to as substance-induced disorders. These include the intoxication and withdrawal syndromes, as well as syndromes such as substance-induced dementia and amnestic, psychotic, mood, anxiety, sleep, and sexual dysfunction disorders. Although all categories of substances produce an intoxication syndrome, the symptoms, signs, and durations of the syndromes vary by substance category. On the other hand, according to DSM-IV-TR, not all categories of substances produce a withdrawal syndrome or all of the other substance-induced disorders. Knowledge of the syndromes characteristic of each category of substances is important in eliciting an accurate history and clinical status.

Content of the Interview

History of the Substance Use Disorder

An understanding of the major categories of the different substances of abuse provides the interviewer with knowledge about their characteristic intoxication and withdrawal syndromes. With this knowledge, the interviewer is better able not only to assess the patient but also to make appropriate treatment recommendations. It is important to ask patients about all categories of substances and not only the patient's primary substance of abuse.

The following are the major categories of substances of abuse:

- *Central nervous system depressants* (e.g., alcohol) and sedative-hypnotics (e.g., barbiturates and benzodiazepines)
- *Stimulants,* such as amphetamines, cocaine, and phencyclidine (PCP)
- *Cannabis* (marijuana and hashish)
- *Opiates,* including heroin, morphine, codeine, oxycodone, methadone, buprenorphine, and fentanyl
- *Hallucinogens,* such as lysergic acid diethylamide (LSD), mescaline, and psilocybin (mushrooms)
- *Nicotine* in the form of cigarettes, chewing tobacco or dip, and snuff
- *Inhalants,* such as paint thinner, gasoline, glue, and cleaning fluids
- *Designer drugs,* including 3,4-methylenedioxymethamphetamine (MDMA, commonly called ecstasy), ketamine, and gamma-hydroxybutyrate (GHB)

A systematic and organized way of collecting information about the patient's history of substance use is to address the following areas:

- Age at first substance use
- Frequency of substance use
- Amount of the substance taken during an episode of use
- Route of administration for the substance
- Consequences associated with substance use
- Treatment history
- Periods of abstinence
- Relapses

The information obtained by asking about the age at first substance use episode serves as the framework for the history and guides the interviewer's subsequent questions. In addition, the patient's age when he or she began using substances has diagnostic and prognostic implications.

Studies have shown that early onset of substance use (before age 15 years) is associated with the subsequent development of substance abuse and dependence (Chen et al. 2005; Hingson et al. 2006; Robins and Przybeck 1985; Sintov et al. 2009; Wills et al. 1996). The early onset of substance use disorders has also been associated with childhood psychopathology that preceded the development of the substance use disorder (Crum et al. 2008; Hahesy et al. 2002; Ostacher et al. 2006; Sintov et al. 2009).

The age at first use of nicotine is also an important component of the history of the substance use disorder. Studies have shown that nicotine use often precedes experimentation with illicit drugs (Adler and Kandel 1981; Warren et al. 1997; Yamaguchi and Kandel 1984a, 1984b) and is more prevalent in individuals with other substance use disorders (Breslau et al. 1991; Budney et al. 1993; DiFranza and Guerrera 1990). Although it is incorrect to assume that all nicotine users have also used illicit drugs or have another substance use disorder, the age at first use of nicotine in a patient who uses other substances helps the interviewer have a more complete picture of the patient's history of substance use.

Once the age at first substance use is established, inquiries about the frequency of substance use as well as the amount of the substance used and the route of administration (oral, inhaled, insufflated or snorted, intravenous, subcutaneous) help the interviewer understand the progression or regression of substance use over time. For example, a patient who says she started snorting (route of administration) one bag (amount) of heroin once a week for 1 year (frequency) and then began using three bags of heroin per day by the intravenous route is reporting her progression of heroin use in all three areas. In addition, the frequency of use, the amount of the substance used, and the route of administration may be related to the development of medical disorders associated with a particular substance and are relevant when discussing the patient's medical history.

General questions about the consequences of substance use focus on changes in academic performance, occupational functioning, and interpersonal relationships, as well as medical and legal problems associated with substance abuse. The history of substance abuse treatment includes questions about hospital admissions for detoxification, as well as admissions to other controlled living situations to support ongoing abstinence. Such programs include residential programs, halfway houses, sober houses, and therapeutic communities. Outpatient programs such as partial hospital programs, as well as group, individual, and pharmacological therapies (e.g., disulfiram, naltrexone, nicotine delivery systems), may also be a part of the patient's prior treatment. Understanding which earlier treatments did or did not help the patient achieve and maintain abstinence can serve as a guide for treatment recommendations. Finally, the interviewer should ask about involvement in self-help groups, such as Alcoholics Anonymous, Narcotics Anonymous, Cocaine Anonymous, Self-Management and Recovery Training, Rational Recovery, and Women for Sobriety. Some patients may express positive or negative feelings about a particular type of self-help group. The interviewer should not support or discredit the patient's feelings about self-help groups but should try to understand the patient's reasons for such reactions, both to educate the patient about self-help groups and to formulate a treatment plan that will be most beneficial to the patient.

Other components of the history of substance use are the patient's periods of abstinence and the circumstances surrounding relapses. The information about abstinent periods and relapses indicates the progression or regression of substance use, the severity of the substance use disorder, and the external factors—such as relationship difficulties, psychiatric symptoms, legal or medical problems, and treatment termination—that may have influenced the patient's return to substance use.

Finally, the interviewer should review other substances of abuse with the patient to ensure that no other substances are being used currently or have been used in the past. For example, a patient may say he only has a problem with cocaine; however, by asking about other substances of abuse, the interviewer may find that the patient has used marijuana daily for the past 10 years but did not mention the marijuana use because he does not consider it to be problematic. Although daily marijuana use may not be significant to the patient, this pattern of use could represent marijuana abuse or dependence that should be addressed with the patient.

Psychiatric History

Research studies have demonstrated an increased prevalence of substance use disorders among patients diagnosed with psychiatric disorders. For example, patients diagnosed with bipolar disorder are six times more likely than the general population to have a co-occurring substance use disorder (Regier et al. 1990). Other psychiatric disorders (Biederman et al. 2006; Hasin et al. 2007; Hesselbrock et al. 1985; Kessler et al. 1997; Krausz et al. 1998; Regier et al. 1990; Rodriguez-Llera et al. 2006; Rounsaville et al. 1991) and personality disorders (Helzer and Pryzbeck 1988; Nock et al. 2006; Rodriguez-Llera et al. 2006; Rounsaville et al. 1991; Weiss et al. 1993) have also been associated with substance use disorders. Conversely, patients diagnosed with substance use disorders are more likely to have a co-occurring psychiatric disorder (Arias et al. 2008; Brady et al. 1991; Currie et al. 2005; Drake and Wallach 1989; Miller et al. 1989; Mueser et al. 1992, 2000). Studies have shown that the co-occurrence of substance use disorders and psychiatric disorders can worsen the prognosis for both disorders (Greenfield et al. 1998; Hides et al. 2006; Najavits et al. 2007; Sonne et al. 1994; Weiss et al. 1988). When coexisting substance use and psychiatric disorders are diagnosed, however, patients can be referred to integrated treatment for both disorders. Increasing evidence shows that integrated treatment improves and enhances outcomes for both disorders (Bellack et al. 2006; Bennett et al. 2001; Mueser et al. 1992; Najavits et al. 1998, 2005; Weiss et al. 2000c). Therefore, clinicians should assess substance use disorders in patients presenting for the treatment of psychiatric disorders, and should assess psychiatric disorders among patients presenting for treatment of substance use disorders.

If a patient reports symptoms consistent with a psychiatric disorder, the interviewer should inquire about the relationship between substance use and the emergence, exacerbation, or regression of psychiatric symptoms. Substance-induced psychiatric disorders occur when the symptoms of the disorder represent a change in affective or cognitive states that arises from the direct physiological effects of a substance. These symptoms generally occur when the patient is intoxicated or is experiencing withdrawal symptoms. Examples of patients with substance-induced psychiatric disorders include a patient who has exhibited symptoms of mania only when intoxicated with cocaine and a patient who has had panic attacks only during benzodiazepine withdrawal. In contrast, a psychiatric disorder is independent of a substance use disorder when the patient reports a history of psychiatric symptoms that predates substance use or that does not resolve after the substance use has been stopped.

A useful way to determine whether psychiatric disorders predate or continue after abstinence from substances is to inquire about the presence or absence of psychiatric symptoms before the patient began using substances and during periods of abstinence. For example, a patient who was diagnosed with major depression 10 years ago and reports having used alcohol daily for the past 6 years in an attempt to ameliorate his untreated depressive symptoms had developed psychiatric symptoms before the initiation of substance use. A patient who says that she continues to have auditory hallucinations 6 months after her last use of marijuana demonstrates psychiatric symptoms that persist during a period of abstinence. Reviewing the patient's history of psychiatric symptoms before the onset of substance use, during episodes of intoxication with or withdrawal from substances, and after cessation of substance use can help the interviewer distinguish between substance-induced psychiatric disorders (which exist because of a substance use disorder) and co-occurring psychiatric and substance use disorders.

Medical History

Evaluating clinicians need to elicit a complete medical history—including current and past medical problems, surgical procedures, and medication allergies—from patients presenting for assessment of a substance use disorder. Regardless of their relationship to substance use, medical problems require treatment, and the interviewer would be remiss if he or she did not make inquiries about medical conditions and recommend treatment or make referrals for further evaluation for any conditions mentioned. In addition, patients with substance use disorders have often neglected their health and routine medical care. The clinician can ask when was the last time the patient had a complete physical examination and follow-up for any medical problems, past or current.

As the patient describes symptoms of a medical disorder, the interviewer should attempt to determine whether the symptoms are related to or independent of substance use. Questions about a reported medical problem should include inquiries about the temporal relationship between the development of the medical condition and substance use. For example, a patient reports that her asthma, which was diagnosed at age 12 years, worsened about 2 years after she began smoking cigarettes at age 18. Other questions for this patient would include a question about the continuation or resolution of symptoms after periods of abstinence. This same patient may report that when she stopped smoking for 2 weeks, she had fewer asthma attacks. The role of pharmacological interventions in the treatment of medical disorders is another way to determine the effect of substance use on a medical disorder. For example, this patient may also report the failure of her previously effective steroid inhalers to treat asthma attacks in the past year. In this case, the patient's cigarette use exacerbated her asthmatic symptoms to the point that steroid inhalers were of limited therapeutic value.

The interviewer should also ask about current and past medical problems that are specific to use of a particular substance. A description of all the medical problems associated with each category of substances is beyond the scope of this chapter; the major medical problems and disorders associated with the more commonly abused substances are listed below (see also Table 1–3).

- *Alcohol.* Alcohol-related medical problems include blackouts, hangovers, withdrawal tremors, withdrawal seizures and delirium tremens, aspiration pneumonia, cardiomyopathy, cerebellar degeneration, gastritis, gastroesophageal reflux disease, hepatitis, pancreatitis, and Wernicke-Korsakoff syndrome.

TABLE 1–3. **Medical problems associated with substance use disorders**

Alcohol
 Aspiration pneumonia
 Blackouts
 Cardiomyopathy
 Cerebellar degeneration
 Delirium tremens
 Gastritis
 Gastroesophageal reflux disease
 Hangover
 Hepatitis
 Pancreatitis
 Wernicke-Korsakoff syndrome
 Withdrawal seizures
 Withdrawal tremors
Nicotine
 Cardiovascular disease
 Chronic obstructive pulmonary
  disease
 Emphysema
 Lung cancer
 Oral cancer
 Peripheral vascular disease
Sedative-hypnotics
 Withdrawal seizures
 Withdrawal tremors
 In overdose:
  Respiratory depression
  Coma
  Death

Cocaine
 Cellulitis (intravenous)
 Cerebral vascular events
 Chest pain
 Dyspnea (intranasal)
 Endocarditis (intravenous)
 Ischemia of gastrointestinal tract
 Myocardial infarction
 Pneumomediastinum (intranasal)
 Pneumothorax (intranasal)
 Pulmonary infarction (intranasal)
 Transient ischemic attacks
Opioids
 Cellulitis (intravenous)
 Constipation
 Endocarditis (intravenous)
 Hepatitis B
 Hepatitis C
 In overdose:
  Respiratory depression
  Coma
  Death
Alcohol and illicit drugs
 HIV infection
 Sexually transmitted diseases
 Tuberculosis

- *Cocaine.* Medical problems related to cocaine use include transient ischemic attacks, cerebral vascular events, ischemia of the gastrointestinal tract, chest pain, and myocardial infarctions. Insufflating or snorting powder cocaine may lead to ischemic necrosis of the nasal septum, whereas smoking crack cocaine may lead to dyspnea, pneumothorax, pneumomediastinum, and pulmonary infarction. Intravenous cocaine use may cause cellulitis or endocarditis.
- *Marijuana.* The evidence for medical disorders associated with marijuana use is sparse and inconclusive. Long-term marijuana use may be associated with the earlier development of respiratory carcinomas in subjects who also use tobacco or alcohol (Taylor 1988), as well as an increased risk of prostate and cervical cancer (Sidney et al. 1997).

- *Opioids.* Intravenous opiate use may result in the same medical disorders as intravenous cocaine use. Other medical problems resulting from opiate use include constipation and, in overdose, respiratory depression, coma, and death.
- *Nicotine.* Use of nicotine can lead to chronic obstructive pulmonary disease, emphysema, cardiovascular disease, peripheral vascular disease, and lung and oral carcinomas.
- *Sedative-hypnotics.* Use of sedative-hypnotics can lead to withdrawal tremors and seizures, as well as a major abstinence syndrome. In overdose, these drugs can lead to respiratory depression, coma, and death.

Patients who abuse substances are at risk of contracting infectious diseases. Intravenous substance use (most commonly heroin and cocaine) with contaminated needles can result in infection with the human immunodeficiency virus (HIV), hepatitis B, and hepatitis C. Individuals under the influence of substances may engage in risky sexual behaviors, resulting in exposure to HIV, hepatitis B, hepatitis C, and the organisms that cause gonorrhea, chlamydia, syphilis, herpes, genital warts, and human papillomavirus infection. Additionally, elevated rates of substance use have been reported among individuals with tuberculosis (Centers for Disease Control and Prevention 2008). In 2007, among approximately 12,000 tuberculosis cases in which information about substance use was available, 2.1% were injection drug users, 8.0% were noninjection drug users, and 13.4% were excessive alcohol drinkers (Centers for Disease Control and Prevention 2008). Because identification and treatment of infectious diseases have important implications for the individual and society, the medical history should include questions about risk factors for infectious diseases, as well as about prior testing and treatment.

In the evaluation of women with substance use disorders, the interviewer should ask about reproductive health history. Relevant history among women of childbearing age includes a menstrual history and ascertaining whether the patient is or may be pregnant. Women who know they are pregnant may wish to obtain additional information on risk to the fetus of the patient's most recent or ongoing substance use. If a pregnancy is in question, the patient can be offered a pregnancy test as well. A pregnancy can serve as a powerful motivator for cessation of substance use, and pregnant women may wish to seek substance abuse treatment that has specialized services (Brady and Ashley 2005). Recent research emphasizes sex differences in all phases of the addiction process, including patterns and levels of use, as well as the progression of the addiction process and relapse (Lynch 2006). Women can experience changes in cravings and substance use during different phases of the menstrual cycle (Allen et al.

1999; Evans and Foltin 2006; Evans et al. 2002; Franklin et al. 2004; Snively et al. 2000), as well as differences in the likelihood of success in stopping their use of substances, such as nicotine, by phase of menstrual cycle (Allen et al. 2008; Franklin et al. 2004, 2008; Perkins 2001). For women who are experiencing perimenopause or for those who are postmenopausal, changes in sleep or symptoms such as hot flashes may be relevant factors in the use of substances.

An understanding of the relationship between the development and exacerbation of medical disorders and substance use provides the interviewer with information that may motivate the patient to change addictive behavior. The medical history will also provide the information necessary to refer the patient to appropriate medical care regardless of the origin of the medical disorder.

Family History

The family history of substance use disorders may reveal a genetic vulnerability to the patient's own development of these disorders. In one study of 1,030 female twin pairs, researchers estimated that the heritability of alcohol dependence liability ranged from 51% to 59%, with the balance being attributable to environmental factors (Kendler et al. 1992, 1994). These results are similar to the estimate reported in studies of male alcohol-dependent twins (McGue 1994; National Institute on Alcohol Abuse and Alcoholism 1997). Compelling evidence for the relationship between genetic determinants and the development of substance use disorders has been provided in family (Bierut et al. 1998; Kendler et al. 1997; Merikangas et al. 1998; Mirin et al. 1991; Prasant et al. 2006), twin (Kendler and Prescott 1998; Kendler et al. 2006), and adoption (Cadoret et al. 1980, 1995) studies. The environment created by families with substance use disorders may also have an impact on the development of substance use disorders in their children. For example, parental modeling of drinking behavior, ethnic differences in drinking customs, parental and familial psychopathology, socioeconomic status, family aggression and violence, and parental cognitive impairment are risk factors that have been shown to affect the development of both alcohol dependence and other mental health problems in the children of alcoholic parents (Ellis et al. 1997). Interviewers can educate patients about genetic vulnerability to substance use disorder and risk factors in the family environment associated with the development of substance use disorder, thereby providing patients with an understanding of their current problems with substances as well as compelling reasons why they should refrain from substance use.

Social and Developmental History

Patient social and developmental histories provide information about factors that may have influenced the development and perpetuation of substance use disorders. An important psychosocial factor to explore is the patient's relationships with others (i.e., family, friends, peers, significant others, authority figures). During adolescence, peer relationships are a powerful influence on both the initiation and the continuation of substance use (van den Bree and Pickworth 2005). The interviewer will also want to know if the patient had any positive influences during adolescence, such as emotionally supportive parents, membership in school organizations, or a focus on academic achievement; such factors are associated with a lower risk for substance use (Brounstein et al. 2007; Kumpfer et al. 2007; Lochman et al. 2007).

Some patients may report both initial and continued use of substances because of the effects of abusive relationships. Several studies have shown an association between self-reported histories of physical and sexual abuse and the development of substance use disorders (Brown and Anderson 1991; Greenfield et al. 2002; Nelson et al. 2006; Rice et al. 2001; Sartor et al. 2007; Wilsnack et al. 1997; Windle et al. 1995). A history of abuse may also be associated with poorer drinking outcomes in alcohol- and cocaine-dependent subjects after treatment (Greenfield et al. 2002; Haver 1987; Hyman et al. 2008). A study of individuals who received intensive substance abuse treatment found that those with a lifetime history of physical and/or sexual abuse had a worse psychiatric status, more psychiatric hospitalizations, and more outpatient treatment at 1-year follow-up than those without an abuse history (Pirard et al. 2005). Conversely, the ability to have meaningful interpersonal relationships can help the patient build a social support network that might support recovery and help the patient remain abstinent (Havassy et al. 1991).

Patients with substance use disorders may report the effects of substance use on their educational attainment and subsequent employment. Studies have shown that substance use may lead to school absenteeism, poor school performance, and dropout (Bray et al. 2000; Lynskey and Hall 2000; Lynskey et al. 2003). In turn, lower educational attainment has been associated with the development of alcohol abuse and dependence in adulthood (Crum et al. 1992, 1993, 2006) and may have effects on abstinence in alcohol-dependent individuals (Curran and Booth 1999; Greenfield et al. 2003). By affecting educational attainment, alcoholism has been associated with lower income and occupational status (Crum et al. 1998; Mullahy and Sindelar 1989).

Finally, the interviewer should inquire about the patient's marital or partner status, because studies have shown that the presence or absence of a spouse or partner can be an important influence on the development and perpetuation of a substance use disorder and may also affect treatment outcomes. For example, women seeking treatment for substance use disorders are more likely than men to be single (Griffin et al. 1989; Weiss et al. 1997), to be involved with an addicted partner (Gossop et al. 1994; Griffin et al. 1989; Hser et al. 1987), or to cite interpersonal factors such as substance use by spouse, partner, or friend as reasons for their own continued substance use (Greenfield 1996; Kandel and Logan 1984). The presence of a supportive partner (Anglin et al. 1987; Eldred and Washington 1976) and the absence of an addicted partner (Nurco et al. 1982) have been shown to be the most consistent factors associated with better treatment outcomes for opiate-dependent women but not for opiate-dependent men.

The social history, therefore, helps both patient and interviewer comprehend which interpersonal relationships, negative experiences, and positive achievements shaped the development and progression of the patient's substance use disorder. These same factors may also affect the outcome of the patient's treatment for substance use disorders.

Physical and Mental Status Examinations

Physical and mental status examinations of patients presenting for an assessment of a substance use disorder are critical parts of the evaluation because, as discussed earlier, both medical and psychiatric disorders are commonly found in this population. Although a mental status examination can and must be performed regardless of the treatment setting, the interviewer may be unable to perform the physical examination. Lack of appropriate space, equipment, and training can interfere with the interviewer's ability to perform the physical examination. Patient factors, such as refusal to undergo an examination or inability to cooperate with the examination due to substance intoxication or withdrawal, may also be reasons to defer the physical examination at the time of evaluation. Under such circumstances, the interviewer should refer the patient to the appropriate person (e.g., primary care physician) or facility (e.g., emergency room) for a complete physical examination.

Specific signs of substance use present during the physical or mental status examination will depend on the type of substance used and the presence of intoxication with or withdrawal from substances (Washburn 2002). According to DSM-IV-TR, patients who are intoxicated with amphetamines or cocaine may exhibit psychomotor agitation or retardation, diaphoresis, evidence of weight loss, and confusion. Alcohol and sedative-hypnotics can cause slurred speech, incoordination, unsteady gait, memory impairment, stupor, or coma in an intoxicated patient. Similarly, opioid intoxication is characterized by slurred speech, drowsiness, and memory impairment. One distinguishing characteristic of opioid intoxication is the appearance of pupillary constriction; severe overdose of opiates can result in pupillary dilation secondary to anoxia in the central nervous system.

Cannabis intoxication can cause motor incoordination, euphoria or anxiety, a sense of slowed time, and impaired judgment. An often obvious sign of cannabis intoxication is conjunctival injection. A patient who is intoxicated with hallucinogens may be anxious, depressed, or paranoid after use; hallucinations, illusions, perceptual distortions, incoordination, diaphoresis, and tremors can also be present. Signs of PCP intoxication include psychomotor agitation, impaired judgment, dysarthria, sensitivity to sounds, ataxia, seizures, and coma. Inhalant use may cause euphoria and impaired judgment, as well as a number of observable physical signs, including incoordination, slurred speech, lethargy, ataxia, psychomotor retardation, stupor, and coma.

Also described in DSM-IV-TR are withdrawal symptoms for the different substances of abuse. Patients withdrawing from either amphetamines or cocaine may present with dysphoria, psychomotor agitation or retardation, and signs of fatigue; they may complain of increased appetite, vivid and unpleasant dreams, insomnia, or hypersomnia. The withdrawal symptoms of alcohol and sedative-hypnotics may include diaphoresis, tremulousness, psychomotor agitation, responsiveness to internal stimuli, and seizures. Patients in withdrawal from CNS depressants may also report anxiety, insomnia, nausea, and vomiting. Lacrimation, rhinorrhea, pupillary dilation, piloerection, and yawning are the observable signs of opioid withdrawal; symptoms that may be reported by patients undergoing opioid withdrawal are dysphoria, fever, nausea, vomiting, muscle aches, and diarrhea. Cannabis, hallucinogens, PCP, and inhalants do not have defined withdrawal syndromes.

Although many physical signs of substance use are easily observed when the interviewer performs the mental status examination, other signs of substance use are best detected by performing a thorough physical examination. For example, small circular lesions representing the point of injection of a drug into both large and small veins, also known as *tracks*, may be found when examining a patient who uses drugs intravenously. If infected, these injection sites may be erythematous, purulent, and warm to the touch. Similarly, a patient with hepatic damage secondary to chronic alcohol use or with hepatitis infection as a result of intravenous drug use may present with scleral icterus or a slightly enlarged liver or, in more advanced cases of hepatic damage, jaundice, abdominal distention secondary to ascites, gynecomastia, spider angiomas, palmar erythema, and caput medusae. A complete description of all the physical findings associated with substance use is beyond the scope of this chapter; these two examples are presented to illustrate the importance of a thorough physical examination to detect other signs of substance-related medical disorders that require immediate treatment.

The physical and mental status examinations of a patient presenting for an evaluation of a substance use disorder can be dramatically affected by states of intoxication or withdrawal. Alterations in mood, affect, psychiatric symptoms, thought processes, thought content, speech, memory, orientation, cognition, insight, and judgment are commonly seen when patients are intoxicated with or are withdrawing from a particular substance. Similarly, substance intoxication or withdrawal can lead to significant changes in the patient's physiological state, causing abnormalities in blood pressure, body temperature, and level of consciousness, and disrupting the stability and functioning of major organ systems, such as the neurological and gastrointestinal systems. In addition, the mental status examination provides important information for the diagnosis of other psychiatric disorders and for the evaluation of the current remission, recurrence, or stability of any other concurrent psychiatric disorder. A comparison of the patient's physical and mental status examinations during different stages of substance abuse treatment is one way to evaluate changes in substance use and in any concurrent medical and psychiatric disorders.

Biological Markers

Biological markers can help in detecting the degree and regularity of the patient's substance use (Kolodziej et al. 2002). Biological markers are most frequently tested and analyzed by sampling breath, urine, blood, hair, and saliva. The highly sensitive and specific breath alcohol testing provides immediate results at low cost and minimal discomfort to the patient. The drawbacks of breath analysis include its narrow window of assessment, which varies from minutes to hours after drinking, depending on the amount of alcohol consumed and on individual differences in alcohol metabolism.

Metabolites of many substances of abuse are excreted in the urine and may be detected by urine toxicology screens. The major disadvantage of urine testing is the variation in detection time for the metabolites of different substances. For example, because cocaine metabolites remain in the urine for approximately 3 days, a urine screening test performed

5 days after the last cocaine use would not detect recent use. Conversely, cannabis metabolites may remain in the urine for a month, resulting in positive urine toxicology screens after several weeks of abstinence. In turn, the detection duration may be affected by dose, frequency of use, cutoff concentration level that results in a positive urine screen, and the patient's rate of metabolism (Cone 1997). Although quantitative urine screening may overcome some of the limitations of urine toxicology screens and reduces the numbers of false-positive and false-negative urine screens, the cost of this test may be prohibitive, and the technology involved in qualitative urine screening requires further evaluation. In addition, adulterants and urine substitutes designed to defeat urine toxicology tests are widely available and can be easily researched and purchased over the Internet, thus increasing the possibility of false-negative results for patients who may use these techniques (Jaffee et al. 2007).

Recent heavy substance use can be detected by serum testing. Alcohol exerts a direct toxic effect on hepatocytes, leading to increased levels of glycoprotein carbohydrate-deficient transferrin (Javors and Johnson 2003), glutamyl transpeptidase (Conigrave et al. 2003), serum aspartate aminotransferase (AST), and serum alanine aminotransferase or ALT). The mean corpuscular volume of red blood cells may also be increased with heavy alcohol use, demonstrating hepatic damage as well as hematological problems, such as deficiencies in vitamin B_{12} and folate. These blood markers can help clinicians monitor changes in the patient's physical health and may be used as a motivator to help the patient decrease or abstain from the use of alcohol. These markers, however, are not specific for alcohol-related medical problems and may be present with other disease states. In addition, blood markers may differ due to individual factors, such as age, body mass index, gender, smoking, caffeine consumption, and the use of certain medications (Aubin et al. 1998; Daeppen et al. 1998).

Hair testing is another method for evaluating biological markers of substance use (Klein et al. 2000). Although it is not fully understood how drugs enter the hair, hair testing may provide a longer time to detect substance use because of the greater stability of the drug in hair samples than in samples of bodily fluids. The disadvantages of hair testing include the possibility of false-positive results due to passive contact with a substance, the possible effect of individual hair characteristics (e.g., hair length) on the test results, and racial bias in hair testing. In addition, hair testing is a recent technology that cannot provide information about the amount of the substance used or the temporal relationship between the presence of the substance in the hair and the use of the substance.

Saliva testing is used primarily to detect very recent substance use and is used to identify substance use in accident victims, automobile operators, and employees before their involvement in activities in which safety is paramount. The detection time for saliva testing is relatively brief, and the technology requires further evaluation to demonstrate its validity (Kaufman and Lamster 2002).

Sweat testing may detect past substance use, and it may act as a cumulative measure of substance use and may extend drug detection times by 1 week or longer compared with urine testing, but it may be less sensitive than urine testing (Huestis et al. 2000). This test is not commonly used because of individual variations in sweat production, possible environmental contamination, and difficulties in collecting and storing sweat samples.

Testing for biological markers can serve an important function in the detection of substance use. The evaluating clinician should consider the substance used, the duration for substance detection, the invasiveness of the technique, and the expense of the test to determine which test is most appropriate for individual patients.

Screening Instruments and Standardized Interviews

Standardized instruments are used for screening, diagnostic assessment, and evaluation of severity (see Table 1–4). A number of short self-report instruments have been developed as screens for the presence of a drug or alcohol use disorder (Allen and Columbus 1995; Kolodziej et al. 2002; Rounsaville and Poling 2000). Such tests do not provide a formal diagnosis but rather provide an indication of the likely presence of substance abuse or dependence.

The CAGE questionnaire (named for its four questions) (Kitchens 1994; Mayfield et al. 1974) asks: "Have you ever 1) felt you should **C**ut down on your drinking? 2) felt **A**nnoyed by criticism of your drinking? 3) felt bad or **G**uilty about your drinking? or 4) taken a drink first thing in the morning (**E**ye-opener) to steady your nerves or get rid of a hangover?" The CAGE is useful because of its brevity and ease of scoring. One positively answered question has a 90% rate of detecting an alcohol-related disorder.

The Alcohol Use Disorders Identification Test (AUDIT; Allen et al. 1997; Babor et al. 1992; Donovan et al. 2006) was designed to screen for hazardous or harmful alcohol consumption as defined by the World Health Organization in a range of clinical and nonclinical settings. This 10-item questionnaire uses a 0–5 score for each question and takes less than 2 minutes to administer and 2 minutes to score (Connors and Volk

TABLE 1–4. Screening measures for substance use

Measure	Target population	Groups used with	Number of items	Problem screened	Cutoff score for harmful use	Time to administer (minutes)
Alcohol Use Disorders Identification Test (AUDIT; Babor et al. 1992)	Adults	Patients seeing primary care physician Patients in ER DWI offenders Employers for workplace screening	10 (3)[a]	Harmful or hazardous alcohol use	8 (range 0–40)	3–5
CAGE (Mayfield et al. 1974)	Adults	Patients in ERs and hospitals Patients seeing primary care physician	4	Alcohol dependence	1 (range 0–4)	<1
CRAFFT (Knight et al. 2002)	Adolescents	Adolescents, young adults Patients in pediatric, medical, or psychiatric settings	6	Alcohol or drug abuse	>1 (range 0–6)	2
Drug Abuse Screening Test (DAST)-10 (shortened DAST) (Yudko et al. 2007)	Adults (also adapted for adolescents)	Patients in medical, primary care, and psychiatric settings	0–10	Drug abuse	Low: 1–2 Moderate: 2–5 Substantial: 6–10 (range 0–10)	1–2

TABLE 1–4. Screening measures for substance use *(continued)*

Measure	Target population	Groups used with	Number of items	Problem screened	Cutoff score for harmful use	Time to administer (minutes)
Fagerström Test for Nicotine Dependence (Heatherton et al. 1991)	Adults, adolescents	Smokers Patients with psychiatric disorders or other SUDs Patients in medical or psychiatric settings	6	Nicotine dependence	High level of dependence: >6 (range 0–10)	2
Michigan Alcohol Screening Test (MAST)	Adults, adolescents	Psychiatric and medical patients Individuals with an AUD	25	Problem drinking	6 (range 0–22)	5
NIDA-Modified Alcohol, Smoking and Substance Involvement Screening Test (NM ASSIST; National Institute on Drug Abuse 2009)	Adults	Patients in general medical settings	12 (prescreen)[b] 63 (self-administered)	Alcohol Tobacco Illicit drug and nonmedical use of prescription drugs	Tobacco: 2 Males consuming alcohol: 5 Females consuming alcohol: 4 Illicit drugs and nonmedical use of prescription drugs: 27	2 (prescreen)[b]
Short Michigan Alcohol Screening Test (SMAST)	Adults (self-administered)	Adult patients in medical and psychiatric settings	13	Alcohol dependence	Probable: >2 Likely: >3 (range 0–13)	1–2

TABLE 1–4. Screening measures for substance use *(continued)*

Measure	Target population	Groups used with	Number of items	Problem screened	Cutoff score for harmful use	Time to administer (minutes)
T-ACE (Sokol et al. 1989)	Adults	Pregnant women	4	Harmful drinking	2 (range 0–5)	<2
TWEAK (Dawson et al. 2001)	Adults	Pregnant women Other adult men and women	5	Harmful drinking	Pregnant women: 2 Nonpregnant adults: 3–4 (range 0–10)	<2

Note. AUD=alcohol use disorder; DWI=driving while intoxicated; ER=emergency room; SUD=substance use disorder.

aThe AUDIT has 10 items; a three-item version is also available.

bThe NM ASSIST has 12 prescreening questions that assess 11 different substance categories, as well as "other" substances. If a patient answers "yes" to all 12 prescreening questions, there may be up to 63 follow-up questions to complete on a self-questionnaire. The time to complete these 63 questions varies depending on the patient.

2004). A score of 8 or more has reasonably good sensitivity in detecting an alcohol use disorder (Conigrave et al. 1995). A three-item version focused on consumption (AUDIT-C) is also available (Gordon et al. 2001; Piccinelli et al. 1997).

The Michigan Alcohol Screening Test (MAST) is useful in assessing the extent of lifetime alcohol-related consequences (Allen and Columbus 1995; Westermeyer et al. 2004b). Commonly used are a 25-item self-test version (Selzer 1971) and the 13-item Short MAST (SMAST; Shields and Caruso 2003, 2004; Shields et al. 2007), and other shortened forms have also been developed (Connors et al. 2004).

The Drug Abuse Screening Test (DAST) (Skinner 1982; Staley and el-Guebaly 1990) is a 28-item self-test designed to detect abuse of or dependence on a wide range of substances other than alcohol. Like the MAST, the DAST has been shortened to a 20-question version and a 10-question version (Yudko et al. 2007).

The National Institute on Drug Abuse (NIDA) has modified the Alcohol, Smoking and Substance Involvement Screening Test (ASSIST), Version 3.0, a validated screening instrument developed by the World Health Organization (World Health Organization 2002) to provide physicians with a screening tool and resources for substance-abusing patients. The NIDA-Modified Alcohol, Smoking and Substance Involvement Screening Test (NM ASSIST; National Institute on Drug Abuse 2009) screens adults age 18 and older using the Five A's of Intervention: *Ask* the patient about substance use, *Advise* the patient strongly and directly to make a change, *Assess* how willing the patient is to make a change, *Assist* the patient to make a change if ready, and *Arrange* to refer the patient for further evaluation and assessment. Unlike other screening instruments, the NM ASSIST screens for alcohol, tobacco, illicit drugs, and nonmedical use of prescription drugs.

The TWEAK test (the name is derived from its five items) was originally designed to screen for high-risk drinking during pregnancy (Bush et al. 2003; Dawson et al. 2001). The T-ACE (Sokol et al. 1989) is a four-item test designed to identify pregnant women at risk for drinking alcohol in quantities that might be dangerous to the fetus (Chang 2001). Neither the TWEAK nor the T-ACE has gender-based items, and the TWEAK has been validated in both male and female populations (Chan et al. 1993).

The six-question CRAFFT is designed for an adolescent population and covers both alcohol and drugs (Knight et al. 2002). Questions focus on whether the adolescent has driven in a car with someone who was using substances, uses drugs and alcohol to relax, uses them alone, forgets things while using, has gotten into trouble while using substances, or has family or friends who have asked the individual to cut back. The CRAFFT is advantageous for use with adolescent and young adult populations because of its brevity, ease of administration, and inclusion of items relevant to this population. It is scored 0–6: a score of 1 provides a high sensitivity, and a score of 2 has reasonably good sensitivity and specificity (Knight et al. 2003).

The Risk Behavior Survey (RBS) is a brief questionnaire that assesses frequency of various HIV sexual and needle-use risk behaviors. It has established construct validity (Deren 1996) and demonstrated test-retest reliability (Needle et al. 1995; Weatherby et al. 1994).

Several structured interviews that are used in research settings (Kolodziej et al. 2002) may also be helpful in some clinical settings. The Timeline Follow-Back (TLFB; Sobell et al. 1992) uses a calendar method that asks patients to reconstruct the type, quantity, and frequency of substance use during a specific time period. The Addiction Severity Index (ASI; McLellan et al. 1992) was developed as a structured interview to assess problem severity in seven areas frequently affected by substance use disorders. Several other questionnaires measure other aspects of severity. These include the Drinker Inventory of Consequences (Miller et al. 1995), which assesses the adverse consequences of alcohol dependence, and the eight-item Clinical Institute Withdrawal Assessment for Alcohol, Revised (CIWA-Ar; Sullivan et al. 1989), which provides a clinical quantification of the severity of alcohol withdrawal syndrome. The Fagerström Test for Nicotine Dependence (Heatherton et al. 1991; Sledjeski et al. 2007) was designed to provide an ordinal measure of nicotine dependence related to cigarette smoking. The Clinical Opiate Withdrawal Scale (COWS) is an 11-item screening tool with a possible score range between 0 and 48; it provides ratings for four levels of withdrawal severity (Center for Substance Abuse Treatment 2004; Wesson and Ling 2003).

Structured interviews are also reliable ways to assess diagnostic information. The Structured Clinical Interview for DSM-IV (SCID; Spitzer et al. 1992) is a clinically based interview that aids in diagnosis of DSM-IV substance-related disorders and other psychiatric disorders. The Psychiatric Research Interview for Substance and Mental Disorders (PRISM) facilitates diagnosis of DSM-IV psychiatric disorders and demonstrates good reliability for establishing psychiatric diagnoses among patients with drug and alcohol use disorders (Hasin et al. 1996).

Involvement of Significant Others

An individual who seeks assessment for a substance use disorder often does so at the prompting of significant others, such as family members, friends, coworkers, or treating clinicians, who are concerned about the person's well-being. Several studies have shown that significant others, serving as collateral informants, can both corroborate and provide additional information about the patient's reported substance use history (Carroll 1995; Maisto et al. 1979; Sobell et al. 1997). By speaking to the patient's significant others, the clinician also allows for their early involvement in treatment planning. As noted in the earlier section "Social and Developmental History," establishing social networks may support the patient's recovery and help him or her remain abstinent (Havassy et al. 1991).

A clinician's contact with collateral informants should occur only with written permission from the patient. If the request for contact with significant others is denied, it is appropriate to explore the patient's reasons for refusal. Some patients cannot provide the name of a collateral informant because they are socially isolated and have no significant supports in their lives (Weiss et al. 2000a). Other patients may be ambivalent about changing their addictive behaviors and therefore do not want significant others involved in their treatment. Other reasons that patients might refuse to authorize communication with certain individuals include involvement of a significant other in substance use; involvement of a significant other in physical, emotional, or sexual abuse of the patient; and the ability of a significant other to cause social consequences, such as unemployment or loss of significant relationships.

The involvement of significant others as both collateral informants and social supports can have either a positive or a negative effect on the patient's initiation of and retention in substance abuse treatment. Because significant others may be a powerful influence in the patient's life, the interviewer should contact only those who will support, rather than hinder, the recovery process.

Stages of Change and Motivational Interviewing

Before discussing treatment options with a patient who has a substance use disorder, the interviewer will want to assess the patient's willingness to stop using substances of abuse. Prochaska et al. (1992) described the five stages of change through which patients proceed before giving up their addictive behavior. Patients are said to be in *precontemplation*, the first stage, if they do not want to change their addictive behavior. These patients may resist change because they do not believe they have a problem or fail to see the seriousness of their problem with substances. The second stage, *contemplation*, occurs when patients are aware of and are thinking about changing their addictive behavior but have not yet committed to change. Patients might remain in this stage for an extended period of time as they weigh both the positive and negative aspects of continued substance use. When patients are in the third stage, *preparation,* they have decided to change their behavior and will do so in the near future. Patients may prepare by reducing the amount of the substance they are using or by seeking a substance abuse treatment facility where they may receive help for their problem. The fourth stage, *action,* occurs when patients are modifying their addictive behavior, such as ceasing substance use. Finally, patients are in the *maintenance* stage when they sustain their changed behaviors and continuously work on relapse prevention. An example of a patient in the maintenance stage is one who has achieved 6 months of sobriety and continues to attend self-help groups to receive support for abstinence and to become better educated about relapse prevention. The University of Rhode Island Change Assessment is a 32-item instrument that can be used to formally assess a patient's readiness to change (McConnaughy et al. 1983).

Understanding the patient's stage of change is important for treatment recommendations. For example, a patient voluntarily seeks an evaluation of marijuana use and says she is ready to stop using marijuana. Recognizing that the patient is in the preparation stage, the interviewer may refer this patient to an appropriate outpatient treatment, such as psychotherapy, group therapy, or a self-help group. Giving this patient a follow-up appointment in 1 month to reevaluate her marijuana use without any other treatment recommendations would be inappropriate because she wants and is ready to change her addictive behaviors. The patient may rethink her decision to abstain from all marijuana use during that month and may choose not to seek treatment at all.

For ambivalent patients in the contemplative stage, the interviewer can use motivational interviewing (Miller and Rollnick 2002). *Motivational interviewing* primarily describes a therapeutic style in which a therapist adopts a nonjudgmental and supportive stance to explore a patient's ambivalence about changing addictive behaviors. This emphasis on therapeutic style (also referred to as adherence to the "spirit" of motivational interviewing) has found strong empirical support that lends increased credence to the importance of the therapist's interpersonal approach to the client, as opposed to specified motivational interviewing techniques (Miller et al. 2005). The desired outcome of motivational interviewing is the resolution of the patient's ambivalence and the facilitation of an increased readiness to consider actual behavior change. This method of interviewing avoids confrontational questions and employs a communicative style that educes the patient's rationale for change and the benefits of change. By using motivational interviewing, the clinician circumvents a patient's defensiveness about substance use and creates an environment in which the patient may speak more freely about the advantages and disadvantages of change. Support for the efficacy of motivational interviewing is mounting, and a variety of meta-analytic integrations yield significant reductions in substance use among clients receiving motivational interviewing or adapted motivational interviewing interventions (e.g., Burke et al. 2003).

Case Illustration

The following case illustrates the principles of assessment outlined in this chapter. The psychiatrist adopts a nonjudgmental style and is able to establish rapport by first exploring the patient's work. The psychiatrist then elicits a full history of the patient's substance use, including age at initiation, progression, periods of heaviest use, periods of abstinence, and adverse consequences. In addition, other drug use history and a history of anxiety symptoms and sleep problems are explored. The patient relates briefly her social, family, and medical history. When the assessment is complete, the psychiatrist formulates a diagnosis and treatment plan and shares this with the patient. Together, they discuss how the patient's anxiety and sleep problems interact with her substance abuse. A menu of treatment recommendations is presented by the psychiatrist, and she and the patient discuss and then agree on the most appropriate course of action that is also acceptable to the patient.

> **Dr. A** is an adult psychiatrist who specializes in the treatment of substance use disorders. For 15 years, she has worked part-time at a large academic hospital, performing psychiatric evaluations and medication management for patients enrolled in the outpatient substance abuse program. She also has a part-time private practice where she provides consultations for patients with substance abuse problems. Patient referrals come from colleagues, insurance companies, and local community mental health programs. She meets **Ms. L** for a 60-minute evaluation in her private office in a suburban medical office building. Ms. L, a 25-year-old single female who works for an area bookstore, has been referred by her primary care physician because of anxiety and marijuana use.
>
> Dr. A starts the interview by asking, "What brought you here to see me today?" Ms. L says her primary care physician recommended Dr. A during a recent appointment when she told him she was anxious "all the time" and liked "a little pot sometimes so I can calm down." Ms. L tells Dr. A that she was promoted to general manager of a local branch of a large chain bookstore 14 months ago. She describes herself as a "lifelong worrier" whose anxiety increased when she received the promotion. She states that she smokes marijuana "sometimes" because it helps her sleep and alleviates the stress of her new job. Dr. A asks, "How often do you smoke marijuana?" Ms. L rolls her eyes and says, "I told you, *sometimes.* The pot is not the problem. It's my job." Sensing that she is reluctant to speak about marijuana use, Dr. A asks Ms. L to tell her more about her job.

Ms. L says she started working at the bookstore right after she graduated from college at age 22. Initially, she was a research specialist—"I found out-of-print copies of books for people"—but her broad knowledge of books and her business sense led to a rapid promotion to book buyer. Dr. A asks if she enjoys working at the bookstore, and Ms. L says she does. "I like the work," Ms. L says, "but I'm always worried that I will make a mistake. I feel really restless and take a lot of small breaks because I can't concentrate." She frequently works later than her assigned hours because she needs so many breaks during the day. When Dr. A asks about her sleep, she says it is "terrible" and has been that way for many years. "That's the main reason why I smoke pot every night," she says.

Dr. A believes that this is a good opening for asking Ms. L more about her marijuana use. She says to the patient, "You smoke pot every night. Has this been going on for a long time?" Ms. L says she first smoked marijuana when she was in college. She attended a prestigious university and double-majored in English literature and business management. Toward the end of her freshman year, she began worrying excessively about her grades and her future career. She also experienced restlessness, poor concentration, and muscle tension. The most troublesome symptom was insomnia: "It took me 2 hours to fall asleep for just 4 hours a night." She says she had to stop working on the college newspaper to help decrease her anxiety. "I was really disappointed because I thought I wanted to go into journalism," she says, "but I just couldn't handle the pressures of school and the paper." Her roommate noticed that she was not sleeping well and suggested that Ms. L smoke marijuana to help her relax before bedtime. With finals approaching, she smoked half a joint with her roommate. She says she slept well and felt less anxious the following day. "I couldn't remember the last time I slept so well," she says. "Did you keep smoking after that night?" asks Dr. A. Ms. L says she smoked a few times during finals but did not smoke marijuana that summer because she did not feel as anxious when classes ended.

Ms. L says she started smoking again when she returned to college for her sophomore year. "Did you smoke more marijuana during your second year than your first year?" asks Dr. A. Ms. L replies by saying, "Maybe a little more" and is vague about how frequently and how much marijuana she smoked. "You said you smoked a few times at the end of your freshman year," Dr. A says. "Did you continue smoking only during times of academic stress or did you start smoking at other times as well?" Ms. L reluctantly admits that she began smoking half a joint three times per week "because my classes were much more difficult during the second year and I really had problems sleeping." She says she "may have" smoked a joint every night during midterms and finals but she's not sure. She says she also smoked half a joint a few times a week during holiday and summer breaks because her worries about school and her insomnia did not improve when she was not attending classes. Dr. A asks if Ms. L's marijuana use continued to increase during her junior and senior years, and Ms. L says no. "I didn't smoke more but I definitely didn't smoke less."

Dr. A then asks the patient if her marijuana use increased after she started working. Ms. L admits that the ongoing anxiety, restlessness, poor concentration, and insomnia resulted in marijuana use four times per week—"Just one joint, though." Her symptoms intensified again when she was promoted to general manager a little over 1 year ago. "I couldn't sleep at all without smoking a joint at bedtime, even if I was off the next day." Dr. A asks if she smoked at any other time during the day. Ms. L says she "never" smoked marijuana before or during work. She admits that she began smoking one half-joint immediately after work in addition to the one joint at bedtime. "Have you had problems at work or in your private life because of your marijuana use?" asks Dr. A. Ms. L says that senior management spoke to her several times about her failure to attend early morning meetings, and several staff members complained about her moodiness and her tendency to "blow up" at staff. She says that since she saw her primary care physician 3 weeks ago, she decreased her marijuana use to one-half joint at bedtime 4 or 5 nights a week. "Did your anxiety get worse?" Dr. A asks. "It did," Ms. L says, "but I have to stop or else I'll lose my job."

Dr. A asks Ms. L to tell about her family. Ms. L says she is the only child of her father, a successful executive, and her mother, "a high-strung homemaker who thinks I don't know that she smokes marijuana when my father is away." Because her paternal grandfather died from alcohol-related liver cirrhosis, her father does not drink and, to the best of her knowledge, he has never used drugs. She says her mother was always worried that some harm would befall her young daughter: "I'm the only person I know who wasn't allowed to trick-or-treat on Halloween." When asked, Ms. L denies a history of childhood physical, emotional, or psychological abuse. She says she does not drink alcohol because she does not like the taste. She was offered cocaine and hallucinogens in college but was too afraid to use them. She denies use of opiates, sedative-hypnotics, inhalants, designer drugs, and nicotine. She has never been in psychiatric or substance abuse treatment. Ms. L says she has no medical problems and, when asked, says her menses occur every 29 days. She became sexually active at age 21 and always used condoms. She has not been sexually active in the past 2 years. She does not take medications and she denies medication allergies.

Dr. A says that she believes Ms. L has generalized anxiety disorder (GAD). Dr. A explains that Ms. L's long history of anxiety, poor concentration, restlessness, and insomnia and the problems these symptoms have caused her are consistent with a GAD diagnosis. Ms. L agrees that these symptoms sound "just like" her. "I also believe you abuse marijuana to help cope with these symptoms," Dr. A says. Ms. L becomes angry when she hears this. "I'm no drug addict!" she says. Dr. A explains that her ongoing use of marijuana despite the problems she has had at work over the past year meets criteria for marijuana abuse. She informs Ms. L that marijuana abuse can be treated and praises her efforts to cut down on her use. She recommends that Ms. L join once-a-week group therapy for young adults who want to stop abusing substances. "Like AA?" she asks. Dr. A explains that the group is not based on the principles of 12-step meetings and is designed to give young adults an opportunity to speak freely about their substance use and their efforts at abstinence. Dr. A also recommends an antidepressant and/or cognitive-behavioral therapy to help treat her GAD, but Ms. L chooses to attend the group before she considers any other treatment options. Ms. L agrees to a follow-up appointment in 3 weeks to discuss her progress.

Conclusion

In this chapter, we have discussed the importance of assessing the use and abuse of substances in all patients seen in the clinical setting. We have outlined the content areas of inquiry of the interview, as well as the adjunctive use of the physical examination, mental status examination, biological markers, reports of significant others, and screening instruments. We have also provided suggestions for the style of interviewing that will support accurate assessment and enhance motivation to change. A careful and accurate assessment of the patient will provide the necessary information for intervention and treatment planning and will increase motivation by beginning to engage the patient in the process of change.

Key Clinical Concepts

- Successful treatment of substance use disorders depends on a careful, accurate assessment and diagnosis.
- Accurate assessment is facilitated by interview settings that provide privacy and patient confidentiality and that permit adequate time to ask key questions, to follow up on positive patient responses, and to give feedback to the patient.
- A substance use history should be obtained from all patients presenting for treatment.
- Patient assessment can be influenced by a number of patient characteristics, including the patient's age; gender; ethnicity; legal, marital, and employment status; degree of insight into the nature of the problem; medical or psychiatric comorbidity; stage in the course of illness (e.g., recovery, recent relapse, first treatment); current phase of use (e.g., intoxication, withdrawing, interepisode); and stage of readiness for change and motivation.
- In addition to diagnosing a substance-related disorder (e.g., a substance use disorder or a substance-induced disorder), it is important to assess individuals for harmful or hazardous use of substances.
- A complete substance use assessment will include eliciting history of use for all the major categories of substances, addressing age at first use, frequency and amount used, consequences of use, and substance abuse treatment history, as well as complete psychiatric, medical, family, and social and developmental histories.

- Biological markers that might be helpful in assessment include sampling of breath, urine, blood, hair, and saliva. The most commonly used biological markers are breath alcohol testing, urine toxicology screens, and serum testing of liver transaminases and carbohydrate-deficient transferrin.

- Assessment can be enhanced by routine use of standardized screening instruments such as the Alcohol Use Disorders Identification Test, Drug Abuse Screening Test, TWEAK or T-ACE, Addiction Severity Index, and Risk Behavior Survey.

- Significant others can both corroborate and provide additional information about the patient's reported substance use history, and their early involvement can be helpful in treatment planning.

- For ambivalent patients who are contemplating their readiness to change, the interviewer can use motivational interviewing techniques that include a nonjudgmental and supportive stance to explore the patient's ambivalence about changing addictive behaviors.

Suggested Reading

American Psychiatric Association: Practice guideline for the treatment of patients with substance use disorders, 2nd edition. Am J Psychiatry 164(4 Suppl):5–123, 2007. Available at: http://www.psychiatryonline.com/pracGuide/pracGuideTopic_5.aspx.

Cummings NA, Cummings JL: The First Session With Substance Abusers: A Step-by-Step Guide. San Francisco, CA, Jossey-Bass, 2000

Johnson SL: Therapist's Guide to Substance Abuse Intervention. San Diego, CA, Academic Press, 2003

Miller WR, Rollnick S: Motivational Interviewing: Preparing People for Change, 2nd Edition. New York, Guilford, 2002

National Institute on Alcohol Abuse and Alcoholism: The Clinician's Guide, Revised, 2005 Edition. Bethesda, MD, National Institutes of Health, 2005

References

Adler I, Kandel DB: Cross-cultural perspectives on developmental stages in adolescent drug use. J Stud Alcohol 9:701–715, 1981

Allen J, Columbus M: Assessing Alcohol Problems: A Guide for Clinicians and Researchers. Rockville, MD, National Institute on Alcohol Abuse and Alcoholism, 1995

Allen JP, Litten RZ, Fertig JB, et al: A review of research on the Alcohol Use Disorders Identification Test (AUDIT). Alcohol Clin Exp Res 4:613–619, 1997

Allen SS, Hatsukami DK, Christianson D, et al: Withdrawal and pre-menstrual symptomatology during the menstrual cycle in short-term smoking abstinence: effects of menstrual cycle on smoking abstinence. Nicotine Tob Res 2:129–142, 1999

Allen SS, Bade T, Center B, et al: Menstrual phase effects on smoking relapse. Addiction 103:808–821, 2008

American Psychiatric Association: Diagnostic and Statistical Manual of Mental Disorders, 4th Edition. Washington, DC, American Psychiatric Association, 1994

American Psychiatric Association: Diagnostic and Statistical Manual of Mental Disorders, 4th Edition, Text Revision. Washington, DC, American Psychiatric Association, 2000

American Psychiatric Association: Practice guideline for the treatment of patients with substance use disorders, 2nd edition. Am J Psychiatry 164(4 Suppl):5–123, 2007. Available at: http://www.psychiatryonline.com/pracGuide/pracGuideTopic_5.aspx.

Anglin MD, Hser YI, Booth MW: Sex differences in addict careers. 4. Treatment. Am J Drug Alcohol Abuse 13:253–280, 1987

Arias AJ, Gelernter J, Chang G, et al: Correlates of co-occurring ADHD in drug-dependent subjects: prevalence and features of substance dependence and psychiatric disorders. Addict Behav 33:1199–1207, 2008

Aubin HJ, Laureaux C, Zerah F, et al: Joint influence of alcohol, tobacco, and coffee on biological markers of heavy drinking in alcoholics. Biol Psychiatry 7:638–643, 1998

Babor TF, Stephens RS, Marlatt GA: Verbal report methods in clinical research on alcoholism: response bias and its minimization. J Stud Alcohol 48:410–424, 1987

Babor T, Fuente J, Saunders J: AUDIT: The Alcohol Use Disorders Identification Test: Guidelines for Use in Primary Health Care. Geneva, World Health Organization, 1992

Babor TF, Higgins-Biddle JD, Saunders JB, et al: AUDIT: Guidelines for Use in Primary Care, 2nd Edition. Geneva, World Health Organization, 2001

Bellack AS, Bennett ME, Gearon JS, et al: A randomized clinical trial of a new behavioral treatment for drug abuse in people with severe and persistent mental illness. Arch Gen Psychiatry 63:426–432, 2006

Bennett ME, Bellack AS, Gearon JS: Treating substance abuse in schizophrenia: an initial report. J Subst Abuse Treat 2:163–175, 2001

Biederman J, Monuteaux MC, Mick E, et al: Young adult outcome of attention deficit hyperactivity disorder: a controlled 10-year follow-up study. Psychol Med 2:167–179, 2006

Bierut L, Dinwiddie S, Begleiter H, et al: Familial transmission of substance dependence: alcohol, marijuana, and habitual smoking. Arch Gen Psychiatry 11:982–988, 1998

Bohn MJ, Babor TF, Kranzler HR: The Alcohol Use Disorders Identification Test (AUDIT): validation of a screening instrument for use in medical settings. J Stud Alcohol 4:423–432, 1995

Brady KT, Casto S, Lydiard RB, et al: Substance abuse in an inpatient psychiatric sample. Am J Drug Alcohol Abuse 4:389–397, 1991

Brady TM, Ashley OS: Women in Substance Abuse Treatment: Results From the Alcohol and Drug Services Study (ADSS). Rockville, MD, Substance Abuse and Mental Health Services Administration, 2005

Bray JW, Zarkin GA, Ringwalt C, et al: The relationship between marijuana initiation and dropping out of high school. Health Econ 1:9–18, 2000

Brems C, Johnson ME, Namyniuk LL: Clients with substance abuse and mental health concerns: a guide for conducting intake interviews. J Behav Health Serv Res 3:327–334, 2002

Breslau N, Kilbey M, Andreski P: Nicotine dependence, major depression, and anxiety in young adults. Arch Gen Psychiatry 12:1069–1074, 1991

Brounstein PJ, Gardner SE, Backer TE, et al: Research to practice: bringing effective prevention to every community, in Preventing Youth Substance Abuse: Science-Based Programs for Children and Adolescents. Washington, DC, American Psychological Association, 2007, pp 41–64

Brown GR, Anderson B: Psychiatric morbidity in adult inpatients with childhood histories of sexual and physical abuse. Am J Psychiatry 1:55–61, 1991

Budney AJ, Higgins ST, Hughes JR, et al: Nicotine and caffeine use in cocaine-dependent individuals. J Subst Abuse 2:117–130, 1993

Burke BL, Arkowitz H, Menchola M: The efficacy of motivational interviewing: a meta-analysis of controlled clinical trials. J Consult Clin Psychol 5:843–861, 2003

Bush KR, Kivlahan DR, Davis TM, et al: The TWEAK is weak for alcohol screening among female Veterans Affairs outpatients. Alcohol Clin Exp Res 12:1971–1978, 2003

Cadoret RJ, Cain CA, Grove WM: Development of alcoholism in adoptees raised apart from alcoholic biologic relatives. Arch Gen Psychiatry 5:561–563, 1980

Cadoret RJ, Yates W, Troughton E, et al: Adoption study demonstrating two genetic pathways to drug use. Arch Gen Psychiatry 1:42–52, 1995

Carroll KM: Methodological issues and problems in the assessment of substance use. Psychol Assess 3:349–358, 1995

Center for Substance Abuse Treatment: Clinical Guidelines for the Use of Buprenorphine in the Treatment of Opioid Addiction. 2004. Available at: http://buprenorphine.samhsa.gov/Bup_Guidelines.pdf. Accessed February 7, 2010.

Centers for Disease Control and Prevention: Reported Tuberculosis in the United States, 2007. September 2008. Available at: http://www.cdc.gov/tb/statistics/reports/2007/default.htm. Accessed February 7, 2010.

Chan AW, Pristach EA, Welte JW, et al: Use of the TWEAK test in screening for alcoholism/heavy drinking in three populations. Alcohol Clin Exp Res 6:1188–1192, 1993

Chang G: Alcohol-screening instruments for pregnant women. Alcohol Res Health 3:204–209, 2001

Chen CY, O'Brien MS, Anthony JC: Who becomes cannabis dependent soon after onset of use? Epidemiological evidence from the United States: 2000–2001. Drug Alcohol Depend 1:11–22, 2005

Cone EJ: New development in biological measures of drug prevalence. NIDA Res Monogr 167:108–129, 1997

Conigrave KM, Hall WD, Saunders JB: The AUDIT questionnaire: choosing a cut-off score. Alcohol Use Disorder Identification Test. Addiction 10:1349–1356, 1995

Conigrave KM, Davies P, Haber P, et al: Traditional markers of excessive alcohol use. Addiction 98 (suppl 2):31–43, 2003

Connors GJ, Volk RJ: Self-report screening for alcohol problems among adults. August 2004. Available at: http://pubs.niaaa.nih.gov/publications/Assesing%20Alcohol/selfreport.htm. Accessed February 8, 2010.

Crum RM, Bucholz KK, Helzer JE, et al: The risk of alcohol abuse and dependence in adulthood: the association with educational level. Am J Epidemiol 9:989–999, 1992

Crum RM, Helzer JE, Anthony JC: Level of education and alcohol abuse and dependence in adulthood: a further inquiry. Am J Public Health 6:830–837, 1993

Crum R, Ensminger M, Ro M, et al: The association of educational achievement and school dropout with risk of alcoholism: a twenty-five-year prospective study of inner-city children. J Stud Alcohol 59:318–326, 1998

Crum RM, Juon HS, Green KM, et al: Educational achievement and early school behavior as predictors of alcohol-use disorders: 35-year follow-up of the Woodlawn Study. J Stud Alcohol 1:75–85, 2006

Crum RM, Green KM, Storr CL, et al: Depressed mood in childhood and subsequent alcohol use through adolescence and young adulthood. Arch Gen Psychiatry 65:702–712, 2008

Cummings NA, Cummings JL: The First Session With Substance Abusers: A Step-by-Step Guide. San Francisco, CA, Jossey-Bass, 2000

Curran GM, Booth BM: Longitudinal changes in predictor profiles of abstinence from alcohol use among male veterans. Alcohol Clin Exp Res 1:141–143, 1999

Currie SR, Patten SB, Williams JV, et al: Comorbidity of major depression with substance use disorders. Can J Psychiatry 10:660–666, 2005

Daeppen JB, Smith TL, Schuckit MA: Influence of age and body mass index on gamma-glutamyltransferase activity: a 15-year follow-up evaluation in a community sample. Alcohol Clin Exp Res 4:941–944, 1998

Dawson DA, Das A, Faden VB, et al: Screening for high- and moderate-risk drinking during pregnancy: a comparison of several TWEAK-based screeners. Alcohol Clin Exp Res 9:1342–1349, 2001

Deitz D, Rohde F, Bertolucci D, et al: Prevalence of screening for alcohol use by physicians during routine physical examinations. Alcohol Health Res World 2:162–168, 1994

Deren S: Sexual orientation, HIV risk behavior and serostatus in a multi-site sample of drug-injecting and crack-using women. Women's Health: Research on Gender, Behavior, and Policy 2:35–47, 1996

DiFranza JR, Guerrera MP: Alcoholism and smoking. J Stud Alcohol 2:130–135, 1990

Donovan DM, Kivlahan DR, Doyle SR, et al: Concurrent validity of the Alcohol Use Disorders Identification Test (AUDIT) and AUDIT zones in defining levels of severity among out-patients with alcohol dependence in the COMBINE study. Addiction 12:1696–1704, 2006

Drake RE, Wallach MA: Substance abuse among the chronic mentally ill. Hosp Community Psychiatry 10:1041–1046, 1989

Drug Addiction Treatment Act of 2000. Public Law No. 106–310, Title XXXV— Waiver authority for physicians who dispense or prescribe certain narcotic drugs for maintenance treatment or detoxification treatment. October 17, 2000. Available at: http://www.naabt.org/documents/DATA200LAWTEXT .pdf. Accessed May 19, 2010.

Eldred C, Washington M: Interpersonal relationships in heroin use by men and women and their role in treatment outcome. Int J Addict 1:117–130, 1976

Ellis D, Zucker R, Fitzgerald H: The role of family influences in development and risk. Alcohol Health Res World 21:218–226, 1997

Evans SM, Foltin RW: Exogenous progesterone attenuates the subjective effects of cocaine in women but not men. Neuropsychopharmacology 31:659–674, 2006

Evans SM, Haney M, Foltin RW: The effects of smoked cocaine during the follicular and luteal phases of the menstrual cycle in women. Psychopharmacology (Berl) 4:397–406, 2002

Frances R, Franklin J: Treatment of Alcoholism and Addictions. Washington, DC, American Psychiatric Press, 1989

Franklin TR, Napier K, Ehrman R, et al: Retrospective study: influence of menstrual cycle on cue-induced cigarette craving. Nicotine Tob Res 1:171–175, 2004

Franklin TR, Ehrman R, Lynch KG, et al: Menstrual cycle phase at quit date predicts smoking status in an NRT treatment trial: a retrospective analysis. J Womens Health 17:287–292, 2008

Gordon AJ, Maisto S, McNeil M, et al: Three questions can detect hazardous drinkers. J Fam Pract 4:313–320, 2001

Gossop M, Griffiths P, Strang J: Sex differences in patterns of drug taking behaviour: a study at a London community drug team. Br J Psychiatry 1:101–104, 1994

Greenfield SF: Women and substance use disorders, in Psychopharmacology of Women: Sex, Gender, and Hormonal Considerations. Edited by Jensvold MF, Hamilton JA. Washington, DC, American Psychiatric Press, 1996, pp 299–323

Greenfield SF, O'Leary G: Sex differences in substance use disorders, in Psychiatric Illness in Women: Emerging Treatments and Research. Edited by Lewis-Hall F, Williams T, Panetta J, et al. Washington, DC, American Psychiatric Publishing, 2002, pp 467–533

Greenfield SF, Shore M: Prevention of psychiatric disorders. Harv Rev Psychiatry 3:115–129, 1995

Greenfield SF, Weiss R, Muenz L, et al: The effect of depression on return to drinking: a prospective study. Arch Gen Psychiatry 3:259–265, 1998

Greenfield SF, Kolodziej ME, Sugarman DE, et al: History of abuse and drinking outcomes following inpatient alcohol treatment: a prospective study. Drug Alcohol Depend 3:227–234, 2002

Greenfield SF, Sugarman DE, Muenz LR, et al: The relationship between educational attainment and relapse among alcohol-dependent men and women: a prospective study. Alcohol Clin Exp Res 8:1278–1285, 2003

Greenfield SF, Brooks A, Gordon S, et al: Substance abuse treatment entry, retention, and outcome in women: a review of the literature. Drug Alcohol Depend 1:1–21, 2007

Griffin ML, Weiss RD, Mirin SM, et al: A comparison of male and female cocaine abusers. Arch Gen Psychiatry 2:122–126, 1989

Hahesy AL, Wilens TE, Biederman J, et al: Temporal association between childhood psychopathology and substance use disorders: findings from a sample of adults with opioid or alcohol dependency. Psychiatry Res 3:245–254, 2002

Hasin DS, Tsai W, Endicott J: The effects of major depression on alcoholism: five-year course. Am J Addict 2:144–155, 1996

Hasin DS, Stinson FS, Ogburn E, et al: Prevalence, correlates, disability and co-morbidity of DSM-IV alcohol abuse and dependence in the United States. Arch Gen Psychiatry 64:830–842, 2007

Havassy BE, Hall SM, Wasserman DA: Social support and relapse: commonalities among alcoholics, opiate users, and cigarette smokers. Addict Behav 5:235–246, 1991

Haver B: Female alcoholics, V: the relationship between family history of alcoholism and outcome 3–10 years after treatment. Acta Psychiatr Scand 1:21–27, 1987

Heatherton TF, Kozlowski LT, Frecker RC, et al: The Fagerström Test for Nicotine Dependence: a revision of the Fagerström Tolerance Questionnaire. Br J Addict 9:1119–1127, 1991

Helzer J, Pryzbeck T: The co-occurrence of alcoholism with other psychiatric disorders in the general population and its impact on treatment. J Stud Alcohol 49:219–224, 1988

Hesselbrock MN, Meyer RE, Keener JJ: Psychopathology in hospitalized alcoholics. Arch Gen Psychiatry 42:1050–1055, 1985

Hides L, Dawe S, Kavanagh DJ, et al: Psychotic symptom and cannabis relapse in recent-onset psychosis: prospective study. Br J Psychiatry 189:137–143, 2006

Hingson RW, Heeren T, Winter MR: Age of alcohol-dependence onset: associations with severity of dependence and seeking treatment. Pediatrics 118:e755–e763, 2006

Horgan C: Substance Abuse: The Number One Health Problem. Key Indicators for Policy. Princeton, NJ, Robert Wood Johnson Foundation, 1993

Horgan C, Skwara K, Strickler G: Substance Abuse: The Nation's Number One Health Problem. Key Indicators for Policy Update. Princeton, NJ, Robert Wood Johnson Foundation, 2001

Hser YI, Anglin MD, McGlothlin W: Sex differences in addict careers, I: initiation of use. Am J Drug Alcohol Abuse 13:33–57, 1987

Huestis MA, Cone EJ, Wong CJ, et al: Monitoring opiate use in substance abuse treatment patients with sweat and urine drug testing. J Anal Toxicol 7:509–521, 2000

Hyman SM, Paliwal P, Chaplin TM, et al: Severity of childhood trauma is predictive of cocaine relapse outcomes in women but not men. Drug Alcohol Depend 92:208–216, 2008

Jaffee W, Trucco E, Levy S, et al: Is this urine really negative? A systematic review of tampering methods in urine drug testing. J Subst Abuse Treat 33:33–42, 2007

Javors MA, Johnson BA: Current status of carbohydrate deficient transferrin, total serum sialic acid, sialic acid index of apolipoprotein J and serum beta-hexosaminidase as markers for alcohol consumption. Addiction 98 (suppl 2):45–50, 2003

Kandel DB, Logan JA: Patterns of drug use from adolescence to young adulthood, I: periods of risk for initiation, continued use, and discontinuation. Am J Public Health 7:660–666, 1984

Kaufman E, Lamster IB: The diagnostic applications of saliva—a review. Crit Rev Oral Biol Med 2:197–212, 2002

Kendler KS, Prescott CA: Cannabis use, abuse, and dependence in a population-based sample of female twins. Am J Psychiatry 8:1016–1022, 1998

Kendler KS, Heath AC, Neale MC: A population-based twin study of alcoholism in women. JAMA 268:1877–1882, 1992

Kendler KS, Neale MC, Heath AC: A twin-family study of alcoholism in women. Am J Psychiatry 5:707–715, 1994

Kendler KS, Davis CG, Kessler RC: The familial aggregation of common psychiatric and substance use disorders in the National Comorbidity Survey: a family history study. Br J Psychiatry 170:541–548, 1997

Kendler KS, Aggen SH, Tambs K, et al: Illicit psychoactive substance use, abuse and dependence in a population-based sample of Norwegian twins. Psychol Med 7:955–962, 2006

Kessler RC, Crum RC, Warner LA, et al: Lifetime co-occurrence of DSM-III-R alcohol abuse and dependence with other psychiatric disorders in the National Comorbidity Survey. Arch Gen Psychiatry 54:313–321, 1997

Kitchens JM: Does this patient have an alcohol problem? JAMA 272:1782–1787, 1994

Klein J, Karaskov T, Koren G: Clinical applications of hair testing for drugs of abuse—the Canadian experience. Forensic Sci Int 107:281–288, 2000

Knight JR, Sherritt L, Shrier LA, et al: Validity of the CRAFFT substance abuse screening test among adolescent clinic patients. Arch Pediatr Adolesc Med 6:607–614, 2002

Knight JR, Sherritt L, Harris SK, et al: Validity of brief alcohol screening tests among adolescents: a comparison of the AUDIT, POSIT, CAGE, and CRAFFT. Alcohol Clin Exp Res 1:67–73, 2003

Kolodziej ME, Greenfield SF, Weiss RD: Outcome measurement in substance use disorders, in Outcome Measurement in Psychiatry: A Critical Review. Edited by IsHak WW, Burt T, Sederer LI. Washington, DC, American Psychiatric Publishing, 2002, pp 207–228

Krausz M, Degkwitz P, Kuhne A, et al: Comorbidity of opiate dependence and mental disorders. Addict Behav 6:767–783, 1998

Kumpfer KL, Alvarado R, Tai C, et al: The Strengthening Families Program: an evidence-based, multicultural family skills training program, in Preventing Youth Substance Abuse: Science-Based Programs for Children and Adolescents. Edited by Tolan P, Szapocznik J, Sambrano S. Washington, DC, American Psychological Association, 2007, pp 159–181

Lochman JE, Wells KC, Murray M, et al: The Coping Power Program: preventive intervention at the middle school transition, in Preventing Youth Substance Abuse: Science-Based Programs for Children and Adolescents. Edited by Tolan P, Szapocznik J, Sambrano S. Washington, DC, American Psychological Association, 2007, pp 185–210

Lynch WJ: Sex differences in vulnerability to drug self-administration. Exp Clin Psychopharmacol 1:34–41, 2006

Lynskey M, Hall W: The effects of adolescent cannabis use on educational attainment: a review. Addiction 11:1621–1630, 2000

Lynskey MT, Coffey C, Degenhardt L, et al: A longitudinal study of the effects of adolescent cannabis use on high school completion. Addiction 5:685–692, 2003

Maisto SA, Sobell LC, Sobell MB: Comparison of alcoholics' self-reports of drinking behavior with reports of collateral informants. J Consult Clin Psychol 1:106–112, 1979

Mayfield D, McLeod G, Hall P: The CAGE questionnaire: validation of a new alcoholism screening instrument. Am J Psychiatry 131:1121–1123, 1974

McConnaughy EA, Prochaska JO, Velicer WF: Stages of change in psychotherapy: measurement and sample profiles. Psychotherapy: Theory, Research and Practice 20:368–375, 1983

McGue M: Genes, environment and the etiology of alcoholism, in The Development of Alcohol Problems: Exploring the Biopsychosocial Matrix of Risk. Edited by Zucker R, Boyd G, Howard J. Rockville, MD, National Institute on Alcohol Abuse and Alcoholism, 1994, pp 1–40

McLellan AT, Kushner H, Metzger D, et al: The fifth edition of the Addiction Severity Index. J Subst Abuse Treat 9:199–213, 1992

Merikangas K, Stolar M, Stevens D, et al: Familial transmission of substance use disorders. Arch Gen Psychiatry 55:973–979, 1998

Miller FT, Busch F, Tanenbaum JH: Drug abuse in schizophrenia and bipolar disorder. Am J Drug Alcohol Abuse 15:291–295, 1989

Miller WR, Rollnick S: Motivational Interviewing: Preparing People for Change, 2nd Edition. New York, Guilford, 2002

Miller WR, Tonigan JS, Longabaugh R: The Drinker Inventory of Consequences (DrInC): An Instrument for Assessing Adverse Consequences of Alcohol Abuse (NIAAA Project MATCH Monograph Series, Vol 4; Mattson ME, Marshall LA, series eds [NIH Publ No 95-3911]). Rockville, MD, National Institute on Alcohol Abuse and Alcoholism, 1995, pp 1699–1704

Miller WR, Moyers TB, Arciniega L, et al: Training, supervision and quality monitoring of the COMBINE Study behavioral interventions. J Stud Alcohol Suppl 15:188–195; discussion 168–169, 2005

Mirin SM, Weiss RD, Griffin ML, et al: Psychopathology in drug abusers and their families. Compr Psychiatry 1:36–51, 1991

Mueser KT, Bellack AS, Blanchard JJ: Comorbidity of schizophrenia and substance abuse: implications for treatment. J Consult Clin Psychol 60:845–856, 1992

Mueser KT, Yarnold PR, Rosenberg SD, et al: Substance use disorder in hospitalized severely mentally ill psychiatric patients: prevalence, correlates, and subgroups. Schizophr Bull 1:179–192, 2000

Mullahy J, Sindelar J: Life-cycle effects of alcoholism on education, earnings, and occupation. Inquiry 2:272–282, 1989

Najavits L, Weiss R, Shaw S, et al: "Seeking safety": outcome of a new cognitive-behavioral psychotherapy for women with posttraumatic stress disorder and substance dependence. J Trauma Stress 11:437–456, 1998

Najavits LM, Schmitz M, Gotthardt S, et al: Seeking Safety plus Exposure Therapy: an outcome study on dual diagnosis men. J Psychoactive Drugs 37:425–435, 2005

Najavits LM, Harned MS, Gallop RJ, et al: Six-month treatment outcomes of cocaine-dependent patients with and without PTSD in a multisite national trial. J Stud Alcohol Drugs 68:353–361, 2007

National Center on Addiction and Substance Abuse: Missed Opportunity: National Survey of Primary Care Physicians and Patients on Substance Abuse. May 2000. Available at: http://www.casacolumbia.org/templates/publications_reports.aspx. Accessed February 9, 2010.

National Center on Addiction and Substance Abuse: Shoveling Up II: The Impact of Substance Abuse on Federal, State and Local Budgets. 2009. Available at: http://www.casacolumbia.org/templates/publications_reports.aspx. Accessed February 9, 2010.

National Institute on Alcohol Abuse and Alcoholism: Ninth Special Report to the U.S. Congress on Alcohol and Health. June 1997. Available at: http://www.eric.ed.gov/ERICDocs/data/ericdocs2sql/content_storage_01/0000019b/80/15/60/de.pdf. Accessed February 9, 2010.

National Institute on Drug Abuse: NM ASSIST [NIDA-Modified Alcohol, Smoking, and Substance Involvement Screening Tool]: screening for drug use in general medical settings. September 2009. Available at: http://ww1.drugabuse.gov/nmassist. Accessed February 9, 2010.

Needle R, Fisher D, Weatherby N, et al: The reliability of self-reported HIV risk behaviors of drug users. Psychol Addict Behav 4:242–250, 1995

Nelson EC, Heath AC, Lynskey MT, et al: Childhood sexual abuse and risks for licit and illicit drug-related outcomes: a twin study. Psychol Med 10:1473–1483, 2006

Nock MK, Kazdin AE, Hirpi E, et al: Prevalence, subtypes, and correlates of DSM-IV conduct disorder in the National Comorbidity Survey Replication. Psychol Med 36:699–710, 2006

Nurco D, Wegner N, Stephenson F: Female narcotic addicts: changing profiles. Journal of Addictions and Health 3:62–105, 1982

Ostacher MJ, Nierenberg AA, Perlis RH, et al: The relationship between smoking and suicidal behavior, comorbidity, and course of illness in bipolar disorder. J Clin Psychiatry 12:1907–1911, 2006

Perkins KA: Smoking cessation in women: special considerations. CNS Drugs 5:391–411, 2001

Piccinelli M, Tessari E, Bortolomasi M, et al: Efficacy of the Alcohol Use Disorders Identification Test as a screening tool for hazardous alcohol intake and related disorders in primary care: a validity study. BMJ 314:420–424, 1997

Pirard S, Sharon E, Kang SK, et al: Prevalence of physical and sexual abuse among substance abuse patients and impact on treatment outcomes. Drug Alcohol Depend 1:57–64, 2005

Prasant MP, Mattoo SK, Basu D: Substance use and other psychiatric disorders in first-degree relatives of opioid-dependent males: a case-controlled study from India. Addiction 3:413–419, 2006

Prochaska JO, DiClemente CC, Norcross JC: In search of how people change: applications to addictive behaviors. Am Psychol 9:1102–1114, 1992

Regier DA, Farmer ME, Rae DS, et al: Co-morbidity of mental disorders with alcohol and other drug abuse: results from the Epidemiologic Catchment Area (ECA) study. JAMA 264:2511–2518, 1990

Rice C, Mohr CD, Del Boca FK, et al: Self-reports of physical, sexual and emotional abuse in an alcoholism treatment sample. J Stud Alcohol 1:114–123, 2001

Robins LN, Przybeck TR: Age of onset of drug use as a factor in drug and other disorders. NIDA Res Monogr 56:178–192, 1985

Robins LN, Regier DA: Psychiatric Disorders in America. New York, Free Press, 1991

Rodriguez-Llera MC, Domingo-Salvany A, Brugal MT, et al: Psychiatric comorbidity in young heroin users. Drug Alcohol Depend 1:48–55, 2006

Rounsaville B, Poling J: Substance use disorder measures, in Handbook of Psychiatric Measures. Task Force for the Handbook of Psychiatric Measures. Washington, DC, American Psychiatric Publishing, 2000, pp 457–484

Rounsaville BJ, Anton SF, Carroll K, et al: Psychiatric diagnoses of treatment-seeking cocaine abusers. Arch Gen Psychiatry 1:43–51, 1991

Sartor CE, Lynskey MT, Bucholz KK, et al: Childhood sexual abuse and the course of alcohol dependence development: findings from a female twin sample. Drug Alcohol Depend 89:139–144, 2007

Schottenfeld R, Pantalon M: Assessment of the patient, in The American Psychiatric Press Textbook of Substance Abuse Treatment. Edited by Galanter M. Washington, DC, American Psychiatric Press, 1999, pp 109–120

Selzer ML: The Michigan Alcoholism Screening Test: the quest for a new diagnostic instrument. Am J Psychiatry 12:1653–1658, 1971

Senay EC: Diagnostic interview and mental status examination, in Substance Abuse: A Comprehensive Textbook. Edited by Lowinson JH, Ruiz P, Millman RB, et al. Baltimore, MD, Williams & Wilkins, 1997, pp 364–369

Shields AL, Caruso JC: Reliability generalization of the Alcohol Use Disorders Identification Test. Educ Psychol Meas 63:404–413, 2003

Shields AL, Caruso JC: A reliability induction and reliability generalization study of the CAGE questionnaire. Educ Psychol Meas 63:254–270, 2004

Shields AL, Howell RT, Potter JS, et al: The Michigan Alcoholism Screening Test and its shortened forms: a meta-analytic inquiry into score reliability. Subst Use Misuse 42:1783–1800, 2007

Sidney S, Quesenberry CP Jr, Friedman GD, et al: Marijuana use and cancer incidence (California, United States). Cancer Causes Control 8:722–728, 1997

Sintov ND, Kendler KS, Walsh D, et al: Predictors of illicit substance dependence among individuals with alcohol dependence. J Stud Alcohol Drugs 70:269–278, 2009

Skinner HA: The Drug Abuse Screening Test. Addict Behav 4:363–371, 1982

Sledjeski EM, Dierker LC, Costello D, et al: Predictive validity of four nicotine dependence measures in a college sample. Drug Alcohol Depend 1:10–19, 2007

Snively TA, Ahijevych KL, Bernhard LA, et al: Smoking behavior, dysphoric states and the menstrual cycle: results from single smoking sessions and the natural environment. Psychoneuroendocrinology 7:677–691, 2000

Sobell LC, Sobell MB, Litten RZ, et al: Timeline Follow-Back: a technique for assessing self-reported alcohol consumption, in Measuring Alcohol Consumption: Psychosocial and Biochemical Methods. Edited by Litten RZ, Allen JP. Totowa, NJ, Humana Press, 1992, pp 41–72

Sobell LC, Agrawal S, Sobell MB: Factors affecting agreement between alcohol abusers' and their collaterals' reports. J Stud Alcohol 58:405–413, 1997

Sokol MS, Pfeffer CR, Solomon GE, et al: An abused psychotic preadolescent at risk for Huntington's disease. J Am Acad Child Adolesc Psychiatry 4:612–617, 1989

Sonne SC, Brady KT, Morton WA: Substance abuse and bipolar affective disorder. J Nerv Ment Dis 6:349–352, 1994

Spitzer RL, Williams JB, Gibbon M: The Structured Clinical Interview for DSM-III-R—Patient Version. New York, Biometrics Research Institute, 1992

Staley D, el-Guebaly N: Psychometric properties of the Drug Abuse Screening Test in a psychiatric patient population. Addict Behav 3:257–264, 1990

Straussner SL: Ethnocultural Factors in Substance Abuse Treatment. New York, Guilford, 2001

Substance Abuse and Mental Health Services Administration: The Confidentiality of Alcohol and Drug Abuse Patient Records Regulation and the HIPAA Privacy Rule: Implications for Alcohol and Substance Abuse Programs. Rockville, MD, Department of Health and Human Services, 2004. Available at: http://www.hipaa.samhsa.gov/Part2ComparisonClearedTOC.htm. Accessed February 9, 2010.

Substance Abuse and Mental Health Services Administration: Treatment Episode Data Set (TEDS) Highlights—2004: National Admissions to Substance Abuse Treatment Services. DASIS Series S-31 (DHHS Publ No SMA-06-4140). Rockville, MD, Department of Health and Human Services, 2006

Substance Abuse and Mental Health Services Administration: Drug Abuse Warning Network, 2006: National Estimates of Drug-Related Emergency Department Visits. DAWN Series D-30 (DHHS Publ No SMA-08-4339). Rockville, MD, Department of Health and Human Services, 2008

Sullivan JT, Sykora K, Schneiderman J, et al: Assessment of alcohol withdrawal: the revised clinical institute withdrawal assessment for alcohol scale (CIWA-Ar). Br J Addict 11:1353–1357, 1989

Taylor FM: Marijuana as a potential respiratory tract carcinogen. South Med J 81:1213–1216, 1988

U.S. Department of Health and Human Services: Health Insurance Portability and Accountability Act of 1996. Available at: http://www.hhs.gov/ocr/privacy. Accessed June 14, 2010.

van den Bree MB, Pickworth WB: Risk factors predicting changes in marijuana involvement in teenagers. Arch Gen Psychiatry 3:311–319, 2005

Warren CW, Kann L, Small ML, et al: Age of initiating selected health-risk behaviors among high school students in the United States. J Adolesc Health 4:225–231, 1997

Washburn P: Substance use disorders: approaching the patient traditional history and physical, or screening? Occup Med 17:67–78, iv, 2002

Weatherby N, Needle R, Cesari H, et al: Validity of self-reported drug use among injection drug users and crack cocaine users recruited through street outreach. Eval Program Plann 4:347–355, 1994

Weiss RD, Mirin SM, Griffin ML, et al: A comparison of alcoholic and nonalcoholic drug abusers. J Stud Alcohol 6:510–515, 1988

Weiss RD, Mirin SM, Griffin ML, et al: Personality disorders in cocaine dependence. Compr Psychiatry 3:145–149, 1993

Weiss RD, Martinez-Raga J, Griffin ML, et al: Gender differences in cocaine dependent patients: a 6 month follow-up study. Drug Alcohol Depend 1:35–40, 1997

Weiss RD, Najavits LM, Greenfield SF, et al: Validity of substance use self-reports in dually diagnosed outpatients. Am J Psychiatry 1:127–128, 1998

Weiss RD, Greenfield SF, Griffin ML, et al: The use of collateral reports for patients with bipolar disorder and substance use disorders. Am J Drug Alcohol Abuse 3:369–378, 2000a

Weiss RD, Griffin ML, Gallop R, et al: Predictors of self-help group attendance in cocaine dependent patients. J Stud Alcohol 61:714–719, 2000b

Weiss RD, Griffin ML, Greenfield SF, et al: Group therapy for patients with bipolar disorder and substance dependence: results of a pilot study. J Clin Psychiatry 5:361–367, 2000c

Wesson DR, Ling W: The Clinical Opiate Withdrawal Scale (COWS). J Psychoactive Drugs 2:253–259, 2003

Westermeyer J: Native Americans, Asians, and new immigrants, in Substance Abuse: A Comprehensive Textbook. Edited by Lowinson J, Ruiz P, Millman RB, et al. Baltimore, MD, Williams & Wilkins, 1997, pp 712–716

Westermeyer J, Tseng WS, Streltzer J: Culture and addiction psychiatry, in Cultural Competence in Clinical Psychiatry. Edited by Tseng WS, Streltzer J. Washington, DC, American Psychiatric Publishing, 2004a, pp 85–106

Westermeyer J, Yargic I, Thuras P: Michigan Assessment-Screening Test for Alcohol and Drugs (MAST/AD): evaluation in a clinical sample. Am J Addict 2:151–162, 2004b

Westermeyer J, Mellman L, Alarcon R: Cultural competence in addiction psychiatry. Addict Disord Their Treat 3:107–119, 2006

Wills TA, McNamara G, Vaccaro D, et al: Escalated substance use: a longitudinal grouping analysis from early to middle adolescence. J Abnorm Psychol 2:166–180, 1996

Wilsnack SC, Vogeltanz ND, Klassen AD, et al: Childhood sexual abuse and women's substance abuse: national survey findings. J Stud Alcohol 3:264–271, 1997

Windle M, Windle RC, Scheidt DM, et al: Physical and sexual abuse and associated mental disorders among alcoholic inpatients. Am J Psychiatry 9:1322–1328, 1995

Woody G, Cacciola J: Diagnosis and classification: DSM-IV and ICD-10, in Substance Abuse: A Comprehensive Textbook. Edited by Lowinson J, Ruiz P, Millman RB, et al. Baltimore, MD, Williams & Wilkins, 1997, pp 361–363

World Health Organization: The ICD-10 Classification of Mental and Behavioral Disorders: clinical descriptions and diagnostic guidelines. Geneva, World Health Organization, 1992/2007. Available at: http://www.who.int/substance_abuse/terminology/ICD10ClinicalDiagnosis.pdf.

World Health Organization: Alcohol, Smoking, and Substance Involvement Screening Test (ASSIST), Version 3.0, 2002. Available at: http://www.who.int/substance_abuse/activities/assist_v3_english.pdf. Accessed February 9, 2010.

Yamaguchi K, Kandel DB: Patterns of drug use from adolescence to young adulthood, II: sequences of progression. Am J Public Health 7:668–672, 1984a

Yamaguchi K, Kandel DB: Patterns of drug use from adolescence to young adulthood, III: predictors of progression. Am J Public Health 74:673–681, 1984b

Yudko E, Lozhkina O, Fouts A: A comprehensive review of the psychometric properties of the Drug Abuse Screening Test. J Subst Abuse Treat 32:189–198, 2007

2 | Testing to Identify Recent Drug Use

Robert L. DuPont, M.D.
Carl M. Selavka, Ph.D.

The diagnosis of substance use disorder, like most other medical diagnoses, is primarily clinical, with the patient's history and the mental status examination playing central roles in the diagnostic process. Nevertheless, laboratory testing to identify recent drug use is increasingly important in clinical settings, ranging from the initial diagnosis to treatment management and from research and epidemiology to health care assessment. Drug testing identifies the recent use of specific abused substances and in some settings can help to differentiate chronic or repetitive ingestions from single or low-frequency uses. Laboratory testing is especially helpful in medical settings as part of the screening process to identify patients for evaluation for substance use disorder.

In this chapter, we review the uses of drug testing. We describe the tests that are now in common practice, including the science on which they rely, the information that these tests can provide to clinicians, and information about some potential strategic considerations when choosing among the wide range of drug tests now available. Drug testing, like all biotechnology, is evolving rapidly. Some tests that we describe are widely available, whereas other testing options are not yet easily obtained. In addition, new drug-testing options will be developed after this chapter is written, although the principles on which drug testing is based and the applications for testing are likely to be more enduring. This is one reason why we emphasize these newer options here.

Drug testing in addiction medicine can identify the recent single and/or repetitive use of drugs of abuse and excessive alcohol consumption, or even the prospective use of particular drugs of abuse. Drug tests cannot detect or measure drug-caused impairment, physical dependence, or addiction to alcohol or other drugs (DuPont 2000). Those clinically important determinations rely, like the diagnosis of addictive illness itself, primarily on clinical assessments, with the laboratory findings often providing complementary data. Drug tests are particularly useful because they identify recent drug use in settings where that information is of diagnostic significance (e.g., in emergency department and other medical care settings) and where the information has value in reinforcing a drug-free standard (e.g., in drug treatment, the criminal justice system, the workplace, family law–based civil jurisdictions, and schools).

Biology of Drug Tests

Two of the hallmarks of addictive disorders are dishonesty about substance use and continued use despite problems caused by that use (DuPont 2000). Addicted people characteristically deny to themselves and to others the negative consequences of their alcohol and other drug use, and they characteristically lie about their alcohol and other drug use to anyone who might interfere with their continued substance use (DuPont 1998). Users of illegal drugs may not know what drugs they are taking, so that even if they wanted to tell their doctors their current drug use history, they may not be able to do so. Many people who have positive test results for recent drug use claim that the use leading to the positive test was isolated or even the first time they used; this is exceedingly unlikely. Rare or occasional use of drugs is unlikely to be detected by drug testing. In fact, the vast majority of positive results on drug tests reflect repeated, continuous drug use (DuPont 1996; DuPont et al. 1995).

Users of alcohol and other drugs consume their substances of choice for the specific effects these substances have on the reward centers of their brains (DuPont and Gold 1995; Volkow and Li 2009). To achieve this brain-rewarding effect, users consume drugs by many routes of administration, including oral ingestion, snorting, smoking, and injecting (Coleman et al. 2005). The common preference of many experienced drug users is to use the routes of administration that produce the most rapid increase in blood levels, because these are most intensely rewarding (DuPont et al. 2009).

Once consumed, the abused drugs are distributed so widely that they can be identified in virtually all parts of the body and in all body fluids and tissues. Drugs are typically metabolized by the liver and in the blood, each drug producing characteristic metabolites that are often longer lasting and detectable at higher levels than the parent drug. Although the pharmacokinetics of this process are complex and substance specific, the general pattern is universal. This common pattern makes testing for all drugs of abuse similar and relatively easy to understand. On the other hand, the pharmacokinetics of each drug are important in the linkage of laboratory results to specific patterns of recent drug use.

Although a wide range of techniques can be used to identify drugs and their metabolites, modern testing for drugs of abuse has settled into a sequence that usually begins with a relatively inexpensive immunoassay screening test, which has high sensitivity but not absolute specificity. This means that the immunoassay screen can detect very low levels of drugs and drug metabolites in the tested specimen, but the results occasionally can be confounded by cross-reactivity with nondrug substances. Most immunoassay drug tests depend on patented monoclonal antibodies that are developed to be highly specific to individual drugs or drug metabolites. For this reason, cross-reactivity with current immunoassay drug tests is seldom a problem (Huynh et al. 2009). The immunoassay screening tests are widely used because they can be automated for laboratory testing and can be used to produce on-site (point-of-collection) test kits.

In the workplace and other settings where results on drug tests must be forensically defensible, presumptive positive results from screening drug tests are confirmed with a highly specific confirmation test, such as a gas chromatography–mass spectrometry (GC/MS) test. This test is not subject to cross-reactivity and is specific to a single drug or drug metabolite. Screening tests can be performed on-site and do not require a clinical laboratory, although confirmation tests are performed only in a laboratory. This picture of a presumptive immunoassay screening test followed by a more sophisticated and expensive confirmation test can be used to produce optimal reliability for all tested specimens, including urine, blood, sweat, saliva (now called *oral fluid* for biological accuracy), and hair.

In many settings where this forensic standard is unnecessary, including most routine, frequently repeated drug testing in addiction treatment and the criminal justice system, an immunoassay test is sufficient without confirmation (DuPont and Selavka 2003). The one exception to this general two-step testing regimen in forensic settings involves the determination of the presence of alcohol. For this volatile substance, breath testing using relatively automated methods and oral fluid tests provide generally reliable results without the need for a separate confirming test to meet forensic standards. Recently, laboratory-based methods for biomarkers produced by drinking alcohol—including ethyl glucuronide (EtG) and fatty acid ethyl esters (FAEEs)—have been employed to differentiate abstinence, social drinking, and chronic, excessive alcohol consumption (Pragst and Yegles 2006, 2008). Over-the-counter drug kits are now available for home use—for example, by parents who use drug tests to deter or detect drug use by their children. In this setting, it is useful for both parents and clinicians to be educated about the benefits and pitfalls of drug tests and to responsibly manage positive test results (DuPont and Bucher 2005).

One common misunderstanding about drug testing relates to the drugs being identified. Virtually all drugs of abuse can be identified with immunoassay screens that are specific to individual drugs. Each targeted drug requires a separate antibody test, which involves separate costs (Selavka 1997). Most laboratories and on-site drug-test kits use limited screens for a small number of drugs in panels that are bundled to keep costs relatively low. When a test subject is thought to be using drugs outside of the narrow list of commonly used drugs, special-order and more comprehensive laboratory tests are needed. In other words, drug tests do not identify "drug use" in a global sense. Rather, they identify recent use of the specific drugs that are targeted on the test panel used for the test. Therefore, when interpreting results from drug tests, it is important to know which specific drugs were targeted in specific test samples. Drugs of abuse other than those on the list of drugs targeted in the particular sample will not be identified, even if their use is recent and has had major behavioral or health effects.

Sample Selection: Blood, Urine, Hair, Oral Fluid, or Sweat

Two decades ago, when drug-testing technology was relatively primitive, the only commonly used sample was urine, in which drugs and drug metabolites are relatively concentrated and easily identified without the need for complex extraction techniques. In earlier years, these initial drug tests were always done at large clinical chemistry laboratories. The one test that has been done outside of laboratories is breath and blood testing for alcohol, which for several decades has commonly employed point-of-collection test methods in the hands of nonscientific personnel.

In more recent years, as drug-testing technology has improved and more reliable procedures for collection and sample handling have been developed, it has become practical to test sweat, oral fluid, and hair to identify recent drug use. Regardless of the sample selected, the drug tests themselves use the same highly reliable science in the same pattern of screening tests, followed, when indicated, by a confirming test. With these technological improvements, toxicology tests in matrices other than those that would be considered "old standards"—such as breath and blood for alcohol, and urine for drugs—have significantly improved the speed, scope, and sensitivity of laboratory data available to assist the medical community in clinical settings, death investigations, and many other traditional and nontraditional venues (Kintz et al. 2009). Modern information technology advances can assist the clinician by providing improvements to the clarity and interpretive usefulness of toxicology reports provided (Kidwell and Riggs 2004).

The sample selected for alcohol and other drug testing reflects many practical factors, including ease of access, cost of the test, and the most appropriate detection window (i.e., the period of time that is sampled to identify drug use). Breath, oral fluid, and hair samples are the most easily collected with high integrity, whereas urine can present logistical and reliability risks. Blood and organ samples (e.g., liver biopsies) are the most invasive and difficult to obtain. When considered as part of a total patient assessment, costs of analysis are similar, although hair and blood testing are somewhat more expensive than urine testing. Oral fluid and sweat testing are more similar to urine testing in cost. Drug tests of sweat, oral fluid, and hair specimens are performed at a limited number of specialized laboratories, whereas urine drug testing is done at most clinical laboratories and dozens of federally accredited specialized drug-testing laboratories.

Urine-testing kits are commonly used for on-site screening, providing results within a few minutes of collection. Oral fluid tests also can be performed on-site. If alcohol and other drug testing is conducted in the workplace, then legal regulations are important considerations, including secure collection with forensic standards of specimen handling and laboratory confirmation (U.S. Department of Health and Human Services 2004). When follow-on laboratory-based methods become essential to meet legal or regulatory expectations related to a testing environment, the stability of drugs and metabolites in urine during storage and shipment could become a concern. Stability of drugs of abuse and metabolites has been the subject of very detailed studies (Zaitsu et al. 2008), and degradation constitutes a real detractor in programs testing urine when compared with hair, and even with oral fluid using stabilized oral fluid collection kits.

Because the level of drug or drug metabolite in urine is strongly influenced by recent fluid consumption, urine levels do not equate with blood levels. For this reason, and because blood and urine levels change rapidly over even short periods of time, urine results are read as either positive or negative at specific cutoff levels. Because both sweat patches and hair tests are not subject to the effects of fluid consumption and because they sample longer time periods, both sweat patch tests and hair tests permit rough quantitation of drug use over the time periods sampled.

Blood has the shortest window of detection, because most drugs are cleared from the blood at measurable levels in 12 hours or less. Urine has a detection window of about 1–3 days, because most drugs are cleared within this time after the most recent use of the drug (Jufer et al. 2000). This is true even for marijuana, unless the tested individual has been a chronic heavy smoker of marijuana, in which case the urine results may remain positive for up to a month after use stops. Even with the availability of today's more potent marijuana, after one or two marijuana cigarettes (in the absence of prior heavy chronic marijuana use), results from urine tests are negative in many subjects within 24 hours, and all results will be negative at the 100-ng/mL cutoff for the target cannabinoid metabolite within 3 days. After one or two marijuana cigarettes, most subjects' results from urine tests will be negative at the more sensitive 15-ng/mL cutoff within 5 days of last marijuana use (Dietz et al. 2007).

Head hair grows at the rate of about 0.5 inch (or a bit more than 1 cm) per month. With each day of drug use, newly created hair cells incorporate drug from the blood on that day, creating a virtual day-by-day "tape recording" of drug use. If a tested person has only a single day of drug use, the incorporation of drug into hair is predominantly localized to the tiny 0.3-mm length of hair representing that day. When surrounded by the "ocean of abstinence" represented by hair growing on days without drug use, this single ingestion is not detected with conventional drug tests of hair. Positive results from hair testing are generally expected only when a person has used a drug at least four to six times (at typical nonmedical doses) per month when conventional hair-test reporting thresholds (cutoffs) are used. For many hair-testing laboratories, even greater frequency of marijuana use is required before a tested person's occasional marijuana smoking becomes detectable at or above common testing cutoffs. For this reason, positive results from hair testing are generally interpreted as reliable indicators of chronic or at least frequently repeated and recent drug ingestion (Morrison et al. 1998). This longer detection window for testing hair, coupled with the ability to distinguish between light, moderate, and heavy use during the prior 90 days or more, makes hair testing especially useful as part of the evaluation for admission to addiction treatment (Charles et al. 2003).

About a week is required for hair to grow from the base of the hair follicle in the scalp or body site to the external skin surface. Thus, a standard 1.5-inch sample of head hair contains drug residuals from the prior 90 days, minus the week immediately before sample collection. Hair testing is particularly useful and superior to urine testing in various situations in which the longer detection window is important (DuPont and Baumgartner 1995). Because preemployment testing of urine for drugs is a scheduled test, a drug user has to refrain from nonmedical drug use for only 3–5 days before submitting a urine sample in order to pass a urine test for abused drugs. It is much harder for most dedicated drug abusers to refrain from drug use for 90 days before preemployment testing, the period covered by a standard hair sample. Longer hair, and therefore longer time periods, also can be tested in special-order tests. If such longer time periods are important, or if a specific time between known periods of abstinence in a longer length of hair is critical, the testing laboratory can work with the clinician to properly segment and/or interpret results to maximize the probative information produced by such examinations.

Hair is always collected by a third party under direct observation, not by the tested person in the absence of observation. Therefore, in contrast to urine samples, with their long history of collection integrity problems (Minakata et al. 2006), hair samples do not pose integrity problems with sample substitution, adulteration, or dilution. However, hair treatments, such as perming, bleaching, and straightening, may reduce drug levels in hair in a way that can convert borderline-positive results to negative results. Conventional hygienic hair treatments have little effect on the detection of drug use with hair tests. Hair is also less invasive to collect than urine and easier to store and transport.

This higher threshold for a positive result in a hair test means that eating poppy seeds will not produce a positive hair laboratory test result for opiates, as it commonly does in urine tests that do not include specific, sensitive testing for unique metabolites of heroin. Positive laboratory results for opiates in urine tests are routinely reversed by medical review officers, making testing of urine samples for opiates in the workplace all but worthless because of the poppy seed problem. More important, high cutoffs for urine opiate detection now in widespread use make it nearly impossible to detect abusers of heroin, a substance for which hair testing is particularly well suited. Similar care must be exercised when addressing positive results for amphetamines, to ensure that illicit drug use is differentiated from legitimate prescriptions (or legitimate metabolite sources).

In recent years, concerns were raised by a few researchers about possible racial bias in hair testing because of the potential for different drug levels to be retained in hair of different colors. This issue originated as a result of a study of drug levels in fur of different colors on the same laboratory mouse. This concern about hair color has sometimes been inappropriately conflated into an issue of racial differences in hair-test results. The claim is not that one race has inherently positive results from hair tests but rather that if people of different races use the same amount of drug (and this debate has usually related to black individuals and cocaine use), one race will have higher levels in the hair than the other race, leading to more positive results from hair tests even if the levels of drug use are the same in the two racial groups.

No data from large samples have demonstrated racial bias in hair testing in human subjects. However, to test the hypothesis that hair tests are biased, both urine and hair were tested in a large sample of police applicants. The results for cocaine are shown in Table 2–1. This study found that among black males, urine tests showed that 11 had positive test results for cocaine and 473 had negative test results; among white males, 5 had positive urine test results for cocaine and 857 had negative test results. For hair tests in this same study, 41 black males had positive test results for cocaine and 443 had negative test results, whereas 20 white males had positive test results and 842 had negative test results. The odds ratio for hair tests compared with urine tests for cocaine for black males was 3.99; for white males, the odds ratio was 3.90, virtually identical. If hair tests were biased compared with urine tests for cocaine, the odds ratio would have been significantly higher for hair than for urine. In fact, in this large real-life study, the odds of positive urine test results for black compared with white individuals were slightly higher than the odds ratio for hair test results (Mieczkowski and Lersch 2002).

The take-home message is that all modern drug tests use the same basic testing science—the immunoassay screen and the GC/MS (or equivalent) confirming test. Drug tests of urine, hair, sweat, and oral fluid use this science to identify individual drugs and drug metabolites reliably and specifically. If this two-step process identifies the drug, then it is present. A person who has not consumed the drug of abuse being tested will have a negative test result whether the test matrix is urine, hair, sweat, or oral fluid. However, innocent exposure may produce a positive test result. (As we describe later in this chapter, poppy seeds can produce a positive result for morphine on urine tests, and hand sanitizers can cause a positive alcohol result with EtG in blood and urine testing.) These are not false-positive results, because morphine is present in urine after poppy seed consumption, and EtG is in the urine after intense use of an alcohol-containing hand sanitizer. These "evidentiary false indicators" are often used as reasons for choosing hair-test strategies for drugs and alcohol-ingestion biomarkers. Hair tests provide evidence of chronic excessive alcohol consumption and repetitive recreational drug use, and do not suffer from these evidentiary false-indicator issues the way urine tests do.

Biological variations in the probability of a positive drug test result are well known to occur despite similar consumption of all drugs. For example, a small woman will have a higher blood alcohol concentration (BAC) for a given amount of alcohol consumed than will a large man. Of course, neither the small woman nor the large man will have positive test results if

TABLE 2–1.   Comparisons by race in preemployment cocaine testing of police applicants

Applicants		Urine test results				Hair test results		
		Black	White	Odds ratio		Black	White	Odds ratio
Males	(+)	11	5	3.99	(+)	41	20	3.90
	(−)	473	857		(−)	443	842	
Females[a]	(+)	1	1	0.8	(+)	10	2	4.1
	(−)	27	22		(−)	26	22	

[a]Too few positive urine test results for meaningful ratio.
Source.   Mieczowski and Lersch 2002.

neither has consumed (or recently been significantly exposed to) alcohol. Decades of experience with alcohol and other drug tests have shown that no clinically valid reason exists to normalize drug test results to mathematically ensure that the same dose of the drug produces the same result across large biological differences, including gender, age, and weight.

Workplace drug testing conducted under federal guidelines unfortunately has been limited for over 20 years to laboratory-based urine tests for a small number of drugs (codeine/morphine, amphetamine and methamphetamine, phencyclidine [PCP], marijuana, and cocaine). This means that testing under current federal guidelines does not detect the use of any other drugs, many of which are commonly abused, such as lysergic acid diethylamide (LSD), methylenedioxymethamphetamine (MDMA; ecstasy) and other stimulants, and synthetic opioids (e.g., hydromorphone, oxycodone, methylphenidate). These limited and out-of-date federal guidelines were written to apply to federally mandated drug testing (for federal workers and for U.S. Department of Transportation–mandated tests). Nevertheless, because the federal standards are often used in other settings, these standards are commonly applied to nonregulated samples as well. For the past two decades, federal standards have not kept up with the rapidly improving science and technology of drug testing. However, the revised federal standards effective October 1, 2010 (U.S. Department of Health and Human Services 2010), include MDMA confirmation and immunoassay screening for the heroin metabolite 6-MAM, as well as more modern confirmation technologies (Feng et al. 2007; Stout et al. 2009).

Non–federally mandated drug testing, including testing in drug treatment programs and in many workplace settings, is not limited by the currently antiquated federal drug-testing standards. Nevertheless, many organizations that use drug tests in settings that are not limited by these regulations are unaware of the wider options available. Unfortunately, such organizations often limit testing to the five drugs in urine tested at federally certified laboratories. Because preemployment drug testing dominates the drug-testing industry, most laboratory offerings and test kits are limited to this regrettably narrow range of abused drugs and use only urine samples for testing.

Urine tests, when used in nonregulated situations, can identify a widely expanded list of controlled substances, thereby offering important diagnostic information. This higher standard characterizes the comprehensive random drug testing routinely used by the United States military. The military drug-test scheme includes testing all samples for the most commonly abused drugs, such as marijuana, cocaine, methamphetamine, and heroin, and then adds a rotation of other drugs to the panel in a random fashion so that the tested person does not know for which other drugs he or she is being tested. This approach preserves the deterrent value of the test but limits the cost of testing. It also permits the military to keep track of the positive rates for many drugs over time so that if a new drug emerges as commonly abused, it can be added to the panel of drugs used to test all service personnel.

New drugs and drug classes of importance are singled out by the military for addition to the rotation drug list, and older target drugs that have lost popularity and do not need to be in the rotation are taken out of the rotation in the military's systematic "prevalence study." Each year, the Department of Defense's toxicology research and development laboratory tests thousands of samples that were found to be negative using current targeted drug tests. These samples that were negative on the routine test panel are anonymized before being sent to the central research and development laboratory at the Armed Forces Institute of Pathology (AFIP). If the AFIP determines that this negative pooled population of military samples has a positive rate greater than a specific level for a given drug, that drug is added to the rotation at all six Department of Defense laboratories. If a drug on the current rotation list falls to a lower prevalence level, it is removed from the list. Commanders are kept informed of the moving drug-test targets and the potential impacts of using specific, including newly added, drugs. However, this target list is not shared with those personnel who are subject to testing. The impact of such military studies is not always globally applicable because of the wide variety of drug-using patterns in different geographical areas (Meririnne et al. 2007). This same sophisticated approach to drug testing is available to commercial drug-testing laboratories, which would benefit from similar intelligent test designs in other settings, including in drug abuse treatment (DuPont and Graves 2005).

Even a single dose of the most commonly abused substances—including inhalants (e.g., nitrous oxide), solvents (involved in "huffing"), and myriad drugs available to medical professionals (e.g., meperidine, fentanyl)—can be detected in urine in the 1–3 days after ingestion. However, the clinician needs to use a reference toxicology laboratory to provide these specialty urine-testing services, often at substantially higher costs.

Cheating, facilitated by the Internet and by determined opponents of drug testing, has long been the Achilles' heel of urine drug tests (Minakata et al. 2006). Cheating can be reduced by direct observation of collection, as used by the military, but cheating is an inherent problem with urine tests. This limitation of the urine test is offset to some extent by several other important factors. Testing urine is generally less expensive than testing hair, oral fluids, or sweat, and this test is far more widely available. When a larger list of drugs is needed in the screen, urine is usually the best choice because a large number of laboratories do urine tests. In contrast, most laboratories doing hair and oral fluid testing offer testing for only a limited range of drugs even though they could test for many more drugs. This limit is not a matter of science. It is a business decision by the laboratories, which reflects the fact that most drug-test clients request the very narrow panels in common use.

Sweat patch testing is relatively new, compared with drug testing of urine, blood, and hair. Early reports suggest relatively limited applicability of sweat patch testing in deterring drug use (Barnes et al. 2008). The tested person wears a patch, similar to a nicotine patch worn by people attempting to quit smoking. Once removed, the patch cannot be replaced without noticeable puckering at the edges of the sweat test collection device. This feature provides reasonable integrity in the sweat patch collection process. Sweat is continuously absorbed into the pad component of the patch; the water in the sweat evaporates through the outer patch membrane, whereas the drugs of abuse and their metabolites accumulate on the absorbent pad. Because skin continuously desquamates, these sweat patches can be worn for periods from a few hours to a few weeks, after which they fall off. During that time, they collect prospective evidence of drug use, rather than the retrospective "historical" data provided by drug tests performed on all other common matrices. Once removed under direct observation, the patches are sent to a laboratory for testing.

Patches are commercially tested to detect cocaine, opiates, marijuana, PCP, and amphetamine and methamphetamine. Sweat patch testing is especially useful for treatment follow-up testing and in return-to-work settings when daily urine testing or intensive random testing for drug use is impractical. Sweat patches are not routinely marketed for the detection of alcohol use; however, alcohol detection patches may find greater application now that EtG and FAEEs have become useful investigative target metabolites for alcohol consumption (Pragst et al. 2004). Patches for alcohol detection will augment traditional blood alcohol ingestion biomarkers, such as liver function and carbohydrate-deficient transferrin laboratory results that can track near-term alcohol intakes in the prior 3–5 days (Bortolotti et al. 2006). Also, in June 2009 the Society of Hair Testing promulgated international consensus standards that recommend interpretation of excessive alcohol consumption over the past 3 months using tests of hair for EtG, and over the past 6 months using hair tests for FAEEs (Society of Hair Testing 2009). See the discussion of EtG and FAEE testing in the "Alcohol Testing" section, later in this chapter (see also Pragst et al. 2010 and Süsse et al. 2010).

Hair testing and sweat patches offer important advantages over urine testing for abused drugs in many settings, including during substance abuse treatment. Both are far more resistant to cheating, offer rough quantitation (enabling the separation of heavy users from light users), and reliably produce positive test results for opiates after heroin ingestion without the complication of possible poppy seed use. Oral fluid testing for drugs of abuse is now commonly used by the insurance industry to detect the use of nicotine (as its metabolite cotinine), cocaine, and other drugs. Oral fluid testing for abused drugs has gained popularity in the workplace and other settings (Barnes et al. 2003). For example, oral fluid tests of impaired drivers can significantly improve the overall detection of ingested drugs in drivers, regardless of whether these impaired drivers also drank alcohol.

An important example of the promise of drug testing using oral fluids was recently demonstrated internationally. In an alpha test by another country's traffic police force (unpublished 2009 study, described in personal communication from A. Lasarow, Principal Director, TrimegLabs Ltd, Cape Town, South Africa), drivers behaving erratically were stopped and subjected to the typical breath tests for alcohol. Drivers who produced negative breath tests had their tongues swabbed using an oral fluid collection strip. The strip gave positive responses when a relatively high concentration of cocaine, amphetamines, opiates, or cannabinoid metabolites was present on the tongue or in the oral fluid. Positive tests gave the police probable cause to collect conventional oral fluid samples and to submit them for laboratory-based analysis. In this alpha test involving hundreds of drivers, over 50% of the erratic drivers who passed the breath tests for alcohol were shown to have recently used drugs that are known to adversely affect driving. The deterrence power of such on-site oral fluid tests in highway settings would be substantial and would make roads and highways safer. Drug tests are seldom done in highway settings in the United States, despite evidence that drugs cause crashes, injuries, and deaths at rates similar to those for alcohol (Compton and Berning 2009; Michael Walsh et al. 2005).

Oral fluid is in equilibrium with blood. For this reason, oral fluid testing using conventional cutoffs detects drug use only within the prior 6–12 hours. Oral fluid testing for alcohol is also available. Because oral fluid is easily obtained (unlike urine and blood) and can be screened on-site (unlike hair samples), it is especially useful in postaccident and highway testing, and in other settings in which easy collection and immediate results are important. One limitation of oral fluid testing is that currently available on-site oral fluid test kits are less sensitive than urine testing and laboratory-based oral fluid testing, especially in detecting recent marijuana use. With modern forensic laboratory–based technologies having lower cutoffs, oral fluid and urine tests provide similar positive rates for other commonly used drugs of abuse in side-by-side testing (Yacoubian et al. 2001). Today's more sensitive generation of on-site oral fluid testing kits promises to raise detection rates closer to those found using laboratory-based oral fluid testing (Kauert et al. 2006; Moore et al. 2007). This will make oral fluid testing, even for marijuana, more practical.

In general, when hair testing and oral fluid testing are performed at the same time on the same individuals as urine testing, more positive results are found with hair testing and fewer with oral fluid testing, as is demonstrated in the comparison of positive results for urine and hair testing on the same subjects in Table 2–1. These different positive drug-test rates are primarily the result of the longer detection window for hair and the shorter detection window for oral fluids compared with urine, which is the drug-test matrix most commonly used today. From the deterrence and drug use detection standpoint, hair drug testing offers superior effectiveness, as shown in the Quest Diagnostics Incorporated (2009) historical test comparison graph (Figure 2–1). Hair drug testing offers clear advantages for identifying drug users, who can then be assisted by clinicians and rehabilitation specialists to abstain from drug use and rebuild their lives.

When testing is done repeatedly on the same individuals, as is typical in drug treatment and the criminal justice system, one way to maximize

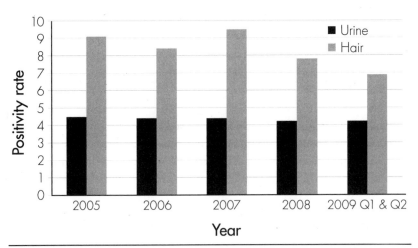

FIGURE 2–1. **Positivity rates for drug use with hair versus urine testing, general U.S. workforce.**

Source. Data from Quest Diagnostics Incorporated 2009.

the benefits of the range of matrices now available is to rotate the testing matrix so the person being tested does not know whether a particular test will use urine, hair, or oral fluids. This strategy dramatically reduces the risk of cheating. It also allows the testing organization to compare the rates of positive test results using these three methods in ways that help to tailor the testing to be more cost-effective (DuPont and Graves 2005).

Table 2–2 lists the commonly used matrices for drug testing and provides a summary of the typical applications of each, including their strengths and limitations.

On-Site Versus Laboratory Drug Tests

Two decades ago, virtually all drug tests were done in large clinical chemistry laboratories. Today, with improved technology, drug tests can be done on-site with test kits and related on-site technology tools developed by many manufacturers. The major advantage of on-site testing is that the results are available within minutes. On-site drug tests have been developed for urine and oral fluids, neither of which requires extraction before testing (Laloup et al. 2006). The on-site tests are commonly based on immunoassays and, therefore, should be used as presumptive screening tests. In settings where forensic standards need to be met (e.g., when major consequences follow a single positive test result), it is important to conduct a confirmation test requiring sophisticated equipment, usually available only at a laboratory. In many clinical settings, especially when the donor admits to the drug use, it is not necessary to conduct a more expensive confirmation test. Because the vast majority of drug tests produce negative results, using on-site kits for screening has tremendous practical advantages. For example, in drug treatment or probation and parole settings, on-site tests permit rapid assessment while the sample donor is at the testing site.

Two limitations need to be considered, however, when using on-site screening tests rather than sending samples to a laboratory for the initial screening test. First, in settings where forensic standards must be met, a positive result on a screening test must be considered a presumptive positive. Therefore, implementation of the consequences for a positive test must be withheld until a confirmation test result is returned from the laboratory, which can take an additional day or longer. In parole and probation settings, flight risk increases dramatically while tested individuals await the confirming result when they know they have created an on-site positive test result. Therefore, duplicate collections should be performed on a subpopulation of all donors within the tested group, in addition to all presumptive positive donors. The people from whom the second sample

TABLE 2–2. Blood, urine, hair, oral fluid, and sweat patch testing for drugs of abuse

Important test features	Blood	Urine	Hair	Oral fluid	Sweat patch
Immunoassay screen	Yes	Yes	Yes	Yes	Yes
Gas or liquid chromatography/mass spectrometry confirmation option (laboratory-based)	Yes	Yes	Yes	Yes	Yes
Chain-of-custody option	Yes	Yes	Yes	Yes	Yes
Retained positive results for retest option	Difficult	Possible	Easy	Difficult	Possible
Medical review officer option	Yes	Yes	Yes	Yes	Yes
Common surveillance window	3–12 hours	1–3 days	7–90 days	3–24 hours	1–21 days
Intrusiveness of collection	Severe	Moderate	None	Slight	Slight
Retest of same sample	Yes	Yes	Yes	Yes	Yes
Compatibility of new sample if original test disputed	No	No	Yes	No	No
Number of drugs screened	Unlimited[a]	Unlimited[b]	Large[c]	≥5 (alcohol)	5[d]
Cost/sample (HHS-5)	~$60–$200	~$15–$30	~$40–$65	~$50	~$35
Can distinguish between light, moderate, and heavy use	Yes, acutely	No	Yes, chronically	No	Yes, prospectively
Resistance to cheating	High	Low	High	High	High

TABLE 2–2. Blood, urine, hair, oral fluid, and sweat patch testing for drugs of abuse *(continued)*

Important test features	Blood	Urine	Hair	Oral fluid	Sweat patch
Best applications	Postaccident and overdose testing for alcohol and other drugs Blood alcohol concentration level	Reasonable cause testing Frequent testing of high-risk groups such as posttreatment follow-up and criminal justice system Unannounced, random tests with observed collection	Preemployment testing Random and periodic testing Testing to determine severity of drug use for referral to treatment Testing subjects suspected of seeking to evade urine test detection Opiate-addicted persons claiming poppy seed false-positive result Differentiation of alcoholics with chronic, excessive alcohol use from social drinkers and abstainers	Postaccident and overdose testing for alcohol and other drugs Blood alcohol concentration level Reasonable cause testing	Posttreatment testing Maintaining abstinence Opiate-addicted persons claiming poppy seed false-positive result Compliance testing in Department of Transportation and criminal justice system applications because of "prospective" nature of the drug ingestion data provided

TABLE 2–2. Blood, urine, hair, oral fluid, and sweat patch testing for drugs of abuse *(continued)*

Note. HHS-5=U.S. Department of Health and Human Services five (5) drug class mandated test panel for cocaine, opiates, PCP (phencyclidine), amphetamines, and THC (marijuana; cannabis).

[a]Blood testing for alcohol is routine, costing about $25 per sample, but blood testing for drugs is done by only a few laboratories in the United States. Blood testing for drugs is relatively expensive, costing about $60 for each drug detected.

[b]Urine tests for nonroutine drugs are available from most reference laboratories, and costs for broad screens are generally less than $200, depending on how many and which drugs are included in the screen.

[c]Hair testing is commonly performed for the HHS-5. However, numerous drugs and metabolites can be detected, and routine "broad testing" is performed in several toxicology reference laboratories. The cost of nonroutine testing of hair is less than $750 in most cases.

[d]Commonly limited to the HHS-5. Tests also can be performed for alcohol, but because nonbeverage alcohol is commonly encountered, interpretation of a positive test result can be problematic. Hair alcohol biomarker testing has clear advantages for rehabilitation compliance testing needs.

is collected should not be told that they produced an on-site positive result. However, all tested donors should be told that a system of negative checks and positive confirmations is built into the program. The delay related to on-site testing must be built into a donor's timing expectations, to maximize effectiveness of such urine-based programs while minimizing flight risks. In many settings, hair testing is superior to on-site urine and oral fluid methods because hair testing is resistant to cheating and because it detects greater drug use frequency. However, the higher costs of hair tests often limit their use, despite these advantages.

The second limitation is that on-site tests may be less sensitive. This means that it is common to get presumptively negative results from on-site samples that laboratories would identify as positive. Because a test sample screened as negative is not routinely sent for a confirmation test, this false-negative problem is serious and is not corrected by the second, confirmation test. Very few on-site positive tests are later confirmed as negative, but this outcome does occur. That is the reason that the confirmation test is critical in forensic settings. Nevertheless, despite these limitations, on-site testing is a valuable option in many settings, including drug abuse treatment.

As discussed for probation and parole applications above, the problem of false-negative results from on-site test kits can be assessed in programs by sending a significant percentage of test samples to the laboratory regardless of whether they screen negative or positive in the on-site test (Cone et al. 2003). With these data, it is possible to determine the probability of a false-negative result on the on-site screen for each specific drug. Usually, marijuana, which is present in lower concentrations in urine and oral fluids, is the drug most likely to produce false-negative results in on-site testing. The testing program can then balance that problem against the obvious benefits of the on-site screen and determine the best course of action.

Dealing With Difficult Results

Most positive drug test results arise from a person's purposeful, nonmedical use of drugs of abuse. However, in some instances, results from drug tests can be difficult to interpret, particularly if the tested individual disputes a positive result. Typically, the tested person admits to the recent drug use when confronted with a positive result. If the result is difficult to interpret and is disputed, it is wise to get help in interpreting the drug test result.

Help can be found in two ways. The first is to contact the laboratory that did the test or, for on-site tests, the manufacturer of the test kits. In today's electronically connected world, laboratories and manufacturers have access to forensic toxicologists who are usually able to provide expert advice on the interpretation of puzzling drug test results immediately. The second strategy when confronted by a difficult drug test result is to contact a local medical review officer, a trained and certified physician who has expertise in interpreting drug test results. Lists of medical review officers can be accessed through the American Association of Medical Review Officers Registry (www.aamro.com/locate). In addition, local drug testing laboratories have lists of medical review officers who can be contacted.

Because drug tests are not always easily understood or well used (Maurer et al. 2006), larger treatment programs and other programs doing drug tests should designate specific staff members to learn how to interpret complex or confusing drug test results, so that each program has in-house expertise. *Principles of Addiction Medicine* (Ries et al. 2009), the textbook of the American Society of Addiction Medicine, is a reliable source with good and up-to-date information about drug tests. The American Society of Addiction Medicine and American Association of Medical Review Officers also offer courses for medical review officer certification and substantial literature resources, which can be helpful for physicians who want to learn more about drug tests and their interpretation.

For help in developing and managing drug testing in specific settings, Hazelden has published three handbooks covering drug tests in drug treatment, the criminal justice system, and schools (DuPont and Brady 2005; DuPont et al. 2005a, 2005b).

Alcohol Testing

Although breath and blood tests for alcohol are common and well understood (having been commonly applied in clinical settings for decades), alcohol also can be detected in urine, along with other drugs of abuse. However, because urine in the bladder has been produced by the kidneys since the prior micturition and because urine concentration of alcohol and other drugs is largely determined by fluid consumption, the alcohol level in the urine sample is not correlated with the blood alcohol level. Alcohol is eliminated from the blood (and therefore from urine and breath) within a few hours of consumption, so urine test results are likely to be negative for alcohol a few hours after drinking stops. This short detection window for alcohol in the urine contrasts with the 1- to 3-day window during which urine is positive for most drugs of abuse following the last drug dose. Because alcohol is rapidly eliminated from the body, testing of the breath, urine, or oral fluids will only detect alcohol consumed within the previous few hours. This biology makes direct alcohol testing useful in detecting recent and potentially impairing alcohol use (because both breath and oral fluid results permit quantification of the current BAC). The standard alcohol tests are of limited value when the standard involves complete abstinence, as is typical for patients in substance abuse treatment.

Within the last few years, a urine test has been developed for EtG, one of the common and relatively stable metabolites of alcohol (DuPont et al. 2007). EtG generally can be identified in the urine 3–5 days following drinking. This test is not useful unless drinking itself (as opposed to heavy drinking or impaired driving) is important to identify, such as in alcohol and other drug treatment programs where abstinence from alcohol consumption is a program requirement. The test is also useful for assessment of people younger than the legal drinking age, as well as people under supervision of the criminal justice system when alcohol consumption is prohibited.

EtG testing in urine is now widely available from drug-testing laboratories. The interpretation of EtG results can be difficult, however, because exposure to nonbeverage alcohol (e.g., in mouthwashes and hand-sanitizing gels) is widespread in the community. Thus, a negative EtG urine test result reliably confirms that no alcohol consumption has occurred during the prior 3–5 days, a finding of great importance in many settings. Conversely, a positive EtG test result may or may not indicate recent consumption of beverage alcohol. One way to handle this confounding problem is to educate the tested person about the environmental exposure to alcohol so that these exposures can be avoided. This is similar to educating the heroin-addicted person in treatment to avoid eating poppy seeds because they might produce a positive result for morphine in urine. When EtG urine testing is used, clinicians must heed the recommendations of the testing laboratory on the interpretation of results because this is a relatively new test, and the applications of the test are rapidly evolving.

Studies of EtG levels in hair have demonstrated their analytical ability to differentiate social alcohol drinkers from problem-generating heavy drinkers. Hair EtG testing can also distinguish beverage consumption from nonbeverage exposure to alcohol in the same way that hair testing separates poppy seed consumption from heroin use, a separation that urine tests cannot achieve. Studies have also demonstrated the value of testing hair for cocaethylene, a unique cocaine metabolite found when alcohol is also consumed (Politi et al. 2006, 2007). Cocaethylene testing is routinely applied in drug testing applications to identify polydrug abusers who consume both cocaine and alcohol.

EtG testing on hair is a forensic examination that is now performed in small numbers of cases in the United States but in large numbers of cases every day internationally. In the United Kingdom and European Union, hair testing for EtG is used to identify patients and other persons exhibiting chronic excessive alcohol ingestion, using World Health Organization standards (Yegles and Pragst 2005).

Another alcohol biomarker system that is being used internationally and has found high acceptability in legal, medical, criminal justice, and family law applications involves testing for four specific FAEEs in hair. FAEE hair testing has been demonstrated to be a highly accurate biomarker to distinguish between abstinent and social drinkers as well as people who are chronic heavy drinkers (Süsse et al. 2010). FAEE hair tests are laboratory based. When coupled with testing of hair for EtG, they are powerful analytical tools to identify alcohol addiction (Pragst et al. 2010).

EtG and FAEE hair tests represent two cutting-edge tools that allow physicians to provide clinical assistance to alcoholic patients in ways that were never before possible. Although firm precedence has not been established in the United States, EtG and FAEEs likely will soon be as widely used in the United States as they are now used in Europe. On-site tests for alcohol in breath and potential detection of EtG in urine can be coupled with laboratory-based testing for EtG and FAEEs in hair. This mix of tests can be enhanced by carbohydrate-deficient transferrin and classical liver function tests when a patient is evaluated for problems caused by chronic excessive alcohol consumption. This battery of tests, some new and some old, gives physicians powerful tools to assist their alcoholic patients.

Drug and alcohol testing requires both knowledge of science and practice. A good example of the skill required in the use of tests for alcohol and other drugs is EtG testing using urine and oral fluid. Because these tests can be positive as a result of the donor's recent use of an alcohol hand sanitizer or an alcohol-containing mouthwash, interpreting a positive EtG test requires clinical judgment, especially if a single positive test can result in severe consequences. People who may undergo urine-based EtG testing for alcohol need to be warned specifically and in detail to avoid alcohol-containing products—which are ubiquitous—or risk getting a positive test result. It is useful to recall that neither hand sanitizers nor mouthwashes confound hair tests for EtG and FAEE, and these products do not affect carbohydrate-deficient transferrin or traditional liver function tests.

Conclusion

Drug testing makes use of the highest levels of modern biotechnology to reliably detect the presence of specific abused drugs and their unique metabolites in a growing number of matrices. Drug tests provide valuable information about the recent use of alcohol and other abused drugs. Drug testing is essential in both the diagnosis of substance use disorders and the evaluation and treatment of these disorders. Drug testing also plays a major role in studying the epidemiology of drug use, because self-reports of the use of alcohol and other drugs are notoriously unreliable. For individuals in drug abuse treatment and those under supervision by the criminal justice system, drug testing encourages treatment adherence and abstinence from alcohol and other drugs. Drug testing also permits the early detection of relapse to alcohol and controlled-substance use, thus enabling timely and appropriate interventions. Understanding the science of drug testing and the practical aspects of how alcohol and other drug testing works, and how to interpret the results of drug tests, has become essential for everyone involved in preventing, treating, and studying substance use disorders. Drug testing is essential in addiction medicine.

Key Clinical Concepts

- Because drugs of abuse are distributed to virtually every part of the user's body, they can be detected in all fluids and tissues.

- Urine is the most commonly used matrix for drug testing, but hair, oral fluid (saliva), and sweat are increasingly being used. No one matrix is best; each has strengths and weaknesses.

- All drug tests, regardless of the matrix used, depend on the same science and are similarly reliable. Nevertheless, the interpretation of drug test results requires specific knowledge.

- Drug tests detect recent drug use. They do not detect dependence, intoxication, impairment, or addiction.

- Most drug test results are confirmed by the sample donor's admission of recent drug use. Difficult and disputed cases benefit from additional help in interpretation, including assistance from the laboratory that conducted the test (or the kit manufacturer for on-site tests) and from a certified medical review officer.

- Smarter drug testing requires the use of all four common test matrices (urine, hair, oral fluid, and sweat) so the donor does not know which matrix will be used. It is desirable to vary the drugs tested for. This approach reduces cheating, improves the deterrent effect of testing, and permits comparison over time of the rates of positive results for the various matrices.

- Drug tests identify only the drug or drug metabolite on the test panel. Many commonly used panels contain a very small number of drugs. Drug testing is improved when a larger panel is used and when the panel is tailored to the drug-using patterns of the specific donor or to the specific population being tested.

Suggested Reading

DuPont RL, Selavka CM: Drug testing in addiction treatment and criminal justice settings, in Principles of Addiction Medicine, 3rd Edition. Edited by Graham AW, Schultz TK, Mayo-Smith MF, et al. Chevy Chase, MD, American Society of Addiction Medicine, 2003, pp 1001–1008

DuPont RL, Newel R, Brethen P: Drug Testing in Drug Abuse Treatment. Center City, MN, Hazelden, 2005

Willette R: Drug testing in the workplace, in Principles of Addiction Medicine, 3rd Edition. Edited by Graham AW, Schultz TK, Mayo-Smith MF, et al. Chevy Chase, MD, American Society of Addiction Medicine, 2003, pp 993–1000

References

Barnes AJ, Kim I, Schepers R, et al: Sensitivity, specificity, and efficiency in detecting opiates in oral fluid with the Cozart Opiate Microplate EIA and GC-MS following controlled codeine administration. J Anal Toxicol 27:402–407, 2003

Barnes AJ, Smith ML, Kacinko SL, et al: Excretion of methamphetamine and amphetamine in human sweat following controlled oral methamphetamine administration. Clin Chem 54:172–180, 2008

Bortolotti F, DePaoli G, Tagliaro F: Carbohydrate-deficient transferrin (CDT) as a marker of alcohol abuse: a critical review of the literature 2001–2005. J Chromatogr B Analyt Technol Biomed Life Sci 841:96–109, 2006

Charles BK, Day JE, Rollins DE, et al: Opiate recidivism in a drug-treatment program: comparison of hair and urine data. J Anal Toxicol 27:412–428, 2003

Coleman JJ, Bensinger PB, Gold MS, et al: Can drug design inhibit abuse? J Psychoactive Drugs 37:343–362, 2005

Compton R, Berning A: Results of the 2007 National Roadside Survey of Alcohol and Drug Use by Drivers (DOT Publ No HS-811-175). National Highway Traffic Safety Facts. July 2009. Available at: http://www.nhtsa.gov/DOT/NHTSA/Traffic%20Injury%20Control/Articles/Associated%20Files/811175.pdf. Accessed February 9, 2010.

Cone EJ, Sampson-Cone AH, Darwin WD, et al: Urine testing for cocaine abuse: metabolic and excretion patterns following different routes of administration and methods for detection of false-negative results. J Anal Toxicol 27:386–401, 2003

Dietz L, Glaz-Sandberg A, Nguyen H, et al: The urinary disposition of intravenously administered 11-nor-9-carboxy-delta-9-tetrahydrocannabinol in humans. Ther Drug Monit 29:368–372, 2007

DuPont RL: Do random workplace drug tests primarily identify casual or regular drug users? MRO Update July/August:5–7, 1996

DuPont RL: Addiction: a new paradigm. Bull Menninger Clin 62:231–242, 1998

DuPont RL: The Selfish Brain: Learning From Addiction. Washington, DC, American Psychiatric Press, 2000

DuPont RL, Baumgartner WA: Drug testing by urine and hair analysis: complementary features and scientific issues. Forensic Sci Int 70:63–76, 1995

DuPont RL, Brady LA: Drug Testing in Schools: Guidelines for Effective Use. Center City, MN, Hazelden, 2005

DuPont RL, Bucher RH: Guide to responsible family drug testing and alcohol testing. Rockville, MD, Institute for Behavior and Health, Inc., September 2005. Available at: http://www.studentdrugtesting.org/FAMGUIDETODRUGTESFINAL.pdf. Accessed February 9, 2010.

DuPont RL, Gold MS: Withdrawal and reward: implications for detoxification and relapse prevention. Psychiatr Ann 25:663–668, 1995

DuPont RL, Graves H: Smarter student drug testing. Rockville, MD, Institute for Behavior and Health, October 2005. Available at: http://www.studentdrugtesting.org/Smarter%20RSDT%20FINAL.pdf. Accessed February 9, 2010.

DuPont RL, Selavka CM: Drug testing in addiction treatment and criminal justice settings, in Principles of Addiction Medicine, 3rd Edition. Edited by Graham AW, Schultz TK, Mayo-Smith MF, et al. Chevy Chase, MD, American Society of Addiction Medicine, 2003, pp 1001–1008

DuPont RL, Griffin DW, Siskin BR, et al: Random drug tests at work: the probability of identifying frequent and infrequent users of illicit drugs. J Addict Dis 14:1–17, 1995

DuPont RL, Mieczkowski T, Newel R: Drug Testing in the Criminal Justice System. Center City, MN, Hazelden, 2005a

DuPont RL, Newel R, Brethen P: Drug Testing in Drug Abuse Treatment. Center City, MN, Hazelden, 2005b

DuPont RL, Skipper GE, White WL: Testing for recent alcohol use. Employee Assistance Digest 28:15–21, 2007

DuPont RL, Goldberger BA, Gold MS: Clinical and legal considerations in drug testing, in Principles of Addiction Medicine, 4th Edition. Edited by Ries RK, Fiellin D, Miller SC, et al. Philadelphia, PA, Lippincott Williams & Wilkins, 2009, pp 1499–1507

Feng J, Wang L, Dai I, et al: Simultaneous determination of multiple drugs of abuse and relevant metabolites in urine by LC-MS-MS. J Anal Toxicol 31:359–368, 2007

Huynh K, Wang G, Moore C, et al: Development of a homogeneous immunoassay for the detection of zolpidem in urine. J Anal Toxicol 33:486–490, 2009

Jufer R, Wstadik A, Walsh S, et al: Elimination of cocaine and metabolites in plasma, saliva, and urine following repeated oral administration to human volunteers. J Anal Toxicol 24:467–477, 2000

Kauert GF, Iwersen-Bergmann S, Toennes SW: Assay of delta9-tetrahydrocannabinol (THC) in oral fluid-evaluation of the OraSure oral specimen collection device. J Anal Toxicol 20:274–277, 2006

Kidwell DA, Riggs LA: Comparing two analytical methods: minimal standards in forensic toxicology derived from information theory. Forensic Sci Int 145:85–96, 2004

Kintz P, Evans J, Villain M, et al: Hair analysis to demonstrate administration of sildenafil to a woman in a case of drug-facilitated sexual assault. J Anal Toxicol 33:553–556, 2009

Laloup M, Del Mar Ramirez Fernandez M, Wood M, et al: Correlation of Delta9-tetrahydrocannabinol concentrations determined by LC-MS-MS in oral fluid and plasma from impaired drivers and evaluation of the on-site Dräger Drug Test. Forensic Sci Int 161:175–179, 2006

Maurer HH, Sauer C, Theobald DS: Toxicokinetics of drugs of abuse: current knowledge of the isoenzymes involved in the human metabolism of tetrahydrocannabinol, cocaine, heroin, morphine, and codeine. Ther Drug Monit 28:447–453, 2006

Meririnne E, Mykkänen S, Lillsunde P, et al: Workplace drug testing in a military organization: results and experiences from the testing program in the Finnish Defence Forces. Forensic Sci Int 170:171–174, 2007

Michael Walsh J, Flegel R, Atkins R, et al: Drug and alcohol use among drivers admitted to a Level-1 trauma center. Accid Anal Prev 37:894–901, 2005

Mieczkowski T, Lersch K: Drug-testing police officers and police recruits: the outcome of urinalysis and hair analysis compared. Policing: An International Journal of Police Strategies & Management 25:581–601, 2002

Minakata K, Gonmori K, Okamoto N, et al: Rapid and sensitive identification and determination of Urine Luck by ESI-MS after reduction of chromate. Forensic Toxicology 24:48–50, 2006

Moore C, Rana S, Coulter C, et al: Detection of conjugated 11-nor-delta9-tetrahydrocannabinol-9-carboxylic acid in oral fluid. J Anal Toxicol 31:187–194, 2007

Morrison JF, Chesler SN, Yoo WJ, et al: Matrix and modifier effects in the supercritical fluid extraction of cocaine and benzoylecgonine from human hair. Anal Chem 70:163–172, 1998

Politi L, Morini L, Leone F, et al: Ethyl glucuronide in hair: is it a reliable marker of chronic high levels of alcohol consumption? Addiction 101:1408–1412, 2006

Politi L, Zucchella A, Morini L, et al: Markers of chronic alcohol use in hair: comparison of ethyl glucuronide and cocaethylene in cocaine users. Forensic Sci Int 172:23–27, 2007

Pragst F, Yegles M: Alcohol markers in hair, in Analytical and Practical Aspects of Drug Testing in Hair. Edited by Kintz P. Boca Raton, FL, CRC Taylor & Francis, 2006, pp 287–323

Pragst F, Yegles M: Determination of fatty acid ethyl esters (FAEE) and ethyl glucuronide (EtG) in hair: a promising way for retrospective detection of alcohol abuse during pregnancy? Ther Drug Monit 30:255–263, 2008

Pragst F, Auwärter V, Kiessling B, et al: Wipe-test and patch-test for alcohol misuse based on the concentration ratio of fatty acid ethyl esters and squalene CFAEE/CSQ in skin surface lipids. Forensic Sci Int 143:77–86, 2004

Pragst F, Rothe M, Moench B, et al: Combined use of FAEE and EtG in hair for diagnosis of alcohol abuse: interpretation and advantages. Forensic Sci Int Jan 8, 2010 [Epub ahead of print]

Quest Diagnostics Incorporated: New hair data validate sharp downward trend in cocaine and methamphetamine positivity in general U.S. workforce, according to Quest Diagnostics Drug Testing Index. November 20, 2009. Available at: http://ir.questdiagnostics.com/phoenix.zhtml?c=82068&p=irol-newsArticle&ID=1357770&highlight. Accessed June 15, 2010.

Ries RK, Fiellin D, Miller SC, et al (eds): Principles of Addiction Medicine, 4th Edition. Philadelphia, PA, Lippincott Williams & Wilkins, 2009

Selavka C: Testing for drugs in hair. The Prosecutor 31:38–44, 1997

Society of Hair Testing: Consensus of the Society of Hair Testing (SOHT) on hair testing for chronic excessive alcohol consumption. Statement adopted June 16, 2009, at SOHT Congress, Rome, Italy. Available at: http://www.soht.org/pdf/Consensus_EtG_2009.pdf. Accessed June 15, 2010.

Stout PR, Bynum ND, Mitchell JM, et al: A comparison of the validity of gas chromatography-mass spectrometry and liquid chromatography-tandem mass spectrometry analysis of urine samples for morphine, codeine, 6-acetylmorphine, and benzoylecgonine. J Anal Toxicol 33:398–408, 2009

Süsse S, Selavka C, Mieczkowski T, et al: Fatty acid ethyl ester concentrations in hair and self-reported alcohol consumption in 644 cases from different origin. Forensic Sci Int Jan 12, 2010 [Epub ahead of print]

U.S. Department of Health and Human Services: Mandatory Guidelines and Proposed Revisions to Mandatory Guidelines for Federal Workplace Drug Testing Programs; Notices (Federal Register, April 13, 2004, Vol. 69, No. 71). 2004. Available at: http://ncadistore.samhsa.gov/catalog/ProductDetails.aspx?ProductID=16833. Accessed February 9, 2010.

U.S. Department of Health and Human Services: Mandatory guidelines for federal workplace drug testing programs: notices (Federal Register, April 30, 2010, Vol 75, No 83). 2010. Available at: http://edocket.access.gpo.gov/2010/2010-10118.htm. Accessed June 15, 2010.

Volkow ND, Li TK: Drug addiction: the neurobiology of behavior gone awry, in Principles of Addiction Medicine, 4th Edition. Edited by Ries RK, Fiellin D, Miller SC, et al. Chevy Chase, MD, American Society of Addiction Medicine, 2009, pp 3–12

Yacoubian GS, Wish ED, Perez DM: A comparison of saliva testing to urinalysis in an arrestee population. J Psychoactive Drugs 33:289–294, 2001

Yegles M, Pragst F: Cut-offs for the detection of alcohol abuse by measurement of fatty acid ethyl esters and ethyl glucuronide in hair. Ann Toxicol Anal 17:121–134, 2005

Zaitsu K, Miki A, Katagi M, et al: Long-term stability of various drugs and metabolites in urine, and preventive measures against their decomposition with special attention to filtration sterilization. Forensic Sci Int 174:189–196, 2008

Cross-Cultural Aspects of Addiction Therapy

Nady el-Guebaly, M.D., D.Psych., D.P.H.

The need for clinicians to have cross-cultural sensitivity and competence increases along with the pace of their contacts with people from other cultures. Clinical cultural competence is a lifelong journey. Most of the recent scientific literature in English addresses culture in the context of modern multiethnic societies in the United States, Britain, Canada, and Australia. In this chapter, I outline the clinically relevant variables of culture and their implications for the assessment, engagement, and retention of patients in therapy.

Concepts and Definitions

The following definitions attempt to explain cross-cultural terminology of relevance to the design of a therapeutic strategy in multiethnic societies (Gonzalez et al. 2001; Keyes 1976).

- *Culture* is the sum total of a group's life ways, including the group's material culture, worldview, social organization, symbols, status, child raising, language, technology, and citizenship. *Subculture* (for the purposes of this chapter) refers to distinct groupings resulting from substance use, abuse, or dependence, as well as other addictions; examples include affiliations with cocktail lounges or crack houses.
- *Ethnicity* refers to a subjective sense of belonging to a given group of persons, held to have a common origin and to share a matrix of cultural beliefs and practices. Ethnicity becomes a component of one's sense of identity and an important source of clinical and social manifestations with respect to one's self-image and intrapsychic life.
- *Acculturation* is the cumulative social learning process that involves assimilating the values of the host culture while retaining the values of the original culture.

- *Race* is a concept under which human beings choose to group themselves, based primarily on their common physiognomy, including physical, biological, and genetic connotations.
- *Cross-cultural* refers to the comparison of characteristics across cultural groups or treatment strategies, addressing both clinician and patient differences in cultures.

Ethnic Groups and Stereotyping

In the United States, epidemiological surveys recognize five major ethnic groups: Whites, African Americans, Hispanic Americans, Asian Americans and Pacific Islanders, and American Indians and Alaska Natives. Clinically, the delineation of these ethnic groups, while a step in the right direction, represents an oversimplification.

Seeking out a review of general ethnic trends may be informative to clinicians unfamiliar with characteristics outside their own community (though such clinicians are becoming, fortunately, a rarer breed). An individual assessment, to gain awareness of a patient's unique cultural pedigree, is a must. So-called Hispanic or Latino ethnic groups have diverse roots traced to more than 20 countries with various phenotypic admixtures, divergent historical origins, diverse social and educational levels, and diverse patterns of use of services. The same can be said of African American, Asian, Native American, and other ethnic groupings traditionally recorded at the introduction of any medical history or clinical presentation. The identification of ethnocultural groups also depends on national political priorities. In Canada, the study of cultures based on English and French languages has been prioritized; in the United Kingdom, particular attention has been paid to religious Muslim groups.

Confounding Variables of Ethnicity

Confounding variables, such as those outlined in the following sections, moderate the impact of ethnicity on the prevalence estimates of substance use and the resulting clinical presentations.

Sociodemographic Variables as Distinct From Culture

It is crucial to control for sociodemographic variables. For example, differences in age distribution must be taken into account. The higher proportion of youth among Native Americans, which are a high-risk group for substance abuse compared with other ethnic groups, influences the prevalence of substance abuse in that ethnic group (Beauvais 1998).

Differences in family stability and the occurrence of domestic violence in a given ethnic group may also be a cause and/or consequence of the prevalence of substance use in that group. The same can be said about differences in socioeconomic status and work history (Westermeyer 1999).

Extent of Acculturation

The extent of recent migration in an ethnic group is viewed as both a risk and a protective factor. For example, first- and second-generation acculturation may create socioeconomic stressors, which increase the vulnerability to addiction. Hawaiian residents of Chinese and Japanese ancestry have lower levels of alcohol use if born in Asia than if born in Hawaii (Johnson et al. 1987).

Legal Frameworks of Home and Host Countries

The traditional use of coca leaves in the Andes and of marijuana and hashish in India and the Middle East adds to the cultural disconnect felt by migrants from these countries arriving in a new community where their drug is illegal but other substances are socially promoted (el-Guebaly and el-Guebaly 1981; Griffiths et al. 1997). The propensity for arrests and imprisonment for alcohol-related offenses differs among aboriginal groups in various countries (Adrian 2002).

Biological Factors and Physical Comorbidities

Studies of the impact of genetic factors on various ethnic groups' predisposition toward substance use and pharmacological treatment have only just started. An early finding is that approximately 50% of Northeast Asians (Chinese, Japanese, and Koreans) have a deficiency in liver aldehyde dehydrogenase, which leads to slower oxidation of acetaldehyde and a resulting "flushing reaction" following ingestion of alcohol. This is considered to be a protective factor against alcohol abuse by Asians (Li 2000). Coping with the reaction, however, can be learned in order to accommodate a Western lifestyle. Socioeconomic disadvantage also leads to differential health outcomes, including fatal and nonfatal overdoses, hepatitis B and C infection, acquired immunodeficiency syndrome (AIDS), and increased risk of pregnancy and perinatal complications (Khalsa and Elkashef 2010).

Psychological Factors

Cultures fostering shame and guilt as means of social control have been reported to facilitate alcohol abuse. Low self-esteem, self-confidence, and assertiveness, as well as a "loss of face," have all been related to the use of substances among adolescents in general and migrant groups in particular (Bhattacharya 1998). The higher rate of suicides among Native American youths following substance use is the ultimate resulting tragedy (Resnick and Dizmang 1971). The typical norms and values in Asian cultures, including traditional values such as responsibility to others, interdependence, restraint, and group achievement, have been shown to have a protective effect (Sue 1987).

Clinical Cultural Formulation

Through a cultural assessment, the clinician can gather a better understanding of the patient's subjective view of the world, the meaning of the illness to him or her, and his or her expected recovery process. In DSM-IV-TR (American Psychiatric Association 2000), the following assessment categories are outlined:

- *Identification of cultural identity.* The patient's overarching ethnic group must be complemented by further descriptors, such as where the patient was raised and by whom, parents' and grandparents' ethnicity, and involvement with both culture of origin and host culture.
- *Explanation for the current illness.* The predominant idioms of distress must be articulated, in addition to the meaning and perceived severity of the symptoms in relation to cultural norms. Traditionally, diagnostic evocation of culture has been associated with rare "culture-bound syndromes" rather than the much more common clinical presentations in daily practice, which include the following factors:
  - *Norm conflict.* When standards held desirable by a culture conflict with the person's behavior.
  - *Normative versus deviant behavior.* As when any substance is used in an abstinence-based group; this would be considered deviant, though not necessarily pathological from a health perspective.
  - *Socially prescribed use.* As when substance use in religious rites is replaced by secular use, often involving new routes of administration (e.g., from eating to smoking opium) and/or new forms of the substance (e.g., from opium to heroin).
  - *Cultural change.* Achieved through migration and exposure to new norms.
- *Cultural environment and function.* The patient's interpretations of social stressors and available social supports are elicited, including religion and levels of functioning and disability.
- *Cultural aspects of the clinician-patient relationship.* Similarities and differences between the clinician's and patient's language, social context,

and beliefs and behaviors of relevance to the clinical onset, course, and treatment create a set of dynamics that should be part of the cultural formulation (see Figure 3–1). Transference and countertransference issues can be understood once underlying mechanisms, such as projection or stereotyping, become visible (Moffic et al. 1988; Westermeyer et al. 2006).

- *Cultural socialization to substance use.* This may occur through several pathways (Westermeyer 2009):
    - Observation of role models (i.e., the type and pattern of use by parenting adults or older siblings)
    - Socialization into use (i.e., who the mentors were, and how the mentoring environment was)
    - Early experience with use (i.e., positive and/or negative effects, helpfulness in coping with daily stressors)
    - Linkage with developmental tasks (i.e., whether the user was attempting courting or an early sexual experience, or was coping with anxiety)
    - Realistic clinical challenges arise when the largely open-ended socioanthropological conversation that is required to assess culture collides with the need for a clinical interview focused on making a diagnosis and establishing a treatment plan. An adequate cultural assessment may require several interviews to get to know the "person

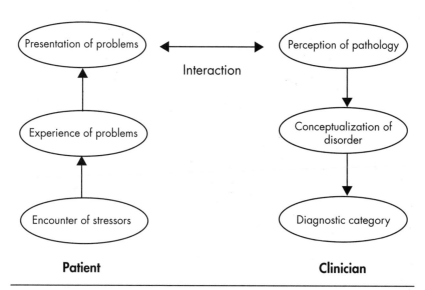

FIGURE 3–1. **Cultural dynamics in clinical assessment.**

behind the illness." Often, belief systems may differ with regard to the nature of the behavior or diagnosis versus treatment compliance, adding to the complexity of clinical care (Bhui and Bhugra 2002). Attempts at bridging the qualitative or quantitative gaps to improve cross-cultural research methodology have included the design of instruments such as the somewhat elaborate Explanatory Model Interview Catalogue (EMIC) (Weiss 1997) or the briefer Short Explanatory Model Interview (SEMI), which uses vignettes (Lloyd et al. 1998).

Case Illustrations

The following case illustrations highlight the challenges of acculturation as a lifelong process (Maria's case); the cross-cultural management of a family's religious values to assist adaptation to the norms of the host society (Ali's case); and lastly, the healing journey required in reintegrating a tribal community (Pam's case).

Maria is a 63-year-old white woman of Dutch descent. She is a retired teacher who has lived alone in her condo since the death of her husband 10 years ago. Her father reportedly sympathized with the Nazi occupation of Holland during World War II and immigrated to South America in 1945. She was born in Uruguay and given the middle name of Adolfina. The parents separated when she was 2 years old, and her mother returned to Holland, leaving Maria to the care of a foster home. She never saw her biological father again. When she was 6, her mother, then remarried, returned to Uruguay to take Maria to Holland. There she was placed in a Catholic residential school, where she was mercilessly teased because of her middle name. Maria also felt that her mother preferred her half-brother born from her second marriage. At age 26, Maria married an Italian geologist in the oil industry, and they lived in several countries prior to finally settling in North America. Maria described her late husband as having been kind and supportive. They had one son and one daughter. Maria collected along the way two bachelor degrees in education and fine arts, as well as a diploma in fashion design from France. She worked as a teacher for about 30 years.

Maria started to drink wine as a young bride accompanying her husband to his post in Algeria during its war of independence, when she feared for their lives. In the 1970s, her drinking escalated and shifted to spirits. In the late 1980s, Maria attended Alcoholics Anonymous (AA) for 8 months at the urging of her husband but was dissatisfied because of its connection with religion: "It reminded me of my Catholic school." After the death of her husband from cancer and her subsequent retirement, Maria escalated her drinking again, to at least half a bottle of spirits a day, to overcome loneliness and depression and to help her sleep. Maria has been hospitalized briefly twice in the last 5 years with depression, along with flashbacks and nightmares about witnessing war scenes in Algeria. These are exacerbated by the daily news or other cues.

During the past year, Maria sought treatment in a residential program but relapsed soon after discharge. An outpatient follow-up also failed to help her become sober. She tried SMART Recovery (Self-Management and Recovery Training) but was not satisfied because "most of the attendants were addicted to drugs and not alcohol."

Maria has a long past history of back pain due to spinal fusion. Currently she is mostly housebound, except for short trips to liquor stores, grocery markets, and occasional movies with her one friend. She has tried various analgesics unsuccessfully in the past and now uses mainly alcohol to deal with her pain.

Maria's current social support consists of her children, who are both doing well but live in other cities. They both phone her once a week and visit her once a year. She has a female companion, originally from Venezuela, who visits her twice a week and helps with housework. Otherwise, her social life is very limited and she passes her time reading.

Her Axis I diagnoses were alcohol dependence, chronic depression, and posttraumatic stress disorder. The clinician also recorded Maria's chronic back pain on Axis III and her isolation on Axis IV.

Engagement and the therapeutic alliance. From the outset, Maria was forthcoming and overtalkative. She detailed her past experiences at length, with a light Dutch accent. Although the patient reported depressed mood, her affect was appropriate and reactive.

To which culture did Maria belong? She spoke Spanish, English, Dutch, French, and Italian. Yet her multiculturalism resulted in a prevailing sense of alienation. She had belonged to her nuclear family, but after the death of her husband and departure of her children, an unbearable sense of aloneness, seeded during childhood, resurfaced.

Establishing a therapeutic alliance meant attempting to meet her needs. Maria felt she no longer fit anywhere, resulting in a pressing need to communicate when given the opportunity. In individual sessions, the clinician could accommodate her constant reminiscing. For her peers in group therapy, however, she lived in another world. She had stories to tell that did not resonate with them. She was variably perceived as being "stuck up" and a nuisance. Both individual and group sessions became a balancing act between validating her perception as a "citizen of the world" and enhancing her acculturation skills for her to feel more at home in her immediate environment (see Lim 2006).

Retention and recovery. Faced with a number of cultural options, Maria finally selected the ethnicity of her South American country of birth, Uruguay, while living in North America. Her friend was from Venezuela, and they both volunteered to teach Spanish courses in a neighboring school to regain a sense of purpose. They were planning a visit back to their lands of birth. Maria's sobriety was maintained, albeit with a couple of lapses, and her reinvolvement with SMART Recovery was episodic. Yearly visits of her son and daughter were coordinated so they could develop a family plan involving summer visits from her growing grandchildren, if she remained sober. She eventually joined a Spanish-speaking seniors group.

Ali is a 25-year-old married man of Pakistani origin. He is currently living in a house with his wife and newborn daughter, his father, his mother, his brother, two sisters, a brother-in-law, a niece, and a nephew. Ali and his wife own another house in the city, but they moved in with Ali's parents after Ali began to experience psychological difficulties. Ali has a high school education and a year of college in business administration. He managed a convenience store franchise for 2 years but was eventually fired because of performance problems. He is currently unemployed.

Ali, raised in the Islamic faith, never tried alcohol or other drugs, except a few cigarettes, until age 22, when he was introduced to cocaine by a friend who simply told him that it was "another kind of cigarette." Around this time, Ali was experiencing symptoms of depression and anxiety stemming from a car accident in which he had thought he was going to die. After the accident, he experienced nightmares and intrusive images, as well as loss of interest, difficulty concentrating, and irritability. He experienced intense anxiety while driving and eventually stopped driving. He found that smoking cocaine provided some relief.

Ali obtained crack cocaine from his friend and from street dealers with increasing frequency, eventually smoking it every 2–3 days. This affected his performance as a manager. A year ago, Ali was voluntarily hospitalized after his parents became concerned about his drug use and paranoid symptoms. He had been observed hiding under his bed and behind a shower curtain and had been preoccupied with the idea that someone was watching him. These symptoms cleared without pharmacological intervention while he was hospitalized, and according to Ali they have not reemerged since his discharge. Nevertheless, he resumed smoking crack about once a month. Ali expressed a strong sense of shame about his drug use and about being supported by his father. He owed some $20,000 to the bank.

Ali was born in Pakistan, where he reportedly had an uneventful childhood. There is no known family history of psychiatric disorder or substance abuse, except that a maternal aunt is rumored to be mentally ill. Ali immigrated to North America with his parents and siblings when he was 12 years old. Four years ago, Ali returned to Pakistan to marry his first cousin; his wife subsequently moved to North America and gave birth to their first child. She reportedly does not know about his drug use. Ali described his relationship with his wife and with his parents and siblings as very supportive. He is especially close to his father. Outside of his family, Ali has only social acquaintances.

Ali has resumed driving and is no longer experiencing anxiety or nightmares. He is still bothered by feelings of depression, guilt, shame, anhedonia, and a sense of personal failure.

His Axis I diagnoses were cocaine dependence, cocaine-induced mood disorder, and posttraumatic stress disorder (in remission). On Axis IV, the clinician recorded employment problems and financial problems.

Engagement and the therapeutic alliance. In view of the significance of Ali's extended family, a follow-up appointment was arranged for Ali, his wife, and his parents. According to his parents, Ali underreported the extent of his drug use. He had also borrowed money from his sisters consistently, without repaying them. His wife, initially silent, soon disclosed awareness of his cocaine intake. The parents had initiated a search for the "best treatment program" in North America, with the help of the extended family. Faced with a range of options, they finally settled on treating Ali in his own community, and the clinician concurred. The family norms were felt to be constructive at this stage and were interwoven with Islamic values (Banawi and Stockton 1993; Hodge 2005). Ali is a faithful Muslim and has shunned drinking since his immigration. Ali's father initiated contact with the local respected imam. The clinician agreed to synchronize therapeutic efforts through regular telephone contacts involving Ali.

Retention and recovery. Ali's therapy had three objectives: achievement of abstinence from cocaine, resumption of an adult constructive role within the family network, and cognitive restructuring within the tenets and values of Islam. For example, his initial belief was that "drugs other than alcohol, not specifically mentioned in the Qur'an, could be experimented with." His acculturation process involved negotiating the tenets of his faith. The Qur'an shuns intoxication, not just alcohol. The use of religious psychotherapy has been demonstrated to be helpful for practicing individuals in several religions (Azhar et al. 1994; Galanter et al. 1991; Koltko 1990).

Therapy focused on the meaning of Ali's religious beliefs to him as he pursued his adaptation to the main host culture. It was recognized that his beliefs could be both a help and a hazard (i.e., fostering shame but boosting his resolve for recovery as well). The enabling behaviors of some family members were clarified, as well as the need for a return to gradual independence for the young parents.

Pam is a 26-year-old single woman who was born into a tribe—a member of the Blackfoot Confederacy—that straddles the western part of the U.S.–Canadian border. The Native American ethnic group encompasses some 500 tribes, many having their own sense of nationhood, language, traditions, and crafts. Pam is currently living with her ex-boyfriend in a rented apartment but is trying to get funding for an apartment of her own. She has a ninth-grade education and is going to school to complete twelfth grade so as to pursue a university education in environmental conservation. She has not worked in several years and is living on social assistance.

Pam started drinking once or twice a month at age 13. At age 18, she binged every weekend but eventually stopped drinking after she witnessed drinking problems in others. When Pam stopped drinking, her doctor prescribed lorazepam and diazepam, both of which she abused seriously for about 2 years. Her physician would write a prescription for about 100 pills of each, and Pam would run out in about 2 weeks. Pam was also using codeine, which she would get from friends, as well as abusing any other pill she "could get my hands on." She experienced seizures and psychosis related to the use of these substances. She last abused these drugs about 5 years ago, with the exception of a suicidal overdose of codeine last year. Her most recent drug use was cannabis 2 months ago, which she has smoked since age 18. Other than a current shoplifting charge, she has no other history of legal problems.

Pam was raised in her tribe in and around a midsize city. She is the oldest child. Her mother had three other children with different fathers. Pam reported that her mother was significantly abusive, emotionally and physically, and had an addiction to substances. Pam was primarily raised by her maternal grandparents, who, until 10 years ago, were both heavy drinkers. Pam knew very little about her father and speculated that he was an alcoholic. Pam reported a history of childhood sexual, physical, and emotional abuse. She also reported that depression and anxiety were very prevalent in her family.

Pam had an extensive list of psychiatric hospitalizations, with a range of diagnoses, including depression, anxiety and adjustment disorders, posttraumatic stress disorder, drug-induced psychosis, substance-induced mood disorder, and borderline personality disorder. Pam also reported taking a variety of medications over the years, including antidepressants, antipsychotics, and benzodiazepines. Currently, Pam is not taking any medication. She has not noticed any mood fluctuation in the last several months. She did experience some anxiety but was able to connect it to her increasing school workload and desire to succeed. Her Axis I diagnoses were alcohol, benzodiazepine, and opioid dependence in remission and cannabis dependence in early remission. A past Axis II diagnosis of borderline personality disorder was noted. On Axis IV, the clinician noted employment, school, housing, financial, and relationship stressors.

Engagement and the therapeutic alliance. Pam started attending counseling at a healing lodge. She felt she had made the changes she needed—that is, becoming abstinent from all substances and learning the skills to assist her in continuing her abstinence. Considering her progress with native counseling, the clinician inquired about the treatment regimen and offered his services on a consultative basis.

The aboriginal healing lodge services are based on the concept of a healing dialogue between mind, body, emotions, and spirit in the Medicine Wheel model. The model is configured as a circle made up of four quadrants, each representing a cardinal direction connected to a part of the person: spirit (east), body (south), emotions (west), and the mind (north). The goal is to keep these parts at the appropriate positioning to help the person find balance, harmony, connection, and wholeness. Traditional processes to facilitate reaching this state of centeredness include the following:

- Sharing circles of 10–20 participants, which provide a safe place to share thoughts and experiences
- Stories through which the narrative of one's experience and understanding is used to discover the traditional values, beliefs, and practices relevant to the narrator
- Rituals such as smudging, naming, and pipe ceremonies (sharing tobacco symbolizes the giver of tobacco asking something of the receiver, such as help with a particular problem and/or emotional support)

- Ceremonies such as the purifying experience of the sweat lodge or connecting with the spirit world in a vision quest through isolation and fasting
- Exploration of dreams, because they may foretell the future or provide new understandings to self or others

Although these approaches have not been tested empirically, their strength is in their relevance to aboriginal traditions and philosophy. They share with Western psychotherapies core therapeutic conditions such as empathy, acceptance, and forgiveness and have more similarities with insight-based rather than cognitive approaches (McCabe 2008). Spirituality is a critical component of the healing process and so is the aboriginal community in seeking help from one another. The counselor is a role model but will often ask for help from the community elders.

Retention and recovery. The origins of the high rates of mental health and social problems among aboriginal populations have been ascribed to the impact of European colonization as well as the legacy of the residential schools teaching children to be ashamed of their heritage. These traumas have resulted in one of three options: 1) adaptation and assimilation with the dominant society; 2) loss of identity characterized by substance abuse, high mortality, and suicide rates; and 3) family disintegration, reaffirmation of culture, and a degree of resistance (Kirmayer et al. 2000). Native women saw their traditional roles eroded by a new patriarchal order sponsored by treaties with governments, but many efforts have been led by women to rebuild their families and communities. Narratives of resistance were inspiring to Pam in her healing journey (Bopp et al. 1984; McCabe 2007, 2008; Shepard et al. 2006).

Management Implications

An often-repeated finding is that treatment resources in Western countries are underused by minority ethnic groups. Encounters with the health-care system and/or the social-welfare system and the intimacy involved in dealing with health issues are fraught with wide-ranging cross-cultural challenges. Examples of perceived barriers to using the health care system include language proficiency, the individual right for confidentiality versus the family expectation for information, the fear of rights being taken away, the ease of disclosure in a therapeutic group involving both sexes, and the use of condoms or needle exchange despite religious taboos.

Models of Care

The increasing multiethnicity of Western English-speaking countries has sparked a debate about optimal models of culturally sensitive delivery of care. In this section, I examine some possible models.

Separate Services for Ethnic Minority Groups

In the United States, separate public and voluntary-sector services for African Americans, Hispanic Americans, and Native Americans are commonplace. Religious denominations sponsor certain hospitals and social services. The creation of separate services is supported by consistent research findings showing that members of ethnic minorities may experience increased coercive treatment and social encounters that promote their distrust in secular hospitals. These experiences are often based on a mutual lack of knowledge of cherished cultural, spiritual, and religious beliefs, as well as a perceived slow pace of change. Arguments against the idea of separate services include fears of promoting ghettoization and further marginalization of those already marginalized (Bhui and Sashidharan 2003).

Cultural Consultation Model

An important issue is how major urban centers in which over 100 languages are spoken should respond to health-care needs. In Montreal, Quebec, for example, a specialized multidisciplinary team brings together clinical experience with cultural knowledge and linguistic skills. Rather than taking on patients for continuing care, the team provides consultations to other clinicians in two or three interviews, which include the family as well. Team members are involved in the training of interpreters and other culture-link workers (Kirmayer et al. 2003).

"Melting Pot" Approach for the Cultural Mosaic

In the melting pot approach, institutional factors promoting ethnic inequalities are addressed. Culturally influenced or capable services are important to the mainstream delivery of services and not only to minority ethnic groups. Culture is not perceived as a problem or disability for minority groups that require specialized interventions. Mainstream services are commonly enriched by responding to the needs of all cultural groups, guaranteeing equality of access and ensuring rights for all individuals (Bhui and Sashidharan 2003).

"Hedge Your Bets" Approach

Advocates of a hedge-your-bets strategy acknowledge, for example, that a combination of prescribed medication and ethnic spiritual therapy may be the best hope to securing patient adherence. This model also encourages a more honest discussion of the other therapies being tried and their interaction, from the reading of sacred texts to the possible ritual infliction of pain.

Culture and Recovery

As presented in the earlier case illustrations, three potent instruments of recovery are commonly recognized in the cross-cultural treatment literature.

First, the significance of the family as the conduit of cultural norms and values is emphasized in most ethnically sensitive programs. Supporting the family foundation and home stability are cherished goals in communities originating from cultures in which there is a strong extended-family network that has been threatened by the reduced family mosaic in many societies. A sensitive family assessment will clarify the individual roles of all members and respect the potential utilization of these roles toward a positive outcome (Delgado 1995).

Second, formal religious affiliation and practice play a major positive role in the development of prevention networks for recovery and treatment compliance in many ethnic groups (Galanter 2006).

Third, the spread of 12-step programs to various parts of the world is an example of the common value placed on spiritual growth as an ingredient of recovery. However, different cultural values have also spurred the growth of various mutual-help movements in addition to AA. In North America, examples of such parallel movements include SMART Recovery (www.smartrecovery.org) for agnostics and Women for Sobriety (www.womenforsobriety.org). Culturally motivated options have developed in other countries as well, including such distinct cultures as Italy, Japan, and Saudi Arabia. All of these approaches promote abstinence as the way to recovery (Allamani and Petrikin 1996; Higuchi and Kono 1994; Patussi et al. 1996; Suwaki 1979). These movements have some major differences from traditional 12-step programs:

- *Alignment with the professional treatment community.* Whereas AA groups have a tradition of autonomy, both Clubs for Alcoholics in Treatment (CATs) in Italy and Danshukai groups in Japan welcome professional participation.
- *Participation of the family.* Although AA and Al-Anon developed as separate but complementary programs, both CAT and Danshukai groups welcome alcoholic individuals with their families. Each CAT group is limited to 12 families; additional recruiting requires splitting of the groups.
- *Tradition of anonymity.* Anonymity is not considered necessary in CATs or in Danshukai. Danshukai also involves a public organizational hierarchy that lobbies for resources.
- *Relative role of religion.* In Italy, CATs are agnostic groups, and in Japan, the Danshukai groups, operating within a primarily nonreligious culture, consider the "higher power" a foreign concept. In Muslim coun-

tries, the concept of "God as we came to know him" clashes with a more preordained perception of God and his 99 attributes described in the Qur'an (Hodge 2005). In German-speaking Europe, the Blue Cross network has close links with the Lutheran Church. These mutual-help movements are not 12-Step based but teach the precepts of the specific religion to attain sobriety.

Cultural recovery may involve regaining a viable ethnic identity and developing a healthy affiliation with an individual's ethnic group, as well as reacquiring a functional social network, regaining a religious or spiritual commitment, rebuilding social status in the recovering as well as the cultural community, and reestablishing vocational and recreational activities. Cultural recovery starts after physical and psychological recovery begin and often takes years (Westermeyer 2009; Westermeyer et al. 2006). Unreasonable cultural expectations, as well as cultural cues to resume the addictive behavior, may delay recovery, whereas cultural abstinence-based programs may facilitate recovery.

Pharmacotherapies can also play an adjunct cultural role. For example, the prescription of disulfiram in recovering alcohol-dependent patients or naltrexone in opioid-dependent patients may provide a plausible excuse for not partaking in situations where a refusal may be misinterpreted as the rejection of a friendly invitation.

Conclusion

The purpose of this chapter has been to advance knowledge of how clinicians can provide optimal clinical care to people from different cultures. The impact of ethnicity is moderated by a number of risk and protective factors. Sometimes clinicians attribute too much to a patient's ethnicity or culture, but at other times, they completely ignore the existence of cultural impact. Cultural sensitivity is not a stereotypical fixation on culture, and it should not be invoked as a ready explanation for the unexplained. Many purported culturally based conclusions range from the subjective to the speculative.

Minority groups underutilize clinical treatment and social services, and making these services more user-friendly should be a first-order concern in multicultural societies. Different culturally sensitive models of care are available: culturally potent instruments of recovery have included a family focus, religious practices, and the development of abstinence-based mutual-help movements. Clinically, a better understanding of the patient can be gained through a systematic cultural formulation that includes the cultural aspects of the clinician-patient relationship.

Key Clinical Concepts

- Culturally sensitive clinical care is required for individuals from different cultures.
- The impact of ethnicity is moderated by both risk and protective factors.
- A cultural assessment improves understanding of the patient's subjective views.
- Culturally sensitive care can be delivered either through separated services, a consultation model, or a sensitized melting pot approach.
- A family focus, religious affiliation, and mutual-help movements have tended to underpin culturally sensitive recovery programs.

Suggested Reading

Adrian M: A critical perspective on cross-cultural contexts for addiction and multi-culturalism: their meanings and implications in the substance use field. Subst Use Misuse 37:853–900, 2002

American Psychiatric Association: Diagnostic and Statistical Manual of Mental Disorders, 4th Edition, Text Revision. Washington, DC, American Psychiatric Association, 2000

Kirmayer LJ, Brass GM, Tait CL: The mental health of Aboriginal peoples: transformations of identity and community. Can J Psychiatry 45:607–616, 2000

Moffic MS, Kendrick EP, Reid K: Cultural psychiatry education during psychiatric residency. J Psychiatr Educ 12:90–101, 1988

Westermeyer J: The role of cultural and social factors in the cause of addictive disorders. Psychiatr Clin North Am 22:253–273, 1999

Westermeyer J, Mellman L, Alarcon R: Cultural competence in addiction psychiatry. Addict Disord Their Treat 5:107–119, 2006

References

Adrian M: A critical perspective on cross-cultural contexts for addiction and multi-culturalism: their meanings and implications in the substance use field. Subst Use Misuse 37:853–900, 2002

Allamani A, Petrikin C: Alcoholics Anonymous and the alcohol treatment system in Italy. Contemp Drug Probl 23:43–55, 1996

American Psychiatric Association: Diagnostic and Statistical Manual of Mental Disorders, 4th Edition, Text Revision. Washington, DC, American Psychiatric Association, 2000

Azhar MZ, Varma SL, Dharap AS: Religious psychotherapy in anxiety disorder patients. Acta Psychiatr Scand 90:1–3, 1994

Banawi R, Stockton R: Islamic values relevant to group work, with practical applications for the group leader. Journal for Specialists in Group Work 18:151–160, 1993

Beauvais F: American Indians and alcohol. Alcohol Health Res World 22:253–259, 1998

Bhattacharya G: Drug use among Asian Indian adolescents: identifying protective/risk factors. Adolescence 33:169–184, 1998

Bhui K, Bhugra D: Explanatory models for mental distress: implications for clinical practice and research. Br J Psychiatry 181:6–7, 2002

Bhui K, Sashidharan SP: Should there be separate psychiatric services for ethnic minority groups? Br J Psychiatry 182:10–12, 2003

Bopp J, Bopp M, Brown L, et al: The Sacred Tree. Lethbridge, Alberta, Canada, Four Worlds Development Press, 1984

Delgado M: Hispanic natural support systems and alcohol and other drug services: challenges and rewards for practice. Alcohol Treat Q 12:17–31, 1995

el-Guebaly N, el-Guebaly A: Alcohol abuse in ancient Egypt: the recorded evidence. Int J Addict 16:1207–1221, 1981

Galanter M: Spirituality and addiction: a research and clinical perspective. Am J Addict 15:286–292, 2006

Galanter M, Larson D, Rubenstone E: Christian psychiatry: the impact of evangelical belief on clinical practice. Am J Psychiatry 148:90–95, 1991

Gonzalez CA, Griffith EEH, Ruiz P: Cross-cultural issues in psychiatric treatment, in Treatments of Psychiatric Disorders, 3rd Edition, Vol 1. Edited by Gabbard GO. Washington, DC, American Psychiatric Press, 2001, pp 47–67

Griffiths P, Gossop M, Wickenden S, et al: A transcultural pattern of drug use: qat (khat) in the UK. Br J Psychiatry 170:281–284, 1997

Higuchi S, Kono H: Early diagnosis and treatment of alcoholism: the Japanese experience. Alcohol Alcohol 29:363–373, 1994

Hodge DR: Social work and the house of Islam: orienting practitioners to the beliefs and values of Muslims in the United States. Soc Work 50:162–173, 2005

Johnson RC, Nagoshi CT, Ahern FM, et al: Cultural factors as explanations for ethnic group differences in alcoholism in Hawaii. J Psychoactive Drugs 19:67–75, 1987

Keyes CF: Towards a new formulation of the concept of ethnic groups. Ethnicity 3:202–212, 1976

Khalsa JH, Elkashef A: Interventions for HIV and hepatitis C virus infections in recreational drug users. Clin Infect Dis 50:1505–1511, 2010

Kirmayer LJ, Brass GM, Tait CL: The mental health of Aboriginal peoples: transformations of identity and community. Can J Psychiatry 45:607–616, 2000

Kirmayer LJ, Groleau D, Guzder J, et al: Cultural consultation: a model of mental health service for multicultural societies. Can J Psychiatry 48:145–153, 2003

Koltko ME: How religious beliefs affect psychotherapy: the example of Mormonism. Psychotherapy: Theory, Research, Practice, Training 27:132–141, 1990

Li TK: Pharmacogenetics of responses to alcohol and genes that influence alcohol drinking. J Stud Alcohol 61:5–12, 2000

Lim RF (ed): Clinical Manual of Cultural Psychiatry. Washington, DC, American Psychiatric Publishing, 2006

Lloyd KR, Jacob KS, Patel V, et al: The development of the Short Explanatory Model Interview (SEMI) and its use among primary care attenders with common mental disorders. Psychol Med 28:1231–1237, 1998

McCabe GH: The healing path: a culture and community derived indigenous therapy model. Psychotherapy: Theory, Research, Practice, Training 44:148–160, 2007

McCabe G: Mind, body, emotions, and spirit: reaching to the ancestors for healing. Couns Psychol Q 21:143–152, 2008

Moffic MS, Kendrick EP, Reid K: Cultural psychiatry education during psychiatric residency. J Psychiatr Educ 12:90–101, 1988

Patussi V, Tumino E, Poldrugo F: The development of the Alcoholic Treatment Club system in Italy: fifteen years of experience. Contemp Drug Probl 23:29–42, 1996

Resnick KH, Dizmang LH: Observations on suicidal behavior among American Indians. Am J Psychiatry 127:882–887, 1971

Shepard B, O'Neill L, Guenette F: Counselling with First Nations women: considerations of oppression and renewal. Int J Adv Couns 28:227–240, 2006

Sue D: Use and abuse of alcohol by Asian Americans. J Psychoactive Drugs 19:57–66, 1987

Suwaki H: Naikan and Danshukai for the treatment of Japanese alcoholic patients. Br J Addict 74:15–19, 1979

Weiss M: Explanatory Model Interview Catalogue (EMIC): framework for comparative study of illness. Transcult Psychiatry 34:235–263, 1997

Westermeyer J: The role of cultural and social factors in the cause of addictive disorders. Psychiatr Clin North Am 22:253–273, 1999

Westermeyer J: Cultural issues, in Addiction Medicine: Principles of Addiction Medicine, 4th Edition. Edited by Ries RK, Fiellin DA, Miller SE, et al. Philadelphia, PA, Lippincott Williams & Wilkins, 2009, pp 493–500

Westermeyer J, Mellman L, Alarcon R: Cultural competence in addiction psychiatry. Addict Disord Their Treat 5:107–119, 2006

4 | Patient Placement Criteria

David R. Gastfriend, M.D.
David Mee-Lee, M.D.

How can a clinician choose the optimal treatment for a patient who is dependent on alcohol or drugs? Is the answer: "Most programs provide 28 days of residential rehabilitation, followed by weekly aftercare meetings modeled on Alcoholics Anonymous, so why not suggest the closest one and hope the patient shows up?" Or is it: "Most approaches fare about as well as the others, so see what the patient will accept and hope it works"? In the modern era of treating addictive diseases, science has provided a better foundation for treatment matching. A broad consensus of experts has reviewed this background and provided a model for choosing optimal treatments for each patient at each given moment in the course of his or her illness. This model is known as patient placement criteria.

Patient placement criteria are decision rules that guide providers and care managers in assigning patients to the optimal clinical and cost-effective level of care. Extensive reviews of the treatment outcome literature demonstrate that treatment for addictive disorders is effective but that no single treatment model or level of care is appropriate for all individuals (Berglund et al. 2003; Institute of Medicine 1990; Miller et al. 2002; Mee-Lee et al. 2010; National Institute on Drug Abuse 1999). However, most programs still deliver services with one predominant ideological model, whether that model is abstinence-mandated 12-step recovery; the Minnesota Model; harm-reduction opioid maintenance treatment; a social model therapeutic community; a behavior therapy model; or a psychiatric and mental health approach. In addition, most treatment and funding systems still provide for only a limited continuum of care. This treatment and funding deficiency continues despite the availability of detailed criteria for a broad array of service levels that has existed for over two decades.

Addiction is multidimensional by nature; this characteristic itself speaks to the need for patient placement criteria. Substance use disorders are heterogeneous in etiology and expression. These disorders cause diverse biopsychosocial problems that vary by population. No single treatment orientation and level of care could effectively and efficiently meet the needs of all patients. Nevertheless, in the minds of the general public and health care providers, drug rehabilitation involves a fixed level of care for all patients (usually residential) for a fixed length of stay (usually 28 days). The placement decision is driven by the diagnosis rather than the assessed needs of the patient. Individuals are fit into fixed length-of-stay programs designed around program specifications, which are often influenced by the available funding or benefit structure.

Beginning in the latter half of the 1980s, cost containment and managed care brought pressure on providers to justify treatment referral for each patient. After a few years of respite from health care inflation, the resurgence of costs at double and triple the general rate of inflation has once again revived pressure for cost containment. Effective use of resources is of great interest in the United States, where a growing number of payers, particularly managed care organizations, are asking or requiring treatment programs to adopt standardized clinical tools such as the American Society of Addiction Medicine Patient Placement Criteria for the Treatment of Substance-Related Disorders (ASAM PPC) (Steenrod et al. 2001). This phenomenon is also occurring internationally, particularly in countries with national health care systems. It is in this larger context of commercial and government payers that patient placement criteria are increasingly being implemented.

Rationale for Patient Placement Criteria

To understand patient placement criteria, one must be aware of the distinction between placement matching and modality matching. *Placement matching* is when one assigns a patient to a treatment setting with certain resource intensity (e.g., a therapeutic community for an opioid-addicted patient with antisocial personality traits). *Modality matching* refers to choosing a type of counseling or pharmacotherapy according to the optimal theoretical model or clinical approach that corresponds to a patient's problems (e.g., motivational enhancement therapy for a patient who is very angry and resistant to accepting a diagnosis of substance abuse disorder) (Gastfriend et al. 2000). Placement matching applies to a setting, such as intensive outpatient or residential care, whereas modality matching focuses, for example, on the suitability in a particular instance of motivational enhancement therapies or 12-step facilitation. Treatment planning involves combining modality matching with placement matching for all pertinent problems and priorities identified in the assessment, which identifies the least intensive level of care that can safely and effectively provide the needed resources to meet the patient's needs (Mee-Lee 1998; Mee-Lee and Shulman 2003).

Level-of-care matching is the basis for cost-effective patient placement criteria. The best opportunity for clinical and cost optimization occurs when level-of-care matching rules are valid and a range of settings is available. In contrast to treatment modalities, levels of care are placement options or settings that offer varying treatment intensities, as well as degrees of 0- to 24-hour structure and medical or nursing management. Levels of care have important cost implications. For example, the following settings represent decreasing levels of expense: hospital treatment, residential treatment, day treatment, and outpatient treatment. In addition to cost implications, levels of care also have treatment effectiveness implications. For instance, detoxification in a hospital level of care is far more expensive and brief compared with utilization of a continuum of five levels of detoxification, which allows a much longer length of monitored withdrawal management for the same or probably lower cost.

Theoretically, certain levels of care might be expected to yield better cost savings than others; however, outcome studies have not shown conclusive benefits for inpatient versus outpatient rehabilitation or detoxification (Annis 1988; Berglund et al. 2003; Hayashida et al. 1989; Litt et al. 1989; Miller and Hester 1986). In fact, studies have consistently failed to prove that more intensive treatment settings offer better outcomes than less intensive ones. Managed care entities have used this pattern to justify eliminating higher levels of care, such as hospital-based detoxification and rehabilitation. A critical point, however, is that investigators in these studies did not attempt to distinguish which patients experienced the best outcomes from which level of care.

The patient placement criteria model is designed to match each patient to treatment by first requiring a multidimensional assessment to identify the patient's problems and priorities within the context of severity of illness and level of function. Next, the patient's specific needs are matched to the appropriate available treatment services and the right intensity of service (which requires a broad continuum of care). Finally, the patient's progress and treatment response are assessed on an ongoing basis. This system of continuous quality improvement employs a cycle of assessment, treatment matching, level-of-care placement, and progress evaluation. Through the careful use of limited resources, the clinician can help the patient stay in ongoing treatment, improving his or her outcome and preventing dropout and relapse.

Organization of the American Society of Addiction Medicine Patient Placement Criteria

The most widely used and researched patient placement criteria for addiction treatment are the ASAM PPC, or ASAM Criteria, first published in 1996 (American Society of Addiction Medicine 1996). The most recent edition, the second edition revised (ASAM PPC-2R), includes criteria for people with co-occurring mental and substance use disorders (Mee-Lee et al. 2001). Managed care cost pressures during the 1980s prompted the development of 40–50 sets of treatment-matching protocols for addictions, many of which were proprietary and conflicting. The result was a haphazard, confusing system that frustrated providers who sought admission for their patients. Eventually, the ASAM PPC emerged, codifying four fundamental levels of care for adult and adolescent treatment. Levels of care are distinguished by the degree to which they provide medical management, structure, security, and treatment intensity. Several important principles guided development of the ASAM PPC. Table 4–1 outlines principles and implications of the ASAM PPC (Mee-Lee et al. 2001, pp. 15–16).

In the ASAM PPC, rules are specified for treatment matching at three time points: admission, continued-stay review, and discharge. To place a patient, the clinician first screens and diagnoses the patient, then assesses patient characteristics in six dimensions. These dimensions encompass all pertinent biopsychosocial aspects of addiction that determine the severity of the patient's illness and level of function, as described in Table 4–2. These problem areas (dimensions) have been identified as essential in the formulation of an individual patient's treatment plan and subsequently in making patient placement decisions.

When performing a comprehensive evaluation, the clinician thinks about a patient's immediate and longer-term needs. Rather than needing a monolithic "program," a given patient may actually need a variety of interventions, of different intensities and modalities (see Figure 4–1). The dose and intensity of these services determine the level-of-care placement decision.

Case Consideration

How the ASAM PPC distinguish between restrictiveness of setting and intensity of services with a depressed patient: On Dimension 3—emotional, behavioral, or cognitive conditions and complications—if the patient is depressed, but not suicidal and impulsive, then the mental health services would not have to be intense and can be delivered at a dose that can safely and efficiently be provided in an outpatient clinic or a therapist's office. However, if the patient is depressed *but also impulsively suicidal*, with a suicide plan and no mitigating factors, then the mental health services should be intensive, with close monitoring, and delivered at a dose that could safely be provided only in a closed psychiatric facility.

Therefore, in clinical practice, the placement decision is the last step in a multidimensional assessment that guides the variety and intensity of services needed in an individualized treatment plan. Where the patient is placed should ideally be determined by the patient's unique treatment plan, not by reimbursement limitations, program ideology, or utilization reviewers. The message to the patient must be that after elucidation of his or her various needs, in a combination that is unique to that patient, a treatment regimen is needed that fits those needs and fosters his or her particular recovery.

The ASAM Criteria describe one prevention level (Level 0.5, or L-0.5) and four basic levels of care, within which there are additional sublevels and modalities:

- *Level 0.5: Early intervention.* Early intervention services are designed to explore and address problems or risk factors that appear to be related to substance use, and to help the individual recognize the harmful consequences of inappropriate substance use.
- *Level I: Outpatient services.* L-I services are provided in regularly scheduled sessions and are designed to help the individual achieve permanent changes in his or her alcohol- and drug-using behavior and mental functioning. These services address major lifestyle, attitudinal, and behavioral issues that have the potential to undermine the goals of treatment or inhibit the individual's ability to cope with major life tasks without the nonmedical use of alcohol or other drugs.
- *Level II: Intensive outpatient/partial hospitalization.* L-II includes organized outpatient services that deliver treatment during the day, before or after work or school, in the evening, or on a weekend. For appropriately selected patients, such programs provide essential education and treatment components while allowing the patients to apply their newly acquired skills in real-world environments. These programs offer to arrange medical and psychiatric consultation, psychopharmacological consultation, medication management, and 24-hour crisis services.
- *Level III: Residential/inpatient services.* L-III encompasses organized services in a 24-hour, live-in setting. Services are provided to individuals who need 24-hour structure and services to prevent imminent danger of negative consequences and to develop sufficient recovery skills to be safely transitioned to less intense levels.

TABLE 4–1. Principles guiding American Society of Addiction Medicine Patient Placement Criteria development, and implications of these principles

Principle	Implications
Objectivity	• The criteria are as objective, measurable, and quantifiable as possible.
	• Certain aspects of the criteria require subjective interpretation.
	• As with other medical or psychiatric conditions, diagnosis, assessment, and treatment form a mix of objectively measured criteria and experientially based professional judgments.
Choice of treatment levels	• Referral to a specific level of care is based on a multidimensional assessment of the patient.
	• The goal is a level of care that is the least intensive but that can accomplish the treatment objectives while providing safety and security for the patient.
	• Levels of care are presented as discrete but represent benchmarks or points along a continuum of treatment services used in a variety of ways, depending on a patient's needs and response.
	• Patients enter the continuum at any level and move through levels of care in consecutive order or skip levels, as needed.
Continuum of care	• Within and across the levels of care, there is a continuum of severity of illnesses treated and intensities of services provided.
	• Funding and reimbursement must match the continuum of care and intensities of service.
	• If only one of many levels of care is offered, movement between levels requires linking the patient with providers of other levels of care whenever indicated by an assessment of the patient's needs and progress.
Length of stay	• No fixed length of stay is required.
	• Length of stay depends on severity of illness and progress/response to treatment.

TABLE 4–2.   **American Society of Addiction Medicine assessment dimensions**

Dimensions	Assessment and treatment planning focus
1. Acute intoxication and/or withdrawal potential	Assess for intoxication and/or withdrawal management. Detoxify in a variety of levels of care and make preparations for continued addiction services.
2. Biomedical conditions and complications	Assess and treat co-occurring physical health conditions or complications. Provide treatment within the level of care or through coordination of physical health services.
3. Emotional, behavioral, or cognitive conditions and complications	Assess and treat co-occurring diagnostic or subdiagnostic mental health conditions or complications. Provide treatment within the level of care or through coordination of mental health services.
4. Readiness to change	Assess stage of readiness to change. If patient is not ready to commit to full recovery, engage in treatment using motivational enhancement strategies. If patient is ready for recovery, consolidate and expand action for change.
5. Relapse, continued use, or continued problem potential	Assess readiness for relapse prevention services and teach, where appropriate. If patient is still at early stages of change, raise awareness of consequences of continued use or continued problems as part of motivational enhancement strategies.
6. Recovery environment	Assess need for specific, individualized, family, or significant other services, as well as need for housing, financial, vocational, educational, legal, transportation, or child care services.

- *Level IV: Medically managed intensive inpatient services.* Staffed by designated physicians with credentials in treating addiction, including psychiatrists and other mental health clinicians, L-IV programs provide 24-hour, medically directed evaluation, care, and treatment of mental and substance use–related disorders in an acute care inpatient setting. Patients' mental health and substance use–related problems are sufficiently severe to require primary biomedical, psychiatric, and nursing care services. Treatment is specific to mental and substance use–related disorders. However, the skills of the interdisciplinary team and the availability of support services allow the conjoint treatment of any co-occurring biomedical conditions that must be addressed.

Case Consideration

How the ASAM PPC sequence alcohol-dependent patients through step-down care: A clinician can use the ASAM PPC-2R to guide the sequence of care for two patients with differing severities of alcohol dependence (Mee-Lee et al. 2001). An alcoholic patient with a history of withdrawal seizures but only mild medical conditions would be matched to L-III.7 (medically monitored inpatient detoxification). After 2–3 days without complications, he would be "stepped down" to L-III.5 (therapeutic community) to deal with problems such as poor adherence; difficulty postponing gratification, with imminent relapse risk; lingering withdrawal discomfort; and lack of a safe place to live. In contrast, a patient who had a supportive family and living environment and was more committed to recovery, even though she was experiencing cravings to use, could be safely treated in a partial hospital or even in an intensive outpatient setting. Self- or mutual-help groups would supplement professional care and provide more extensive daily recovery support. Such flexible use of levels of care would employ the least intensive and least costly settings that could be expected to address the patient's needs in both phases of treatment.

Assessment Tools for Clinical Use and Research

The ASAM PPC clinical decision tree is complex and sophisticated. Although a clinician usually tends to conduct psychosocial assessments partly via a general outline structure and partly by intuition, the systematic approach of the ASAM PPC can potentially benefit from the use of some structured assessment questionnaires or interviews (Gastfriend et al. 1994). Such instruments include the Addiction Severity Index (ASI; McLellan et al. 1992), the Recovery Attitude and Treatment Evaluator (RAATE; Gastfriend et al. 1995; Mee-Lee 1988; Mee-Lee et al. 1992; Najavits et al. 1997), the Clinical Institute Withdrawal Assessment (CIWA; Sullivan et al. 1989), and the Clinical Institute Narcotics Assessment (CINA; Fudala et al. 1991). The CIWA and CINA are standardized scales

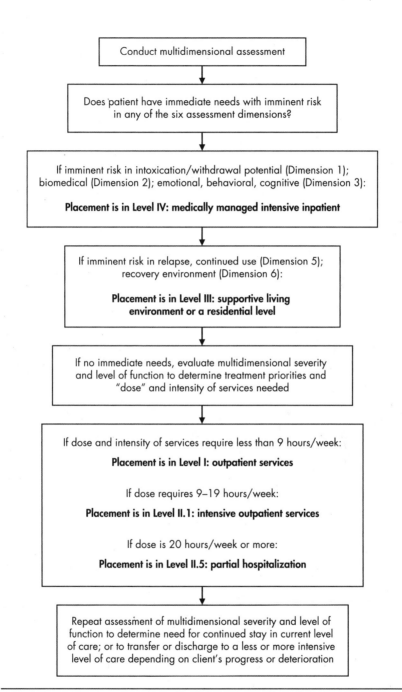

FIGURE 4–1. **Overview of the sequence for patient assessment and matching to treatment/placement.**

For full sequence of decision rules, see Mee-Lee et al. 2001.

that can be used to evaluate the ASAM PPC's first assessment dimension, acute intoxication or withdrawal. The ASI and the RAATE can be used to evaluate patients on several dimensions. The ASI is a widely used, structured interview tool designed to assess patients with substance abuse on seven dimensions: medical status, employment/support status, drug use, alcohol use, legal status, family/social relationships, and psychiatric status. The RAATE was initially developed by Mee-Lee (1988) and later modified and adapted for use in research on the ASAM PPC. Typical items from the RAATE include the following questions: "Does the patient demonstrate a commitment to seeking help or treatment?" "Does the patient realize that recovery is an ongoing process requiring personal responsibility?" "Does the patient have a chronic physical condition or disability which interferes with treatment or recovery efforts?" "Is the patient able to focus on addictions treatment even if he/she has psychiatric/ psychological symptoms?" "Is the work/school system accommodating or supportive of the treatment/recovery program?" The instruments listed above are the main feeders of an automated decision tree created to facilitate the use of the first edition of the ASAM PPC (Turner et al. 1999). A new assessment software package (ASAM PPC-2R Assessment Software; Recovery Search, Inc., Newton, MA) is being used in research and utilizes these instruments or similar types of questionnaires or items to yield objective, quantitative level-of-care determinations according to the ASAM PPC-2R.

Research Findings and Automation

Publication of these nonproprietary matching criteria raised considerable interest, which ranged from creation of continuing education courses on the criteria to adoption of the assessment tools by managed care entities covering 50 million people and public agencies in approximately 30 U.S. states (Mee-Lee 2005). A shortcoming existed, however, because no process of field trial testing preceded the publication of the criteria. This led scientists to subject the ASAM PPC to the crucial process of research testing (Gastfriend and Mee-Lee 2003). The literature, in general, strongly supports the need for patient placement criteria based on multidimensional assessment in treatment planning (Gastfriend et al. 2000; Hser et al. 1999; McLellan et al. 1997). Numerous studies have shown that treatment models based on the ASAM PPC's dimensions and levels of care can validly predict patient outcomes and can also reduce costs (Alterman et al. 1994; Annis 1988; Gastfriend and McLellan 1997; Hayashida et al. 1989; Mechanic et al. 1995). More specifically, a considerable body of work exists on the ASAM PPC itself, including at least nine evaluations involving a total of 3,641 subjects. Federal agencies, including the National Institute on Drug Abuse, the National Institute on Alcohol Abuse and Alcoholism, and the Center for Substance Abuse Treatment, have invested more than $7 million in research on the various assessment tools and placement guidelines of the ASAM PPC (Gastfriend 2001).

In the earliest evaluation of the 1991 ASAM PPC, the Boston Target Cities Project used a one-page version of the ASAM Criteria in a large, urban, public population. Compared with direct self-referred admission to treatment programs, patients who were referred via centralized intake centers using standardized assessment with this coarse implementation of the ASAM Criteria were 38% more likely to make the transition to longitudinal treatment within 30 days and were significantly less likely to return for repeat detoxification within 90 days (Plough et al. 1996). These findings suggested that use of the PPC can be feasible, because even this shortened version was associated with improved retention. An incomplete implementation of the original ASAM Criteria by McKay et al. (1997) was used to retrospectively test their psychosocial dimensions (i.e., Dimensions 4, 5, and 6). This study suggested some areas of validity but highlighted a need for further revision. A prospective, naturalistic study examined the validity and impact of the PPC, comparing the placement of 287 adults in Washington State with 240 adults in Oregon, where a statewide PPC training model was fully implemented. Results showed that in Oregon, with use of the PPC, patients had more individualized lengths of stay and were more likely to utilize the intensive outpatient level of care (Deck et al. 2003).

To help deal with the complexity of the multidimensional branching logic of the ASAM PPC, researchers at the Massachusetts General Hospital Addiction Research Program implemented the ASAM Criteria as a comprehensive computerized interview (Turner et al. 1999). With this real-time, computerized method, different providers assessing the same patient had a good likelihood of arriving at the same level-of-care recommendation (i.e., interrater reliability; intraclass correlation coefficient= 0.77; $P<0.01$) (Baker and Gastfriend 2003), comparing favorably with the literature on evaluations such as DSM diagnosis and severity rating (Endicott et al. 1976; Hall 1995; Regier et al. 1994).

To date, three prospective studies have tested the computer-assisted ASAM PPC Assessment Software (Turner et al. 1999) in three different samples (public system Medicaid and uninsured patients, insured patients, and veterans) using three different outcomes (acute no-show to treatment, 90-day drinking rates, and long-term hospital utilization). The first prospective study, a multisite trial in Massachusetts, is the only randomized, controlled trial of placement criteria to be conducted to date. In this project, 700 subjects were randomly selected to receive L-II or L-III treatment, either matched or mismatched, according to the recommendation of the ASAM PPC algorithm. Results showed that the ASAM PPC recommendations fit well with other valid assessments such as the ASI (i.e., showed good concurrent validity) (Turner et al. 1999). The study also found evidence that the ASAM PPC Assessment Software was valid for predicting treatment outcomes (i.e., showed good predictive validity), because patients who were mismatched to a lower level of care than was recommended by the computer ended up having higher acute no-show rates (Gastfriend 2001). The same findings as in the overall study cohort were observed in patient subgroups with high-frequency cocaine use (Kang et al. 2002) and patients with comorbid symptomatology; the latter subgroup also had higher no-show rates when mismatched to a higher level of care than recommended (Angarita et al. 2007). Thus, compared with matching patients to the recommended ASAM PPC Assessment Software level of care, patients have been found to have adverse outcomes both with undermatching and overmatching.

In the second trial, a naturalistic study of 248 newly admitted, primarily alcohol-dependent subjects in New York City, Magura et al. (2003) showed that outpatients who had received a lower level of care than that recommended by the ASAM PPC (e.g., patient received L-I, outpatient care, whereas L-II, intensive outpatient care, was recommended) had significantly and substantially poorer alcohol-use outcomes 90 days later. Also of note is that this study revealed that overtreatment, according to the ASAM PPC Assessment Software, did not improve outcome.

In the third trial, a naturalistic study of 95 U.S. Department of Veterans Affairs patients near Boston, Massachusetts, initial ASAM PPC matching was associated with reductions in subsequent hospital utilization. Patients who were judged by the algorithm as needing L-IV (i.e., hospital) care but who were undermatched to L-III care (residential rehabilitation), however, used significantly and substantially more hospital bed days over the next 12 months than did patients who were judged to be appropriately matched (Sharon et al. 2003).

These results support the predictive validity and cost-effectiveness of the use of the ASAM PPC Assessment Software. The ultimate goal of this ongoing research is revision of the ASAM PPC that will emerge not -simply from the current expert consensus process but also through the findings of multiple national and international research studies.

Revision of the ASAM PPC

The way that services were grouped or "bundled" in the original ASAM Criteria did not allow for ample flexibility to meet individual patient needs (e.g., the need for more than four levels of care, for criteria on methadone treatment, and for outpatient detoxification). The latest revision, the 2001 ASAM PPC-2R (Mee-Lee et al. 2001), separated or "unbundled" pharmacotherapies such as detoxification, and created five levels of detoxification that encompassed two levels of ambulatory detoxification: social detoxification and medically monitored and managed detoxification. Opioid maintenance therapy (e.g., methadone) was included, and the treatment continuum was expanded to describe multilevel criteria for both outpatient and inpatient settings. For L-II (intensive outpatient) care, new criteria were described to distinguish between evening care or day treatment programs (L-II.1) and partial hospitalization (L-II.5). For L-III (residential inpatient) care, criteria were added to distinguish between clinically managed, low-intensity residential treatment (e.g., L-III.1, supervised domiciliary or working halfway house); clinically managed, medium-intensity residential treatment (e.g., L-III.3, modified, individualized treatment for cognitively impaired patients); clinically managed, high-intensity residential treatment (e.g., L-III.5, therapeutic community or residential treatment center); and medically monitored, intensive, inpatient treatment (e.g., L-III.7, residential rehabilitation with on-site nursing supervision). Criteria were added for a new level of care: L-0.5, early intervention, which was defined as professional services for individuals who are at risk of developing substance use–related problems but who may not yet qualify for a diagnosis.

Using Multidimensional PPC Assessment to Focus Treatment Priorities

The ASAM PPC-2R can help a clinician address the needs of patients with dual diagnoses (i.e., co-occurring mental disorder and substance use–related disorder). The clinician evaluates the patient in detail *within* each of the six dimensions and then *across* the six dimensions, and finally *constructs the treatment plan* given the available options along the continuum of mental health and substance-use service sublevels. The following case provides a detailed example of this iterative review process.

> **Ann,** a 32-year-old divorced white woman, has been diagnosed with alcohol dependence, marijuana abuse, and major depressive disorder. She has been abstinent from alcohol for 48 hours and has been able to abstain periodically for only up to 72 hours because of sweats, internal tremors, and nausea (but never hallucinations, delirium tremens, or seizures).
>
> She was hospitalized just 1 week ago for alcoholic hepatitis. She smokes up to two or three joints a day but stopped yesterday. In addition, she reports two past suicide attempts using sleeping pills, but the most

recent attempt was 3 years ago. She sees a psychiatrist once a month for fluoxetine, which she takes as prescribed for depression.

Ann lives in a rented apartment and has very few friends since moving after her divorce a year ago. Currently unemployed after being laid off when the department store at which she worked closed, she has worked as a waitress, checkout person, and salesperson. She has never lost a job due to addiction.

Ann appears slightly anxious, but her vital signs are normal and she manifests no sweats, tremor, or nausea. She speaks calmly and is cooperative. Ann shows awareness of her consequences from chemical use but tends to minimize them and blame others, including her ex-husband, who left her without warning. She does not know much about chemical dependency but wants to learn more. She says her 11-year-old son doesn't see any problems with her drinking and doesn't know about her marijuana use.

Considerations within each dimension. Dimension 1—Ann has been abstinent from alcohol for 48 hours and shows no current withdrawal signs. With her past history of no more than moderate withdrawal symptoms and even considering her use of marijuana (which would not mask withdrawal symptoms in the same way that benzodiazepines would), it is unlikely that withdrawal would just begin 48 hours after her last drink. Dimension 2—Ann's recent episode of alcoholic hepatitis is a problem of possibly high severity, considering that she was released from the hospital 1 week ago and she has drunk in the intervening days. Dimension 3— Given Ann's history of two past suicide attempts and depression, perhaps her mental health should be assessed as severe. Dimension 4—Ann's readiness to change is characterized by ambivalence, given her tendency to minimize and blame, but also current willingness to learn more about chemical dependency. Thus, she is in the contemplation stage of change (Prochaska et al. 1992) with moderate severity, because she will need active education and engagement strategies to ensure that her initial willingness does not tilt back toward unreadiness to change. Dimension 5— Ann would be rated as having a very high continued use potential based on her inability to abstain beyond 72 hours and her drinking upon her recent hospital discharge. Dimension 6—Given her many stressors, the recovery environment is one of Ann's highest-priority problems, because being an unemployed single mother lacking a support system represents multiple stressors. Her son's response to her substance use is a bit incongruous and calls for a session with him. [Note that each patient's needs and risks are evaluated individually; Ann's risks might seem to be less than those of someone who is homeless, but the ASAM PPC-2R requires individualized consideration of her own problems relative to her function.]

Considerations across the dimensions. Dimension 1 needs to be considered in light of Dimension 2 concerns about possible liver dysfunction due to Ann's hepatitis. Because insufficient information is available to make a determination about her liver function, more information is needed from her referring physician. Nevertheless, this combination may not pose any serious withdrawal risk.

In Dimension 3, Ann's history of past suicide attempts and her depression should cause concern. However, her suicide attempts were 3 years ago and interacted with a Dimension 6 psychosocial stressor that was unique at that time (i.e., her husband leaving her without warning). She is being treated for her depression and is compliant with her medication, except for the admonition not to drink. Severity in this dimension is low, but she should be observed because of the following: 1) she has many Dimension 6 stressors that have the potential for increasing severity in Dimension 3, and 2) she has been apparently stable, in terms of her depression, on a "cocktail" of fluoxetine, cannabis, and alcohol, and it is unclear what effect a change in the formula would have. However, she may not need additional mental health services in the next few weeks, and it may help to observe her depression once she is detoxified and in recovery.

Dimension 4, in which she is ambivalent and unskilled in recovery activities, must be considered in light of her Dimension 5 high risk for relapse and Dimension 6 lack of supports. Ann may not have time to learn recovery skills during the 72-hour window in which she previously tended to resume alcohol and/or marijuana use.

Dimension 5 presents a very significant problem. On the basis of Ann's last 3-month history, her concurrent use of cannabis and the fact that she drank soon after hospitalization for alcoholic hepatitis indicate that her potential for continued use of alcohol and marijuana is very high. Dimension 6 interacts seriously with Dimension 5, because Ann's stressful environment may exacerbate her urges for continued use, and the lack of structure in her environment is unlikely to help her protect herself.

Constructing the treatment plan. Ann's treatment plan should include strategies and supports to maintain near-term abstinence, especially in the next 24–48 hours. This can give her an initial success and spur her to develop a short-term treatment goal, which is conceivable by her and achievable. Ann's two highest-severity dimensions are therefore 5 and 6. Her immediate service needs are for close support, especially over the next 48 hours as she deals with marijuana withdrawal, cravings, and relapse impulses. If Ann is willing and able to use frequent Alcoholics Anonymous or similar meetings in conjunction with their volunteers, especially any sober companionship over the next 24–48 hours, intensive outpatient treatment (L-II.1) would be most appropriate.

Given Ann's current Dimension 3 issues, dual diagnosis–capable intensive outpatient treatment is needed. Furthermore, because most intensive outpatient treatment programs operate in the evening, if daytime intensive outpatient treatment is unavailable, consideration should be given to the need for child care for her son and the relative merits of her attending an intensive outpatient evening program and not being with her son. If evening treatment is ruled out and no day programs are available, or if community and program supports are not easily available, a partial hospitalization program (L-II.5) can be considered. In exploring the options with Ann, if she is deemed to be too impulsive with cravings to abstain, a 24-hour clinically managed residential detoxification service (L-III.2-D; i.e., detoxification) or clinically managed low-intensity residential

(L-III.1) service in combination with L-II.5 may meet Ann's needs. However, any 24-hour setting raises child care complications.

In cases such as Ann's, gaps in the continuum of care are often exposed. Such gaps lead addiction treatment providers to use only the most intensive levels of care, such as Level III.7, medically monitored intensive inpatient treatment, or Level IV, medically managed intensive inpatient treatment, to meet the patient's needs. In such cases, these levels of care are not clinically necessary; they use resources inefficiently and decrease access to care for those who do need those levels of intensity.

Additional Features of the ASAM PPC-2R

Below, we highlight other specific features of the ASAM PPC-2R and the ways in which they help practitioners and programs retool services.

- Adolescent criteria use a broad continuum of care, with eight levels. This change expanded the assessment of emotional, behavioral, and cognitive conditions and complications by adding criteria for five subdomains (dangerousness/lethality, interference with addiction recovery efforts, social functioning, capacity for self-care, and course of illness). These changes reflect the needs of adolescents who have co-occurring mental health and addiction problems.
- L-I outpatient treatment criteria were expanded to promote greater access to care for dual-diagnosis patients, unmotivated patients mandated into treatment, and others who previously had access to care only if they agreed to periods of intensive primary treatment. Knowledge and application of cognitive-behavioral therapies, such as motivational interviewing, motivational enhancement, solution-focused therapy, and stages-of-change work, greatly increased between the PPC editions. The ASAM PPC-2R increased options for patients who previously would have been turned away as not ready for treatment or as "in denial," requiring coerced intensive treatment levels. These improvements were designed to increase access to care and hopefully engage clients earlier, utilize resources more efficiently, and improve effectiveness of recovery efforts.
- Expansion of criteria in Dimension 3 to "emotional, behavioral, or *cognitive* conditions and complications." Also, with the addition of the new subdomains of assessment that address co-occurring mental and substance use–related disorders, services can now focus on multiple needs, not only on the addiction.
- Dimension 4 was changed from "treatment acceptance/resistance" to "readiness to change." This expanded the field's understanding of Di-

mension 4 to include assessment of the patient's readiness to change. The change also helped to make treatment more readily available to all, not only those ready to embrace abstinence and recovery.

- Dimension 5 was expanded to "relapse, continued use, or *continued problem* potential" to encompass mental health clinical presentations. Also, Dimension 5 was enhanced with an expanded "sequence of factors" that are known to contribute to relapse potential. The sequence involves the historical pattern of relapse, the acute pharmacological response to substance(s), second-order behavioral responsivity that may mediate the preceding factors, and third-order personality or learned responses that may modify the preceding factors.

- "Continued-service and discharge/transfer criteria" were reduced and simplified. General continued-service and transfer/discharge criteria guidelines applicable to all levels of care were developed to replace separate continued-service and discharge criteria for each separate level of care. These changes facilitated reassessment and modification of the individual's treatment and services plan, allowing clinicians to focus more on the individual treatment plan, rather than on the patient's achievement of preset program goals.

- New criteria and descriptions of services were provided for the management of the patient with co-occurring mental and substance use disorders. Dual diagnosis–capable services typically can meet a patient's needs as long as the patient's psychiatric disorders are sufficiently stabilized and the individual is capable of independent functioning to such a degree that his or her mental disorders do not significantly interfere with participation in addiction treatment. Dual diagnosis–enhanced services encompass the ability to screen for and address a wide variety of mental health levels of function that co-occur with the patient's addiction-treatment needs. Dual diagnosis–enhanced programs are specifically designed and enhanced to meet those needs on-site for patients with significant and unstable or disabling dual-diagnosis needs. With addiction-only services, the admission criteria and policies and procedures for ongoing services and program content do not accommodate co-occurring mental disorder. For example, individuals taking psychotropic medications are not generally accepted, coordination or collaboration with mental health services is not routinely present, and mental health issues are not usually addressed in treatment planning. In a study of 453 providers, 65% of the programs were identified as dual diagnosis capable, 23% as addiction-only services, and 12% as dual diagnosis enhanced (McGovern et al. 2007).

Significance

As the ASAM Criteria have evolved, support has broadened and resulted in adoption by payers, single-state agencies, and state Medicaid programs. In 1997, the criteria were adopted by the U.S. Department of Defense for worldwide use and by the U.S. Department of Veterans Affairs for its 171 hospitals nationwide. A multisite study funded by the government of Norway has translated the software into Norwegian (Recovery Search, Inc., Newton, MA) and is developing it for eventual implementation across that country. International collaboration has been initiated to implement the use of the criteria in European, Asian, and South American countries.

A majority of U.S. outpatient treatment programs (57%) report that they routinely use the ASAM Criteria to assess and place their clients (Chuang et al. 2009). According to findings from this analysis of the National Drug Abuse Treatment System Survey, financial and accreditation pressures appear foremost among the influences on ASAM PPC adoption. For every percentage point increase in a program's population covered by Medicaid or private managed care, the odds that the program routinely uses the ASAM PPC increases by 1%–2%. Also, compared with unaccredited programs, programs approved by the Commission on Accreditation of Rehabilitation Facilities have triple the rate of ASAM PPC adoption (Chuang et al. 2009). Consistent with these financial pressures, a survey of 450 private substance abuse treatment agencies conducted by the National Treatment Center revealed that ASAM PPC adoption was associated with program survival. Specifically, programs that had not survived 24 months after an earlier survey were less likely to have adopted the ASAM PPC, and those that closed within 6 months of the initial survey had even lower adoption rates. ASAM PPC adoption may confer a possible competitive advantage with managed care organizations ("Treatment Matching Interest Group" 2004).

One challenge, however, is that the continuum of care is still not sufficiently available for effective ASAM PPC implementation. One-third (31%) of U.S. outpatient treatment programs do not offer any levels of care that are more resource intensive than ASAM L-I (Chuang et al. 2009). Also, although private managed care was associated with programs using the ASAM PPC, only public managed care was associated with a greater likelihood of offering more resource-intensive services. Thus, it is not at all clear that the current health care financing system is successfully influencing development of the continuum of care via the ASAM PPC. Despite the support shown for the ASAM PPC, a desirable continuum of care is still only in the planning stages in many regions. Although the cost of using the ASAM PPC itself to place clients is quite low (Chuang et al.

2009), some levels of care mandated by the ASAM continuum, such as L-IV and L-III.7, are costly, and treatment programs may be reluctant to invest in developing the full continuum of care (Ducharme et al. 2007). Many areas lack options such as methadone treatment access for halfway house residents or office-based detoxification programs. Methadone programs are the most segregated of all program categories in terms of types of services provided (Chuang et al. 2009), which contradicts the recommendations of the ASAM PPC. Benefit plans and public funding often remain restricted to a limited continuum of care, even though a broader range of options could provide longer lengths of care and monitoring using the same or even fewer resources; for example, a flexible use of five levels of detoxification would likely be less expensive and allow a longer period of withdrawal management than a few days of high-cost detoxification at the hospital level of care.

Nevertheless, these criteria are useful guides for improving the quality and reducing the cost of patient care, particularly for capitated systems. Hypotheses about matching services to particular patient characteristics or needs (Table 4–3) should also serve as strategic guidelines for health care networks during program development and acquisition.

Conclusion

In psychotherapy, every clinician understands that the patient is unique and that his or her particular constellation of strengths, vulnerabilities, problems, and resources dictates how the treatment will be formed and delivered. Treatment for addiction must similarly be individualized. No single treatment model or program serves the purposes of every patient. With the help of patient placement criteria, providers can address patients' unique substance use problems on a rational basis. Adoption of formal rules, such as the ASAM PPC-2R, is under way in numerous states, managed care entities, professional provider societies, and provider groups, and interest in the criteria has increased internationally. Initially, such criteria relied more heavily on consensus recommendations than on empirical matching data, but outcome research data drive their continuous revision. The technology for conducting psychosocial treatment-matching studies has been rapidly increasing in sophistication and has been demonstrated to yield adequate reliability and concurrent validity. Although predictive validity continues to be studied, the national research portfolio on placement criteria is expanding. Given the push for evidence-based practices and recent dramatic cost pressures, there is an essential public health need for further research in this area if addiction services are to continue to grow in quality and availability.

TABLE 4–3. Matrix for matching services to needs

Risk rating and description	Types of services and modalities needed	Intensity of service/level of care/setting
Assess severity and level of function to identify needs for services in all six ASAM assessment dimensions.	Identify the specific variety of services required to address priority needs, based on the risk assessment in each dimension.	Determine what type of service setting and level of care can efficiently and safely provide necessary intensities of service.
Risk ratings are benchmarked on a scale of 0–4, with 0 indicating full function and no risk in this assessment dimension.	If 0, no specific services are needed in this assessment dimension.	Intensity of services is benchmarked on a scale of 0–4, with 0 indicating that no specific level of care or treatment setting is needed in this assessment dimension.
In whatever dimension is being assessed, if risk rating is 1–4, the severity and risk levels rise with the higher number.	Specific services in an individualized treatment plan are designed to match the severity, level of function, and risk in this assessment dimension.	The intensity of services will rise with the higher risk rating in Dimensions 1–3, but will be variable for Dimensions 4–6, depending on the mix of services selected from the middle column.

Note. ASAM=American Society of Addiction Medicine.
Source. Adapted from Mee-Lee et al. 2001.

Key Clinical Concepts

- Treatment outcome research demonstrates that treatment for addictive disorders is effective but that no single model or level of care is appropriate for all individuals. The services themselves and where they are delivered should therefore be individualized to each patient's assessed needs.

- The most widely used and researched patient placement criteria tool for addiction treatment is the ASAM PPC. The most recent edition, published in 2001, includes criteria for people with co-occurring mental and substance use disorders.

- The ASAM PPC incorporates multidimensional assessments of severity of illness and level of function; problem and priority identification; treatment matching of needs to services; and level-of-care placement within a broad continuum of care. On-going assessment of progress and treatment response determines movement to less or more intensive levels of care.

- The ASAM PPC describes a broad range of levels of care. However, benefit plans, public funding, and provider programs are frequently restricted to a limited continuum of care, even though a broader range of options could provide longer lengths of care and monitoring using the same or even fewer resources.

- More than a decade of research on the ASAM PPC supports the tool's predictive validity and cost-effectiveness. Based on this research, a variety of computer-assisted assessment and placement tools are in development.

Suggested Reading

Gastfriend DR (ed): Addiction Treatment Matching—Research Foundations of the American Society of Addiction Medicine (ASAM) Criteria. Binghamton, NY, Haworth Medical Press, 2004

Mee-Lee D: ASAM patient placement criteria: implications for assessment and treatment of patients with co-occurring disorders. Counselor Magazine 5:28–33, 2005

Mee-Lee D: ASAM's placement criteria: what's new. Behavioral Health Management 3:32–34, 2005

Mee-Lee D, Shulman GD: The ASAM placement criteria and matching patients to treatment, in Principles of Addiction Medicine, 4th Edition. Edited by Ries RK, Fiellin D, Miller SC, et al. Philadelphia, PA, Lippincott Williams & Wilkins, 2009, pp 387–399

Miller SD, Mee-Lee D, Plum B, et al: Making treatment count: client-directed, outcome informed clinical work with problem drinkers, in Handbook of Clinical Family Therapy. Edited by Lebow J. New York, Wiley, 2005, pp 281–308

TIPS & TOPICS [A monthly newsletter of clinical knowledge and skills tips on person-centered services and application of PPC principles]. Available at: http://www.DavidMeeLee.com

References

Alterman AI, O'Brien CP, McLellan AT, et al: Effectiveness and costs of inpatient versus day hospital cocaine rehabilitation. J Nerv Ment Dis 182:157–163, 1994

American Society of Addiction Medicine: Patient Placement Criteria for the Treatment of Substance-Related Disorders, 2nd Edition (ASAM PPC-2). Chevy Chase, MD, American Society of Addiction Medicine, 1996

Angarita GA, Reif S, Pirard S, et al: No-show for treatment in substance abuse patients with comorbid symptomatology: validity results from a controlled trial of the ASAM Patient Placement Criteria. J Addict Med 1:79–87, 2007

Annis H: Patient-treatment matching in the management of alcoholism. NIDA Res Monogr 90:152–161, 1988

Baker SL, Gastfriend DR: Reliability of multidimensional substance abuse treatment matching: implementing the ASAM Patient Placement Criteria. J Addict Dis 22 (suppl 1):45–60, 2003

Berglund M, Thelande, S, Jonsson E (eds): Treating Alcohol and Drug Abuse: An Evidence-Based Review. Weinheim, Germany, Wiley-VCH Verlag, 2003

Chuang E, Wells R, Alexander JA, et al: Factors associated with use of ASAM criteria and service provision in a national sample of outpatient substance abuse treatment units. J Addict Med 3:139–150, 2009

Deck D, Gabriel R, Knudson J, et al: Impact of patient placement criteria on substance abuse treatment under the Oregon Health Plan. J Addict Dis 22 (suppl 1): 27–44, 2003

Ducharme LJ, Mello HL, Roman PM, et al: Service delivery in substance abuse treatment: reexamining "comprehensive" care. J Behav Health Serv Res 34:121–136, 2007

Endicott J, Spitzer R, Fleiss JL, et al: The Global Assessment Scale: a procedure for measuring overall severity of psychiatric diagnosis. Arch Gen Psychiatry 33:766–773, 1976

Fudala PJ, Berkow LC, Fralich JL, et al: Use of naloxone in the assessment of opiate dependence. Life Sci 49:1809–1814, 1991

Gastfriend DR: Placement criteria come of age. Paper presented at the annual medical-scientific meeting of the American Society of Addiction Medicine, Los Angeles, CA, April 20, 2001

Gastfriend DR, McLellan AT: Treatment matching: theoretic basis and practical implications. Med Clin North Am 81:945–966, 1997

Gastfriend DR, Mee-Lee D: The ASAM patient placement criteria: context, concepts and continuing development. J Addict Dis 22 (suppl 1):1–8, 2003

Gastfriend DR, Baker SL, Najavits LM, et al: Assessment instruments, in Principles of Addiction Medicine. Edited by Miller N, Doot M. Chevy Chase, MD, American Society of Addiction Medicine, 1994, pp 1–8

Gastfriend DR, Filstead WJ, Reif S, et al: Validity of assessing treatment readiness in patients with substance use disorders. Am J Addict 4:254–260, 1995

Gastfriend DR, Lu SH, Sharon E: Placement matching: challenges and technical progress. Subst Use Misuse 35:2191–2213, 2000

Hall R: Global Assessment of Functioning: a modified scale. Psychosomatics 36:267–275, 1995

Hayashida M, Alterman AI, McLellan AT, et al: Comparative effectiveness and costs of inpatient and outpatient detoxification of patients with mild-to-moderate alcohol withdrawal syndrome. N Engl J Med 320:358–365, 1989

Hser YI, Polinsky ML, Maglione M, et al: Matching clients' needs with drug treatment services. J Subst Abuse Treat 16:299–305, 1999

Institute of Medicine: Broadening the Base of Treatment for Alcohol Problems. Washington, DC, National Academy Press, 1990

Kang SK, Sharon S, Pirard S, et al: Predictors for Residential Rehabilitation and Treatment No-Show in High Frequency Cocaine Users: Validation of the American Society of Addiction Medicine (ASAM) Criteria. Las Vegas, NV, American Academy of Addiction Psychiatrists, 2002

Litt M, Boca F, Cooney N: Matching Alcoholics to Aftercare Treatment by Empirical Clustering. Farmington, CT, University of Connecticut Health Center, 1989

Magura S, Staines GL, Kosanke N, et al: Predictive validity of the ASAM Patient Placement Criteria for naturalistically matched vs. mismatched alcohol-dependent patients. Am J Addict 12:386–397, 2003

McGovern MP, Xie H, Acquilano S, et al: Addiction treatment services and co-occurring disorders: the ASAM-PPC-2R taxonomy of program dual diagnosis capability. J Addict Dis 26:27–37, 2007

McKay JR, Cacciola JS, McLellan AT, et al: An initial evaluation of the psychosocial dimensions of the American Society of Addiction Medicine criteria for inpatient vs. intensive outpatient substance abuse rehabilitation. J Stud Alcohol 58:239–252, 1997

McLellan AT, Kushner H, Metzger DS, et al: The fifth edition of the Addiction Severity Index. J Subst Abuse Treat 9:199–213, 1992

McLellan AT, Grissom GR, Zanis D, et al: Problem-service "matching" in addiction treatment: a prospective study in 4 programs. Arch Gen Psychiatry 54:730–735, 1997

Mechanic D, Schlesinger M, McAlpine DD, et al: Management of mental health and substance abuse services: state of the art and early results. Milbank Q 73:19–55, 1995

Mee-Lee D: An instrument for treatment progress and matching: the Recovery Attitude and Treatment Evaluator (RAATE). J Subst Abuse Treat 5:183–186, 1988

Mee-Lee D: Use of patient placement criteria in the selection of treatment: overview of addiction treatment, in Principles of Addiction Medicine, 2nd Edition. Edited by Graham AW, Schultz TK. Chevy Chase, MD, American Society of Addiction Medicine, 1998, pp 363–370

Mee-Lee D: ASAM's placement criteria: what's new. Behavioral Health Management 25:32–34, 2005

Mee-Lee D, Shulman GD: The ASAM Patient Placement Criteria and matching patients to treatment: overview of addiction treatment, in Principles of Addiction Medicine, 3rd Edition. Edited by Graham AW, Schultz TK, Mayo-Smith MF, et al. Chevy Chase, MD, American Society of Addiction Medicine, 2003, pp 453–465

Mee-Lee D, Hoffmann NG, Smith M: Recovery Attitude and Treatment Evaluator (RAATE) Manual. St Paul, MN, CATOR/New Standards, 1992

Mee-Lee D, Shulman GD, Fishman M, et al: ASAM Patient Placement Criteria for the Treatment of Substance-Related Disorders, 2nd Edition, Revised (ASAM PPC-2R). Chevy Chase, MD, American Society of Addiction Medicine, 2001

Mee-Lee D, McLellan AT, Miller SD: What works in substance abuse and dependence treatment, in The Heart and Soul of Change, 2nd Edition. Edited by Duncan BL, Miller SD, Wampold BE, et al. Washington, DC, American Psychological Association, 2010, pp 393–417

Miller WR, Hester RK: The effectiveness of alcoholism treatment: what research reveals, in Treating Addictive Behaviors: Processes of Change. Edited by Miller WR, Heather N. New York, Plenum, 1986, pp 121–174

Miller WR, Wilbourne PL, Hettema JE: What works? A summary of alcohol treatment outcome research, in Handbook of Alcoholism Treatment Approaches: Effective Alternatives. Edited by Hester RK, Miller WR. New York, Allyn & Bacon, 2002, pp 13–63

Najavits LM, Gastfriend DR, Nakayama EY, et al: A measure of readiness for substance abuse treatment: psychometric properties of the RAATE research interview. Am J Addict 6:74–82, 1997

National Institute on Drug Abuse: Principles of drug addiction treatment: a research-based guide (NIH Publ No 00-4180). Rockville, MD, National Institute on Drug Abuse, 1999

Plough AL, Shirley L, Zaremba N, et al: CSAT Target Cities Demonstration Final Evaluation Report, Boston Office for Treatment Improvement. Boston, MA, Massachusetts Bureau of Substance Abuse Services, 1996

Prochaska JO, DiClemente CC, Norcross JC: In search of how people change: applications to addictive behaviors. Am Psychol 9:1102–1114, 1992

Regier DA, Kaebler CT, Roper M, et al: The ICD-10 clinical field trial for mental and behavioral disorders: results in Canada and the United States. Am J Psychiatry 151:1340–1350, 1994

Sharon E, Krebs C, Turner W, et al: Predictive validity of the ASAM Patient Placement Criteria for hospital utilization. J Addict Dis 22 (suppl 1):79–93, 2003

Steenrod S, Brisson A, McCarty D, et al: Effects of managed care on programs and practices for the treatment of alcohol and drug dependence, in Services Research in the Era of Managed Care: Organization, Access, Economics, and Outcomes. Edited by Galanter M. New York, Springer, 2001, pp 51–70

Sullivan JT, Sykora K, Schneiderman J, et al: Assessment of alcohol withdrawal: the revised Clinical Institute Withdrawal Assessment for Alcohol Scale (CIWA-Ar). Br J Addict 84:1353–1357, 1989

Treatment Matching Interest Group (TMIG) study finds growing use of placement criteria and an association with program survival. National Institute on Drug Abuse Clinical Trials Network Bulletin, Vol 4–5, Mar 10, 2004. Available at: http://ctndisseminationlibrary.org/bulletin/20040310.pdf. Accessed June 25, 2010.

Turner WM, Turner KH, Reif S, et al: Feasibility of multidimensional substance abuse treatment matching: automating the ASAM Patient Placement Criteria. Drug Alcohol Depend 55:35–43, 1999

5 | Motivational Enhancement

Carlo C. DiClemente, Ph.D., A.B.P.P.
Miranda Garay Kofeldt, M.A.
Leigh Gemmell, Ph.D.

Patient motivation is a necessary ingredient in substance abuse treatment and recovery. Because of the reinforcing nature of addictive substances and the physiological and psychological reliance they engender, individuals with problematic and dependent patterns of substance use often refuse to acknowledge problems or seek treatment. Even when substance abusers arrive at a treatment program, many are ambivalent about the need to modify their substance use and resist any consideration of reducing use or abstaining completely. Going to treatment is not a panacea that turns ambivalence and lack of readiness into commitment to change; a significant number of individuals who enter a treatment facility fail to complete the treatment and many drop out after intake or a single session (Simpson and Joe 1993; Wickizer et al. 1994). Even those who comply with and complete treatment do not always achieve stated goals. Patient reluctance to seek help, attrition, and relapse cause significant problems for all types of treatment providers (therapists, nurses, clinicians, and other health care providers) as they try to help individuals who abuse drugs and alcohol along the path to recovery. All of these barriers are connected to patient motivation.

Earlier in the history of substance abuse treatment, motivation for recovery and treatment was viewed almost completely as the responsibility of the patient. Treatment professionals believed that interventions could not work until each alcohol- or drug-dependent individual reached his or her personal "bottom" and brought the needed motivation to change into treatment. Little was done to help the unmotivated other than confronting them vigorously about "denial" or waiting until they experienced sufficient losses or consequences to admit problems and seek help from treatment providers. Unmotivated individuals often were turned away from treatment or simply told to attend mutual-help meetings, such as Alcoholics Anonymous and Narcotics Anonymous, in the hope that the testimony of peers would stimulate motivation to change. Societal systems became frustrated with this lack of motivation and began to use incarceration or mandated treatment to manage substance abuse problems (Loue 2003). Such coercion increased treatment attendance but not necessarily motivation to change.

Since the late 1980s, a significant shift has occurred in how society and the treatment community understand and address the problem of motivation in patients with substance abuse. Public health approaches have encouraged aggressive screening and brief interventions with vulnerable populations in medical settings (DiClemente 2005; Fleming et al. 2002). Courts, employers, and professional sports have begun to screen for substance abuse and to refer users to intervention and treatment providers for help in managing substance abuse in the legal and employment systems (Turner et al. 2002). More and more frequently, treatment providers are being asked to motivate and not merely educate or medicate substance-abusing patients.

Fortunately, demands on treatment providers to become more involved in patient motivation have been accompanied by advances in treatment perspectives and strategies. The developers of one more recent model of behavior change outlined a series of stages of change and identified preaction (precontemplation, contemplation, and preparation) tasks that need to occur before individuals begin to take action and maintain change (DiClemente 2003; Prochaska et al. 1992). Consistent with the focus on preaction tasks and motivation, addiction treatment professionals began to develop strategies for addressing substance abusers' lack of motivation (Miller and Rollnick 2002; Petry 2006; Smith and Meyers 2004). Evidence for this shift in perspective includes the fact that motivational considerations are now viewed as critical for engagement in treatment and modification of substance use (e.g., American Society of Addiction Medicine Patient Placement Criteria) and motivational enhancement approaches are becoming an integral part of most outreach, detoxification, and treatment programs. This chapter offers an overview of motivational considerations, highlights how motivational enhancement approaches are being used, and briefly reviews research regarding the application and efficacy of these approaches in the management and treatment of alcohol and drug abuse problems.

Defining Motivation

Motivation is a complex phenomenon and should not be likened to a mechanism that has an "on-off" switch. Most patients are not truly unmotivated to quit their drug or alcohol use but are simply more motivated to engage in behaviors other than those desired by treatment providers. The challenge is to engage substance abusers in treatment and assist them in moving through a multidimensional intentional process of behavior change that leads to recovery. This process, as described in the stages of change, involves five distinct steps that individuals take to create a sustainable behavior change (DiClemente 2003). Once individuals become addicted or develop a pattern of abuse, they are not interested in change and are in a *precontemplation* stage; the treatment provider's task is to help the patients become interested in and concerned about the need for change. Once interested, individuals move through a *contemplation* stage by engaging in a risk-reward analysis that leads to a firm decision to change. Decision making is followed by a *preparation* stage, in which the patient creates an effective and acceptable change plan while increasing commitment for implementing the plan. All of the mentioned preaction tasks must be accomplished to some degree for a substance abuser to move through early stages before actually taking successful action to modify substance use. The *action* stage includes implementing and revising the action plan and stopping the problematic pattern of behavior while beginning to establish a new pattern of abstinence or of modified drinking or drug use. *Maintenance*, the final stage and task of the process, involves the integration of abstinence or significant reduction into the lifestyle of the recovering substance abuser. Patient motivation involves completion of multiple tasks to an extent that is sufficient to support and sustain successful recovery (Carbonari and DiClemente 2000; DiClemente 2003).

It should be acknowledged that there are many other perspectives on motivation. Some envision motivation as following behavior change, in which case individuals can engage in a behavior without being completely motivated or "fake it until they make it." Often, patients use this strategy to deal with ambivalence, but eventually the intrinsic or internal tasks of the change process will need to be completed as the individual moves from faking to making the change a personal process. Another perspective looks at change as the product of a number of motivational influences that appear better viewed as a chaotic and nonlinear process and not as sequenced and reasoned, as described in the stages-of-change model (West and Sohal 2006). Behavioral economics perspectives view motivation as elicited by reinforcement and use contingency management techniques, such as rewarding drug-free urine tests to get people to stop engaging in a behavior, that have been shown to be effective in achieving abstinence from drugs and alcohol (Vuchinich and Heather 2003). In this perspective, however, individuals ultimately need to find or identify some personally meaningful contingencies or reasons to maintain abstinence once external contingencies are terminated (Petry 2006).

Motivational Enhancement Interventions

Although a number of interventions and strategies that focus on internal and external dimensions of motivation have been designed to influence patient engagement in and movement through the process of recovery, the most well-known approach, called *motivational interviewing*, was developed by Miller and Rollnick (1991, 2002). Motivational interviewing concentrates primarily on preparing people for change and focuses on preaction tasks, but because motivation is also needed to sustain action and prevent relapse, motivational interviewing also includes a second phase that encourages development of a change plan and support for the implementation of that plan (Miller and Rollnick 2002). Motivational enhancement approaches that include motivational interviewing and its adaptations have been used primarily for engagement and briefer interventions (Substance Abuse and Mental Health Services Administration 1999). Increasingly, however, motivational interviewing interventions are being attached to more traditional treatment approaches, such as cognitive-behavioral therapy (CBT), twelve-step, medication, interpersonal, and network/systems approaches. One important lesson learned about change of substance abuse behaviors from motivational enhancement and brief interventions is that many individuals accomplish some or all of these tasks on their own prior to, during, or subsequent to treatment, and sometimes even without the assistance of treatment (DiClemente 2006). Although treatment providers have to be prepared to assist unmotivated patients' progress though each of the stages of change, they do not necessarily have to assist individuals in accomplishing each and every one of the tasks of the stages.

In this chapter, *motivational interviewing* and *enhancement interventions* refer specifically to those that use a motivational style and set of interviewing strategies and approaches that have been designed to focus on helping patients resolve reluctance and ambivalence to change, promote decision making, and support change language (i.e., expressions of desire, ability, reasons, and need to change) and commitment (see Table 5–1; Miller and Rollnick 2002). Motivational interviewing encompasses a style of patient-provider interaction that is characterized by collaboration, evocation, and autonomy. It includes a number of strategies and techniques to enhance decision making and the resolution of ambivalence. Initially, motivational interviewing approaches were used in brief interventions (recalled using the acronym FRAMES) that gave Feedback to patients about the problem, emphasized personal Responsibility, offered Advice and a Menu of options, used an Empathic approach, and supported the patients' sense of Self-efficacy or confidence that they could make the change. In interventions such as the Drinker's Check-Up program, for example, individuals with alcohol problems were evaluated and given feedback and advice over short periods of time or in one or two sessions of consultation (Bien et al. 1993; Miller and Rose 2009; Miller et al. 1988).

Motivational enhancement approaches have been incorporated into more formal treatment programs and interventions in a number of ways. Adaptations of motivational interviewing include brief interventions in opportunistic settings, such as emergency departments (Longabaugh et al. 2001); treatment engagement strategies to be used prior to more extensive treatment (Carroll et al. 2006); and a four-session motivational enhancement therapy (MET) that was developed, manualized, and first used in outpatient and aftercare settings in the large multisite alcoholism treatment trial called Project MATCH (Matching Alcoholism Treatment to Client Heterogeneity; Miller et al. 1994). Other researchers and clinicians have developed interventions that integrate motivational interviewing approaches into stage-based approaches, thereby matching the interventions to stages of change (Substance Abuse and Mental Health Services Administration 1999b; Velasquez et al. 2001). In an effort to incorporate family members into the process, Smith and Meyers (2004) have created family- and community-based motivational interviewing approaches to increase motivation and encourage treatment entry with patients in the early stages of change. Additionally, the ARISE approach (A Relational Intervention Sequence for Engagement; Landau et al. 2004) uses family members to assist in engaging patients in treatment and promoting change. Finally, contingency management approaches use monetary and other rewards to reinforce abstinence behaviors, thereby creating incentives for movement toward change and initiation of abstinence (Petry 2006; Vuchinich and Heather 2003).

Although there are a number of ways to manipulate and increase patient motivation, the focus in this chapter is primarily on stimulating changes through stage-based approaches because these approaches have become widespread across the treatment community and have been studied in a variety of intervention settings. We use the term *motivational enhancement* to describe the various types of intervention and treatment strategies that use motivational interviewing and stage-based approaches.

TABLE 5–1. Key elements for Motivational Enhancement Treatment

Style	Strategies (OARS)	Techniques
Collaboration	Open-ended questions	Rolling with resistance
Equal power between patient and provider	Elicit longer responses	Reframe
Patient input on decisions	Affirm the patient	Shift focus
Evocation	Provide tailored support	Enhance discrepancy
Share belief in patient's ability to change	Reflective listening	Asking open-ended questions
Empathize with patient's experience	Clarify client's meaning	Begin with "how"
Autonomy	Summarize	"Tell me about…"
Positive regard for client	Reflect deeper understanding	Affirming the client
Respect client choice	Show empathy	Acknowledge efforts/strengths
	Acceptance supports change	Reflective listening
	Elicit change talk	Reflect feelings, ambivalence about change
	Highlight and resolve ambivalence	Summarizing statements
	Roll with resistance	Collect information
	Come alongside client	Make transitions
		Additional skills
		Ask permission to give advice
		Present a menu of options

Motivational counseling *strategies*:
Methods to enhance patient engagement in the change process

A motivational *style of* counseling:
A "style for eliciting patient motivation to change behavior"

Strategies of Motivational Enhancement

The core of motivational enhancement lies in the style of the interaction between provider and patient. Providers create an atmosphere of trust, collaboration, respect, and openness by being empathic and believing in the patient's ability to change. The key strategies of motivational interviewing are represented by the acronym OARS: Open-ended questions, Affirmations, Reflective listening, and Summarizing (see Table 5–1). Through open-ended questions, the provider invites the patient to share his or her perspectives and views. Affirmations are comments, reflections, and summaries made by the provider to highlight the patient's strengths and successes and to increase self-efficacy and create a trusting provider-patient relationship. By reflecting back what he or she is hearing, seeing, and experiencing in the interaction, the provider conveys to the patient a sense of being listened to and ensures accuracy of understanding. Through summaries, the provider can collect and link together several themes, make transitions to other topics, and make sure that the picture he or she is getting is complete. Providers use these strategies to elicit self-motivational statements that reflect a patient's verbalizations of any desire, ability, reasons, or need related to changing substance abuse behavior. Reflecting these verbalizations will ideally increase the patient's commitment to make a change.

Even though motivational interviewing fosters patient autonomy and collaboration, and providers are taught to avoid the "expert" trap of simply providing answers to patient questions, this approach is directive. Providers are trained to guide the conversation toward change talk, to avoid confrontations, and to roll with resistance. Effective ways to roll with resistance include reframing and shifting the focus. *Reframing* involves helping the patient to see something in a new light. For example, if a patient reports feeling that his loved ones are "nagging" him to quit, a provider can focus on how much the family must care about the person to keep asking the client to change. *Shifting the focus* involves directing the client to attend to something other than what is causing the resistance. If he says something like, "There is no way I will stop drinking!" the provider could slow things down by saying, "Let's talk about what problems you are experiencing now, before we start to think about changing your alcohol use."

In motivational interviewing, the clinician is expected to provide objective feedback, offer options and advice carefully, and promote choice. Numerous books and manuals describe this approach (Arkowitz et al. 2008; Miller and Rollnick 2002; Rollnick et al. 2008; Rosengren 2009; Substance Abuse and Mental Health Services Administration 1999a);

however, the practitioner would be well served to have more extensive, experiential training to use these strategies and techniques, because they require practice and significant shifting of some of the prototypical ways that providers interact with patients during intake and in other situations that usually employ closed-ended questions to obtain specific information. Training is also necessary to learn how to use the strategies to direct the conversation and manage time constraints imposed by treatment settings. Adaptations of this approach that have been developed for use in group therapy would also require training. For example, Velasquez and colleagues (2001) have created a manual for group therapy that emphasizes the use of motivational enhancement in the treatment of substance abuse. Additionally, the Clinical Trials Network (CTN) supports several studies that are currently examining the efficacy of manualized MET interventions (Carroll et al. 2002) in community settings, among pregnant substance abusers, and among Spanish-speaking individuals seeking treatment for substance abuse (www.drugabuse.gov/CTN/research .html). The CTN represents the collaboration between the National Institute on Drug Abuse (NIDA), treatment researchers, and community-based service providers who conduct substance abuse treatment efficacy studies and ensure effective treatment is translated into practice. We highlight some of the key techniques in the following case examples and then review the literature about usefulness and efficacy of motivational approaches with various types of substances of abuse.

Case Illustrations

Macy is a 36-year-old single woman who is a marketing project manager at an advertising agency. Macy can drink many of her male counterparts and customers under the table, which is generally advantageous in her business. However, at times, the behavior is met with disgust, and it interferes with intimate friendships. Macy has always been headstrong but has experienced periods of depression and considered suicide during adolescence. Her history includes having become popular in high school because she drank with the guys, which made her feel better temporarily. However, she has often questioned her self-worth and her ability to love someone.

Her romantic relationships often consist of dating someone for a number of years, then ending the relationship when marriage is discussed. She currently lives with a boyfriend of 3 years, Shawn, who works in product design at the same agency. Her boyfriend is tolerant of her drinking and uses marijuana recreationally, but wants her to commit to their relationship more seriously. Her parents have lectured her about her drinking and failure to get married. Although her father had been a heavy drinker for most of his life, he recently quit and is pressuring Macy to join Alcoholics Anonymous.

In the past 3 months, Macy has coped with these increasing stressors by spending more time at the bar. She was charged with driving while intoxicated. Her lawyer asked her to go to an alcohol treatment program to help her case, and her father became more aggressive about her participation in Alcoholics Anonymous. She began to stay home from work and drink all day. Eventually, she went to the treatment program for evaluation. She explained away all of her problems, describing how none of the problems were due to her alcohol use, and how drinking was functional in her life, because it increased her success at work.

Motivational approaches. [The clinician working with Macy used the key strategies of motivational interviewing, which are represented by the acronym OARS.]

Open-ended questions: Macy, tell me about your drinking. What is going on at work? Are there any concerns that you might lose your job due to your current drinking levels? In what ways do you think drinking might be related to your feeling down? How might your drinking be affecting your current job performance?

Affirmations: I hear you saying that you don't think that you need to be here, but I am impressed that you have come nonetheless. I see that you have given this all a lot of thought and you have some good insights. It takes courage for you to begin dealing with these problems.

Reflections: It seems like everyone is pressuring you to make changes you are not certain you want to make. Quitting drinking doesn't seem to be an option for you at the present time. Relationships are complicated and difficult.

Summarizing: I'd like to take a moment to summarize what we've talked about so far. You feel that right now you are being forced into treatment by your lawyer, father, and boyfriend because of a mistake related to drinking. They are concerned about your drinking, and you believe they care about you. However, you feel that your drinking is not really the problem; it makes you seem like "one of the guys," which helps your job. When it comes to your feelings of depression, you aren't sure how these feelings are related to your drinking. Did I miss anything?

Discussion. The goal is that these approaches would reduce Macy's resistance to discussing her drinking, depression, and work problems. Accepting her perspective and making sure that she is heard and understood may begin to produce change language. Eliciting change language would ideally increase Macy's concern and commitment to change and, ultimately, increase the chances that she would remediate the problem by reducing excessive use or abstaining.

Sam, a 40-year-old divorced father of two, began using illicit drugs in college and became a heavy marijuana user in his late 20s. He became a freelance computer consultant after he was fired from his job at a software development firm due to poor job performance. His wife became intolerant of his use and insisted that he quit when they began to have children. Sam hid his habit, pretending to quit. He began to come home later at night. This behavior, his inconsistent income, and refusal to go to counseling led to his divorce. When his parents asked about the divorce, Sam explained that he and his wife had grown apart, that she wanted someone making money, and that he refused to share those values. When they asked about his drug use, he exploded with anger and shouted that he was responsible for his own life and that his wife blamed his drug use as an excuse to divorce him.

Over the past 5 years, Sam had increased his heroin use and begun to associate with and provide complex computer-programming services for individuals dealing drugs. This lifestyle led to further alienation from his children, family, and friends. His sister, with whom he generally had a close relationship, continuously conveyed her concerns, despite his beliefs that she was overreacting. However, he did have doubts at times that his lifestyle was acceptable, particularly when coming down off heroin and when considering the consequences of being with his acquaintances if a police raid ever occurred. When he was using heroin, these concerns disappeared.

Motivational approaches. [The clinician working with Sam used the key strategies of motivational interviewing, as represented by the acronym OARS.]

Open-ended questions: Do you have any concerns about your current lifestyle? What goals do you have for the future? Are there some things you want to do that are difficult to achieve in your current way of living? What are the good and not so good aspects of heroin for you? What concerns, if any, do you have about the people with whom you spend time now?

Affirmations: You are not sure about whether you want to change or not, but you are making a good effort to find out. I see that you are concerned about being a good provider for your children. You have some very good technical skills that are a real asset.

Reflections: You seem to have had a number of losses recently. It's hard for you to imagine a life without any drug use, but at the same time, you'd like to get your family back. You aren't sure you can be successful.

Summarizing: I'd like to take a moment to summarize what we've talked about so far. You feel that you should be able to make your own life choices, but you realize the ones you have made have hurt your family financially and emotionally. The choices you have made up to now also make it hard for you to feel safe. You have some sense that your drug use may also affect your mood and lead to angry outbursts. Right now you are feeling a bit trapped and trying to figure out what to do. Is that about right? Did I miss anything?

Discussion. These strategies are geared to activate motivation and offer some help and direction only when Sam begins to indicate with change talk that he might be ready to do something about his heroin use. However, the questions, reflections, and summaries are couched in terms that accentuate the potential for change and highlight change language in an attempt to direct the conversation toward change and away from sustaining the problematic behavior.

Motivational Enhancement in Alcohol Treatment

To date, two very large multisite randomized controlled trials with alcohol-abusing and -dependent participants have examined the effectiveness of MET compared with other nonpharmacological interventions. The first of these, Project MATCH, consisted of two parallel studies, each consisting of 12 weeks of treatment delivered as outpatient care or aftercare, that were designed to examine the differential effects of three manualized treatments with alcohol-dependent or alcohol-abusing participants (Project MATCH Research Group 1997a). Participants were randomly assigned to receive 12 sessions of CBT, four sessions of MET, or 12 sessions of an individual therapy called 12-step facilitation (TSF), delivered over 12 weeks. All participants were followed for 1 year posttreatment, and outpatients also received follow-up at 3 years posttreatment. Although there was little support for matching, which would have indicated differential effects of treatments based on participant characteristics, all three of these treatments improved alcohol consumption and consequence outcomes at follow-up, and there were no substantial differences across the three treatments. With this alcohol-dependent population, a four-session MET intervention performed as well as the more comprehensive 12-session treatments in improving drinking outcomes, although patients in MET drank more during the treatment period (DiClemente et al. 2001). The most substantive support for matching did involve a match between individuals in MET. Drinkers higher in state/trait anger had better outcomes in MET than in the other two treatments. Retrospective studies conducted with MATCH data show that MET intervention benefits can differ based on population. For example, MET performed better than CBT and TSF for increasing the proportion of days abstinent and decreasing drinking intensity in Native American participants at both short- and long-term follow-up assessments (Villanueva et al. 2007), and some evidence suggested that minority women who were pregnant benefited more from MET than other styles of intervention (Winhusen et al. 2008).

The second large, multisite, randomized controlled study was the United Kingdom Alcohol Treatment Trial (UKATT), which compared the effects of MET and social behavior and network therapy (SBNT) on alcohol-related outcomes in alcohol-dependent or alcohol-abusing participants (UKATT Research Team 2001). Treatment for the SBNT group consisted of eight sessions using cognitive-behavioral strategies and techniques to help participants create positive social support networks that were meant to help change drinking behaviors. The MET group received three sessions over an 8-week period. Participants were followed for 1 year. The results of this study indicated that both MET and SBNT were effective interventions in producing reductions in drinking and improving abstinence outcomes (UKATT Research Team 2005).

The findings from Project MATCH and UKATT are consistent in demonstrating that participants who received three or four sessions of MET did as well as participants who received cognitive-behavioral or social support types of treatment for a longer period of time. In MET, the clinician begins with an assessment of alcohol history, patterns, problems, and consequences; provides objective feedback using empathy; engages the patient in a discussion of drinking and lifestyle using motivational interviewing techniques (reflection, affirming, summarizing, rolling with resistance, and avoiding argumentation); and works with the patient to overcome ambivalence and to create a patient-driven change plan. This type and amount of support and direction appears to be sufficient to engage the change process and motivate modification of drinking behavior. It should be noted that this approach may be more helpful when patients are high in state/trait anger (hostility and anger control) and that patients with drinking-saturated environments may need more long-term support for sobriety from mutual-help groups (Project MATCH Research Group 1997b, 1998).

The role of motivation and the use of motivational enhancement strategies are being explored in alcohol-related pharmacotherapy trials as well. The COMBINE (Combining Medications and Behavioral Interventions) study was a randomized controlled trial that examined the independent and combined effects of medication and behavioral therapy on alcohol-related outcomes, such as abstinence from alcohol (Anton et al. 2006). The behavioral therapy component, called a combined behavioral intervention, included components of motivational interviewing, CBT, and TSF. The results of this study indicated that the combined behavioral intervention was a useful addition to medication management and naltrexone in improving drinking outcomes. Although the study did not examine the effects of MET alone, it provides initial support for the use of motivation-based interventions in conjunction with medication management to improve alcohol-related outcomes. Some brief adherence enhancement strategies that incorporate motivation-enhancing strategies are also being developed and used in some trials (Volpicelli et al. 2001).

Brief Motivational Interventions for Alcohol Use Disorders

Brief interventions for individuals with alcohol problems have become respected and empirically supported strategies for reaching large numbers of individuals with hazardous, abusive, and dependent patterns of drinking. These interventions are generally conducted in a variety of settings, can occur in person or by telephone, and can be implemented in 10–15 minutes or extended to include several (e.g., two to four) contacts. Patients discuss their drinking, complete some assessment measures, and are given feedback and advice about their drinking (Miller et al. 1998), designed to be an incentive for altering problematic drinking (Babor et al. 2001). Although this type of proactive therapy has been used with a wide range of drinking patterns, from hazardous to dependent, most research has been done with individuals who abuse alcohol and have not yet developed a pattern reflecting alcohol dependence (U.S. Department of Health and Human Services 1997). Unlike more traditional treatments for problematic drinkers, this technique does not involve overtly confrontational tactics (Miller and Rollnick 2002). The lack of explicit confrontation is thought to reduce the defensiveness of targeted individuals, who tend not to be self-referred and may not see any need for substance use treatment. Often, the goal of brief interventions is harm reduction rather than complete abstinence (U.S. Department of Health and Human Services 1997).

Overall, brief interventions generally have been found to be effective (Substance Abuse and Mental Health Services Administration 1999a; U.S. Department of Health and Human Services 1997). A meta-analysis of controlled studies comparing baseline with posttreatment alcohol measures found that brief interventions were quite effective and yielded high mean effect sizes (Cohen's $d=0.70–0.80$) for problem drinkers (Bien et al. 1993). When brief intervention groups were compared with control groups that were assessed and advised, the effect size fell to 0.38, indicating that merely asking individuals about their drinking and related correlates may result in less drinking for some individuals (Bien et al. 1993). Moreover, this meta-analysis revealed that brief interventions were comparable to more extensive treatment in terms of treatment success. In fact, Miller et al. (1998) conducted a large meta-analysis of the effectiveness of treatments and found that brief motivational interventions had some of the best effect sizes in comparison with a large number of alternative treatments. Nevertheless, additional research is warranted to determine which individuals benefit most from these interventions, because there is some evidence that for men, brief interventions may be more beneficial than merely screening for alcohol problems (this effect has not been found for women) (Babor and Grant 1992; U.S. Department of Health and Human Services 1997).

A number of studies have examined brief interventions with problem drinkers, including drinkers with hazardous, binge, and abusive patterns of use. In much of their research on the Drinker's Check-Up, a brief evaluation and consultation program for problem drinkers from the community, Miller et al. (1988) excluded drinkers who met criteria for alcohol dependence and focused on problem drinkers. However, in a more recent meta-analysis that evaluated high-quality randomized controlled trials in primary care settings, Wilk et al. (1997) concluded that heavy drinkers had better outcomes with brief alcohol interventions than with no intervention, with an odds ratio of almost 2:1 (1.91). Some of the reviewed studies also suggested lower mortality and morbidity and decreases in health-care costs (Edwards and Rollnick 1997; Miller et al. 1988). The success of brief interventions has led many groups to call for including brief interventions in many different health-care settings. For example, the College of Surgeons is making screening and brief intervention for alcohol a part of the accreditation criteria for Level I trauma units (Committee on Trauma 2006), and other settings are recommending a stepped-care approach for working with problem drinkers who do not respond to brief interventions (Joseph et al. 1999).

Brief interventions targeting vulnerable populations of drinkers require appropriate screening. One of the issues that must be addressed in implementing these programs is how to define the problem that would trigger the intervention. *Problem drinking* has been defined in a variety of ways in various settings and studies. Some use "at-risk drinking in the previous month or an alcohol use disorder in the past 12 months" as the screen, whereas others use screening instruments such as the CAGE questions (Ewing 1984) or the Alcohol Use Disorders Identification Test (AUDIT; Babor et al. 2001), either in part or in their entirety. The effectiveness of a single question, "On any single occasion during the past 3 months, have you had more than five drinks containing alcohol?" has been compared with responses to the AUDIT. Findings indicated that the question had a 74% positive predictive ability for problem drinking (sensitivity=62%; specificity=93%). Thus, this single question appears useful in screening for problem drinking, but does not necessarily capture drinkers engaged in what are called hazardous drinking patterns, as defined by daily or weekly levels of drinking (for additional information, visit the National Institute on Alcohol Abuse and Alcoholism Web site: www.niaaa.nih.gov/Publications/AlcoholAlerts).

A second concern and difficulty in studies examining brief interventions is whether they reach the population of individuals who most need interventions. Edwards and Rollnick (1997), for instance, reviewed all published studies of brief interventions for drinking conducted in primary care settings and found high levels of attrition in these studies. Although researchers rarely publish attrition analyses that describe how participants who dropped out or who were lost during study follow-up may differ from those who completed the study, this study found some evidence to suggest that the two groups are very different from each other: those who dropped out tended to be younger, less educated, and heavier drinkers.

Motivational Enhancement and Drug Abuse

Although less research has been done exploring the use of motivational interviewing and MET approaches to reduce drug use, a growing body of empirical studies supports their efficacy in motivating change and enhancing treatment entry and engagement for patients experiencing problems with multiple substances and drugs other than alcohol. Much of the research finding positive effects suggests that when motivation-enhancing components precede more intense substance abuse treatment, retention in treatment increases (Martino et al. 2000; Saunders et al. 1995; Stotts et al. 2001; Swanson et al. 1999).

Carroll et al. (2006) reported that compared with a standard intake interview, integrating motivational techniques and strategies was associated with significantly better rates of retention across four substance abuse treatment centers where marijuana, cocaine, and methamphetamines were often the most frequently used drugs. Although three of the four sites demonstrated that motivational techniques used at intake resulted in fewer days of drug use in the 28 days postintake, the results were not statistically significant.

A manual for implementing MET as a precursor to outpatient drug treatment has been evaluated for the National Institute on Drug Abuse Clinical Trials Network. This treatment consists of three sessions based on Miller et al.'s (1994) manual, which focuses on problem identification and feedback, resolving ambivalence, and creating a change plan. A study testing the efficacy of this three-session MET compared with counseling as usual demonstrated no differences between groups in program retention, self-reported use of primary drug of choice, and percentage of positive urine tests during the 4 weeks postintervention (Ball et al. 2007). However, at the 16-week follow-up, MET participants were significantly more likely to have sustained the reductions in self-reported days of drug use per week. This study was complicated by the presence of interaction effects, such that superior outcomes due to MET were present only for participants with alcohol as their primary drug of choice. Drug users experienced no significant benefits from MET. The three-session treatment was also used in a multisite randomized trial for Spanish-speaking substance users (Carroll et al. 2009). Similar to the results of Ball et al.'s (2007) study, MET and counseling as usual produced changes in substance use, but there were no significant differences by treatment type.

Also, although significant benefits of MET were not present for users of drugs other than alcohol, benefits were present for those with alcohol as their primary drug of choice; a significant effect of modest magnitude was apparent for days of alcohol use per week.

Although some would argue that brief MET is effective as a stand-alone treatment for substance use disorders, others object because of findings that link longer drug treatment to better outcomes (Simpson et al. 1997). However, MET is consistent with long-term treatment approaches; its philosophy can guide intervention and its techniques can be used during longer-term treatment, as long as the provider remains cognizant of an individual's stage of change and the fact that motivation is needed throughout the process of change. The Haight Ashbury Free Clinics have developed a manual for high-dose motivational enhancement consisting of 12 sessions (Polcin et al. 2004). The first three sessions are congruent with those mentioned above as part of the National Institute on Drug Abuse study. The final nine sessions continue to employ motivational enhancement techniques and provide help in resolving continued ambivalence, reinforce accomplishments and progress, address drug use and temptations to use, and allow for revision of the change plan. Longer-term use of MET could be particularly beneficial if an individual does not move quickly from early (e.g., precontemplation) to later (e.g., action) stages of change.

Nicotine

Although more research needs to be done in the area of nicotine addiction, a few studies support the potential that MET has for reducing smoking. The use of MET with patients by home-health-care nurses has led to more quit attempts and greater reductions in the number of cigarettes smoked daily than when patients received the standard care for smoking cessation (Borrelli et al. 2005). These benefits were maintained at 1 year posttreatment, and the percentage of individuals in the MET condition who quit smoking was double that of the standard care group. Other research compares adaptations of motivational interviewing and MET, termed *adapted motivational interviewing* (AMI), to the provision of authoritarian advice to quit smoking (Butler et al. 1999; Colby et al. 1998). Adults in an AMI group used fewer cigarettes in the 24 hours prior to assessment, increased the time between waking up and the first cigarette of the day, had more attempts to quit that lasted 1 week or more, and were more likely to move into a later stage of change (Butler et al. 1999). In an adolescent population, a 30-minute AMI session resulted in two-thirds of the sample attempting to quit smoking, as well as significant reductions in smoking rate and dependence (Colby et al. 1998). Although AMI results were not significantly better than results following 5 minutes of brief advice, the effectiveness of AMI was supported and may be preferred due to its less confrontational nature. However, these types of interventions are not always effective with individuals with multiple problems (Velasquez et al. 2000), and even a four-session MET intervention with drug-abusing pregnant women was not found to be sufficient to motivate changes in smoking (Haug et al. 2004).

Marijuana

The use of MET components has led to significant reductions in marijuana use by adults (Marijuana Treatment Project Research Group 2004; Sinha et al. 2003) and adolescents (Colby et al. 1998; Monti et al. 1999). In studies of adults, MET and skills-based relapse prevention interventions both demonstrated decreases in marijuana-related problems and symptoms of dependence (Stephens et al. 2000). Although neither intervention outperformed the other, only 3 hours of MET was as effective as 28 hours of relapse prevention in increasing abstinence. The brevity of MET supports its use as a cost-effective alternative to more extensive care, particularly if an opportunity for lengthy care is not likely (e.g., with homeless populations not seeking treatment). Finally, in a study comparing two sessions of MET, nine sessions of MET plus CBT, and a delayed-treatment control group, the nine-session treatment performed best, but the two-session MET condition produced significant reductions in marijuana use among dependent adults and was as effective as MET plus CBT in increasing the use of coping skills (Litt et al. 2005).

Findings in adolescent populations have not been as convincing but reflect that continued research is important and that stronger effects may be found if more intensive treatment is provided. A one-session MET intervention to address alcohol and marijuana use in homeless adolescents did not affect the use of these two substances, but the use of other illicit drugs at the 1-month follow-up had decreased significantly (Peterson et al. 2006). Similarly, Walker et al. (2006) reported that while adolescents significantly reduced marijuana used 3 months after 2 sessions of MET, the change was not significantly better than the decrease of use in the wait-list control group. However, the authors felt the MET approach was effective in attracting heavy-using, non–treatment-seeking, voluntary student participants.

Cocaine

Motivational enhancement is likely to be useful, particularly as a precursor to more intensive treatment, for individuals seeking help for cocaine misuse (DeLeon et al. 1997). Level of motivation has been found to influence success in treatment for cocaine abusers, suggesting that increasing motivation will increase success. In fact, those with low initial motivation to change who received MET reported lower rates of relapse to cocaine use and fewer days of cocaine use at 1-year follow-up than did those with high initial motivation (Rohsenow et al. 2004). Although benefits were not immediately observable (i.e., at the 3–6 month follow-up periods), effects may emerge up to 1 year posttreatment. In this study, MET was also predictive of decreased alcohol use and of increases in motivation, treatment expectations, perceived negative effects of cocaine, and self-efficacy to deal with high-risk situations. However, for individuals with high initial motivation to change, those receiving MET reported higher frequencies of cocaine use and more severe alcohol problems than did those with low motivation and those not receiving MET. Thus, it is possible that MET should only be used when motivation for change is low; this is reflective of the need to match intervention strategies to stage of change (Booth et al. 1998; DiClemente 2003). The type of change to which patients commit also has effects on treatment success. Specifically, those who commit to complete abstinence are less likely to relapse than are those who commit to reduction of use (Rohsenow et al. 2004). Thus, with cocaine users, it may be helpful not only to encourage change in MET but also to stress the importance of committing to complete abstinence.

Methamphetamine

Thirty treatment-seeking methamphetamine users were enrolled in a nine-session MET treatment program (Galloway et al. 2007). The manualized treatment was associated with good treatment retention; participants attended 78% of the MET sessions, and 73% completed treatment. In addition, there was a significant decrease in positive urine screens (64% to 44%). The lack of any comparison group limited the interpretability of this study. However, the relatively high treatment retention rates and decrease in positive drug screens for a difficult-to-treat group support the utility of the approach and the further study of the manual with methamphetamine users in randomized controlled trials.

Opiates and Polydrugs

Research on the effectiveness of MET for treating patients with addiction to opiates and multiple drugs is lacking. We found only one study on opiate addiction that used an intervention based on motivational interviewing, and the intervention did not contain all of the components necessary to define it as MET (Saunders et al. 1995). Nevertheless, this study found that one intervention session plus one follow-up session resulted in decreased opiate-related problems and greater compliance with treatment 6 months later. Significant reductions in actual use were not found. Individuals who injected multiple drugs were included in a study that provided five 30-minute sessions of MET/AMI or risk reduction sessions of equivalent intensity (Booth et al. 1998). The outcome, successfully completing the intake procedure for treatment entry, did not differ between groups. Although MET/AMI interventions have been shown to increase treatment entry in a number of drug use studies, strong support for the use of these methods has not been found for the use of opiates and multiple drugs, perhaps due to a lack of research.

Although numerous studies have shown support for motivational techniques, some have not found effects on drug use outcomes (Booth et al. 1998; Donovan et al. 2001; Miller et al. 2003; Schneider et al. 2000). For example, Schneider et al. (2000) found that motivational interviewing was no more effective than confrontational interviewing in an employee assistance program for substance abuse, and thus concluded that both would afford similar benefits; however, motivational techniques provide an alternative for practitioners and patients who prefer to avoid a confrontational approach. Nonsignificant effects in these studies could be attributed to mismatching strategies with a patient's stage of change. When treatment is incongruent with an individual's stage of change (e.g., an individual is further along in the process of change than the intervention), resistance to treatment and change and/or dropout is more likely (Booth et al. 1998; Rollnick et al. 2008). Stage status could also serve as an alternative outcome variable, because behavior change is not the only outcome one would expect from motivational enhancement approaches.

Positive effects on substance abuse have emerged when interventions based on this model are provided by clinicians who are not substance abuse treatment specialists (Dunn et al. 2001). However, as with any other psychosocial treatment, MET "must be provided with fidelity and skill" (Madson and Campbell 2006, p. 67). Clinicians planning to implement MET are encouraged to attend training and refer to primary sources of information about MET (Mid-Atlantic Addiction Technology Transfer Center 2009; Miller and Rollnick 2002; Miller et al. 1994).

Integrating MET into the treatment plan of new patients entering treatment for any combination of drug problems is likely to demonstrate benefits, especially among those who report low motivation for change (Dunn et al. 2001) and are unready, unwilling, or unable to change (DiClemente 2003). Additionally, MET has been found to maintain its effects regardless of length of follow-up (Dunn et al. 2001), and effects can emerge at time points subsequent to initial posttreatment assessments.

Motivational Enhancement With Dually Diagnosed Populations

Based on the potential for increased severity of illness and impairment for individuals with co-occurring substance abuse and mental illness, concerns and skepticism exist regarding the efficacy of motivational enhancement techniques with dually diagnosed patients. However, motivational enhancement interventions have often produced improved outcomes compared with control conditions in a range of alcohol- and drug-abusing patients who have had coexisting psychiatric problems of varying degrees (Bien et al. 1993; Stotts et al. 2001). Techniques based on motivational interviewing principles have been viewed as promising in a systematic literature review of interventions for improving medication adherence and are viewed as superior to more traditional psychoeducational approaches for dually diagnosed individuals (Ziedonis and Trudeau 1997; Zygmunt et al. 2002). Swanson et al. (1999) found that adding motivational interviewing techniques to initial assessment increased attendance at outpatient appointments by psychiatric patients overall and by dually diagnosed patients. Steinberg et al. (2004) found that motivational interviewing and personalized feedback increased tobacco treatment engagement and attendance for individuals with serious mental illness. In innovative proactive programs that reach out to homeless, drug-abusing individuals with serious mental illness, treatment providers have gone onto the streets to discuss behavior change using motivational interviewing principles (Fisk et al. 2006). In a pilot study, Martino et al. (2000) found that integrating MET into intake procedures for individuals with psychotic or severe mood (e.g., bipolar) disorders increased treatment retention. Significant effects were not found for motivational levels, commitment to abstinence, medication adherence, or short-term drug use outcomes. Brief motivational interventions prior to treatment do not always improve treatment engagement and outcomes, particularly in populations of drug abusers who are poor, are of minority status, are less educated, and have multiple problems (Donovan et al. 2001; Miller et al. 2003).

Many of these findings are promising, but more extensive evaluation is needed of how to use both brief interventions and motivation-enhancing approaches with dually diagnosed individuals (particularly those with serious mental illness and substance abuse). Nevertheless, initial findings indicate that dually diagnosed individuals can be motivated through assessment and intervention to move through the process of modifying substance use in ways that are similar to those described above, with some modifications and attention to the special needs of this population (DiClemente et al. 2008).

Conclusion

Motivation is critical for individuals to make changes in substance-abusing behaviors. To overcome the common difficulties and barriers to successful modification of problematic patterns of substance use and to recover from alcohol and drug dependence, individuals must negotiate a multidimensional path of change that requires decision-making, choice, commitment, and coping activities. Motivation is needed to stimulate and negotiate accomplishment of these tasks. A number of highly self-motivated individuals negotiate this path on their own without treatment. Others seem to benefit from brief motivational interventions to help them to activate the process. However, many others need treatment and assistance to consider, decide about, plan, and commit to changing their problematic substance-using behaviors. Motivational enhancement approaches could be very helpful for all health-care providers who treat problems related to substance abuse or who treat substance abuse directly.

Motivational enhancement techniques are being incorporated in a number of ways into interventions to assist individuals with problematic patterns of alcohol and drug use. Screening and brief interventions are being used to address problematic use more proactively in a variety of health-care and opportunistic settings. Particularly for alcohol abuse, screening and brief motivational interventions are being offered in primary care offices, emergency departments, trauma centers, college health and student services, employee assistance programs, and other venues. At the same time, substance abuse treatment providers are developing pretreatment motivational enhancement approaches, delivered in both individual and group formats, that prepare patients for treatment, increase engagement, and accelerate movement through the process of change. Some treatment programs are using MET as one option for patients, either as stand-alone treatment or as part of a more comprehensive, multicomponent treatment delivered as a package or in a stepped-care manner (offering more extensive treatments to individuals unable to change with less intensive motivational approaches). Clearly, there are many ways to incorporate motivational enhancement and motivational interviewing approaches into substance abuse interventions (Wagner and Conners 2007).

It is important to note that motivational enhancement approaches actually have two key components. The first represents a style or way of interacting with the patient that is patient-centered, nonconfrontational, empathic, respectful, and reflective in its advice giving (Miller et al. 1993). The second component consists of the techniques and strategies that are designed to influence motivation, resolve ambivalence, and elicit self-motivational statements and activities. These techniques include complex reflections, use of summaries to frame motivational messages, techniques to manage and roll with resistance, offering advice with permission, maximizing opportunities to affirm and build the patient's sense of efficacy with regard to implementing change, and assisting the patient to create a realistic change plan rather than attempting to control the patient change process. Although the techniques are focused on the tasks that generally occur in the earlier stages of change, the style of motivational interviewing and MET can be integrated into most treatment approaches and is compatible with use of pharmacotherapy, mutual-help, and intensive psychosocial treatments.

Over the past 15 years, major advances have occurred in treatment options that have extended the reach and effectiveness of interventions for patients with alcohol and drug abuse problems. Motivational enhancement represents one of these advances. The reach and impact of motivational enhancement approaches are only beginning to make a difference in the behaviors of substance abuse treatment providers.

Key Clinical Concepts

- The clinician should assess to determine the patient's current stage: precontemplation, contemplation, preparation, action, or maintenance.
- Motivational interviewing is a collaborative style of patient-provider interaction in which the clinician uses an empathic approach to provide feedback and to offer advice and a menu of options while encouraging the client to take personal responsibility for change.
- The motivational interviewing approach helps the clinician avoid the "expert" trap of becoming someone who provides answers to the patient in a directive manner.
- Successful outcome studies of motivational interviewing have been carried out in relation to a variety of drugs, including alcohol, nicotine, marijuana, cocaine, and methamphetamine.

Suggested Reading

Arkowitz H, Westra HA, Miller WR, et al (eds): Motivational Interviewing in the Treatment of Psychological Problems. New York, Guilford, 2008

Miller PM: Evidence-based Addiction Treatment. Burlington, MA, Academic Press, 2009

Miller WR, Rollnick S: Motivational Interviewing: Preparing People to Change Addictive Behavior. New York, Guilford, 1991

Miller WR, Rose GS: Toward a theory of motivational interviewing. Am Psychol 64:527–537, 2009

Rollnick S, Miller WR, Butler CC: Motivational Interviewing in Health Care: Helping Patients Change Behavior. New York, Guilford, 2008

Rosengren DB: Building Motivational Interviewing Skills: A Practitioner Workbook (Applications of Motivational Interviewing Series). New York, Guilford, 2009

References

Anton RF, O'Malley SS, Ciraulo DA, et al: Combined pharmacotherapies and behavioral interventions for alcohol dependence: the COMBINE study: a randomized controlled trial. JAMA 295:2003–2017, 2006

Arkowitz H, Miller WR, Westra HA, et al (eds): Motivational Interviewing in the Treatment of Psychological Problems. New York, Guilford, 2008

Babor TF, Grant M (eds): Programme on Substance Abuse: Project on Identification and Management of Alcohol-Related Problems. Report on Phase II: A Randomized Clinical Trial of Brief Interventions in Primary Health Care. Geneva, World Health Organization, 1992

Babor TF, Higgins-Biddle JC, Saunders JB, et al: The Alcohol Use Disorders Identification Test: guidelines for use in primary care. Geneva, World Health Organization Department of Mental Health and Substance Dependence, 2001

Ball SA, Martino S, Nich C, et al: Site matters: multisite randomized trial of motivational enhancement therapy in community drug abuse clinics. J Consult Clin Psychol 75:556–567, 2007

Bien TH, Miller WR, Tonigan JS: Brief interventions for alcohol problems: a review. Addiction 88:315–336, 1993

Booth RE, Kwiatkowski C, Iguchi MY, et al: Facilitating treatment entry among out-of-treatment injection drug users. Public Health Rep 113:116–128, 1998

Borrelli B, Novak S, Hecht J: Home health care nurses as a new channel for smoking cessation treatment: outcomes from project CARES (Community-nurse Assisted Research and Education on Smoking. Prev Med 41:815–821, 2005

Butler CC, Rollnick S, Cohen D, et al: Motivational consulting versus brief advice for smokers in general practice: a randomised trial. Br J Gen Pract 49:611–616, 1999

Carbonari JP, DiClemente CC: Using transtheoretical model profiles to differentiate levels of alcohol abstinence success. J Consult Clin Psychol 68:810–817, 2000

Carroll KM, Farentinos C, Ball SA, et al: MET meets the real world: design issues and clinical strategies in the Clinical Trials Network. J Subst Abuse Treat 23:73–80, 2002

Carroll KM, Ball SA, Nich C: Motivational interviewing to improve treatment engagement and outcome in individuals seeking treatment for substance abuse: a multi-site effectiveness study. Drug Alcohol Depend 81:301–312, 2006

Carroll KM, Martino S, Ball SA, et al: A multisite randomized effectiveness trial of motivational enhancement therapy for Spanish-speaking substance users. J Consult Clin Psychol 77:993–999, 2009

Colby SM, Monti PM, Barnett MP, et al: Brief motivational interviewing in a hospital setting for adolescent smoking: a preliminary study. J Consult Clin Psychol 66:574–578, 1998

Committee on Trauma, American College of Surgeons: Resources for Optimal Care of the Injured Patient: 2006. Chicago, IL, American College of Surgeons, 2006

DeLeon G, Melnick G, Kressel D: Motivation and readiness for therapeutic community treatment among cocaine and other drug abusers. Am J Drug Alcohol Abuse 23:169–189, 1997

DiClemente CC: Addiction and Change: How Addictions Develop and Addicted People Recover. New York, Guilford, 2003

DiClemente CC: The challenge of change. J Trauma 59:1–2, 2005

DiClemente CC: Natural change and the troublesome use of substances: a life-course perspective, in Rethinking Substance Abuse: What the Science Shows, and What We Should Do About It. Edited by Miller WR, Carroll KM. New York, Guilford, 2006, pp 81–96

DiClemente CC, Carbonari J, Zweben A, et al: Motivation hypothesis causal chain analysis, in Project MATCH Hypotheses: Results and Causal Chain Analyses (NIH Publ No 01-4238). NIAAA Project MATCH Monograph Series, Vol 8. Edited by Longabaugh R, Wirtz PW. Rockville, MD, 2001, pp 206–222

DiClemente CC, Nidecker M, Bellack AS: Motivation and the stages of change among individuals with severe mental illness and substance abuse disorders. J Subst Abuse Treat 34:25–35, 2008

Donovan DM, Rosengren DB, Downey L, et al: Attrition prevention with individuals awaiting publicly funded drug treatment. Addiction 96:1149–1160, 2001

Dunn C, DeRoo L, Rivara FP: The use of brief interventions adapted from motivational interviewing across behavioral domains: a systematic review. Addiction 96:1725–1742, 2001

Edwards AG, Rollnick S: Outcome studies of brief alcohol intervention in general practice: the problem of lost subjects. Addiction 92:1699–1704, 1997

Ewing JA: Detecting alcoholism: the CAGE questionnaire. JAMA 252:1905–1907, 1984

Fisk D, Rakfeldt J, McCormack E: Assertive outreach: an effective strategy for engaging homeless persons with substance use disorders into treatment. Am J Drug Alcohol Abuse 32:479–486, 2006

Fleming M, Mundt M, French M, et al: Physician advice for problem drinkers: long-term efficacy and benefit-cost analysis. Alcohol Clin Exp Res 26:36–43, 2002

Galloway GP, Polcin D, Kielstein A, et al: A nine session manual of motivational enhancement therapy for methamphetamine dependence: adherence and efficacy. J Psychoactive Drugs Nov (suppl 4):393–400, 2007

Haug NA, Svikis DS, DiClemente CC: Motivational enhancement therapy for nicotine dependence in methadone-maintained pregnant women. Psychol Addict Behav 18:289–292, 2004

Joseph J, Breslin C, Skinner H: Critical perspectives on the transtheoretical model and stages of change, in Changing Addictive Behavior: Bridging Clinical and Public Health Strategies. Edited by Tucker JA, Donovan DM, Marlatt AG. New York, Guilford, 1999, pp 160–190

Landau J, Stanton MD, Brinkman-Sull D, et al: Outcomes with the ARISE approach to engaging reluctant drug- and alcohol-dependent individuals in treatment. Am J Drug Alcohol Abuse 30:711–748, 2004

Litt MD, Kadden RM, Stephens RS; Marijuana Treatment Project Research Group: coping and self-efficacy in marijuana treatment: results from the Marijuana Treatment Project. J Consult Clin Psychol 73:1015–1025, 2005

Longabaugh R, Woolard R, Nirenberg TD, et al: Evaluating the effects of a brief motivational intervention for injured drinkers in the emergency department. J Stud Alcohol 62:806–816, 2001

Loue S: The criminalization of the addictions. J Leg Med 24:281–330, 2003

Madson MB, Campbell TC: Measures of fidelity in motivational enhancement: a systematic review. J Subst Abuse Treat 31:67–73, 2006

Marijuana Treatment Project Research Group: Brief treatments for cannabis dependence: findings from a randomized multisite trial. J Consult Clin Psychol 72:455–466, 2004

Martino S, Carroll KM, O'Malley SS, et al: Motivational interviewing with psychiatrically ill substance abusing patients. Am J Addict 9:88–91, 2000

Mid-Atlantic Addiction Technology Transfer Center: Motivational interviewing: resources for clinicians, researchers, and trainers. November 2009. Available at: http://www.motivationalinterviewing.org. Accessed February 13, 2010.

Miller WR, Rollnick S: Motivational Interviewing: Preparing People to Change Addictive Behavior. New York, Guilford, 1991

Miller WR, Rollnick S: Motivational Interviewing: Preparing People for Change. New York, Guilford, 2002

Miller WR, Rose GS: Toward a theory of motivational interviewing. Am Psychol 64:527–537, 2009

Miller W, Sovereign R, Krege B: Motivational interviewing with problem drinkers, II: the Drinker's Check-Up as a preventive intervention. Behavioural Psychotherapy 16:251–268, 1988

Miller WR, Benefield RG, Tonigan JS: Enhancing motivation for change in problem drinking: a controlled comparison of two therapist styles. J Consult Clin Psychol 61:455–461, 1993

Miller WR, Zweben A, DiClemente CC, et al: Motivational enhancement therapy manual: a clinical research guide for therapists treating individuals with alcohol abuse and dependence (NIH Publ No 94-3723). NIAAA Project MATCH Monograph Series, Vol 2. Edited by Mattson ME. Rockville, MD, National Institute on Alcohol Abuse and Alcoholism, 1994

Miller WR, Andrews NR, Wilbourne P, et al: A wealth of alternatives: effective treatments for alcohol problems, in Treating Addictive Behaviors. Edited by Miller WR, Heather N. New York, Plenum, 1998, pp 203–216

Miller W, Yahne CE, Tonigan JS: Motivational interviewing in drug abuse services: a randomized trial. J Consult Clin Psychol 71:754–763, 2003

Monti PM, Colby SM, Barnett NP, et al: Brief intervention for harm-reduction with alcohol-positive older adolescents in a hospital emergency department. J Consult Clin Psychol 71:754–763, 1999

National Institute on Drug Abuse: National Drug Abuse Treatment Clinical Trials Network: research studies. Updated May 2010. Available at: http://www .drugabuse.gov/CTN/research.html. Accessed June 15, 2010.

Peterson PL, Baer JS, Wells EA, et al: Short-term effects of a brief motivational intervention to reduce alcohol and drug risk among homeless adolescents. Psychol Addict Behav 20:254–264, 2006

Petry NM: Contingency management treatments. Br J Psychiatry 189:97–98, 2006

Polcin DL, Galloway GP, Palmer J, et al: The case for high-dose motivational enhancement therapy. Subst Use Misuse 39:331–343, 2004

Prochaska JO, DiClemente CC, Norcross JC: In search of how people change: applications to addictive behaviors. Am Psychol 47:1102–1114, 1992

Project MATCH Research Group: Matching alcoholism treatments to client heterogeneity: Project MATCH posttreatment drinking outcomes. J Stud Alcohol 58:7–29, 1997a

Project MATCH Research Group: Project MATCH secondary a priori hypotheses. Addiction 92:1671–1698, 1997b

Project MATCH Research Group: Matching alcoholism treatments to client heterogeneity: treatment main effects and matching effects on drinking during treatment. J Stud Alcohol 59:631–639, 1998

Rohsenow DJ, Monti PM, Martin RA, et al: Motivational enhancement and coping skills training for cocaine abusers: effects on substance use outcomes. Addiction 99:862–874, 2004

Rollnick S, Miller WR, Butler CC: Motivational Interviewing in Health Care: Helping Patients Change Behavior. New York, Guilford, 2008

Rosengren DB: Building Motivational Interviewing Skills: A Practitioner Workbook (Applications of Motivational Interviewing Series). New York, Guilford, 2009

Saunders B, Wilkinson C, Phillips M: The impact of a brief motivational intervention with opiate users attending a methadone programme. Addiction 90:415–424, 1995

Schneider RJ, Casey J, Kohn R: Motivational versus confrontational interviewing: a comparison of substance abuse assessment practices at employee assistance programs. J Behav Health Serv Res 27:60–74, 2000

Simpson DD, Joe GW: Motivation as a predictor of early dropout from drug abuse treatment. Psychotherapy 30:357–368, 1993

Simpson DD, Brown BS, Joe GW: Treatment retention and follow-up outcomes in the Drug Abuse Treatment Outcome Study (DATOS). Psychol Addict Behav 11:294–307, 1997

Sinha R, Easton C, Renee-Aubin L, et al: Engaging young probation-referred marijuana-abusing individuals in treatment: a pilot trial. Am J Addict 12:314–323, 2003

Smith JE, Meyers RJ: Motivating Substance Abusers to Enter Treatment: Working With Family Members. New York, Guilford, 2004

Steinberg ML, Ziedonis DM, Krejci JA, et al: Motivational interviewing with personalized feedback: a brief intervention for motivating smokers with schizophrenia to seek treatment for tobacco dependence. J Consult Clin Psychol 72:723–728, 2004

Stephens RS, Roffman RA, Curtain L: Comparison of extended versus brief treatments for marijuana use. J Consult Clin Psychol 68:898–908, 2000

Stotts A, Schmitz JM, Rhoades HM, et al: Motivational interviewing with cocaine dependent patients: a pilot study. J Consult Clin Psychol 69:858–862, 2001

Substance Abuse and Mental Health Services Administration, Center for Substance Abuse Treatment: Brief interventions and brief therapies for substance abuse. Treatment Improvement Protocol (TIP) Series 34 (DHHS Publ No SMA-99-3353). Rockville, MD, Substance Abuse and Mental Health Services Administration, 1999a

Substance Abuse and Mental Health Services Administration, Center for Substance Abuse Treatment: Enhancing motivation for change in substance abuse treatment. Treatment Improvement Protocol (TIP) Series 35 (DHHS Publ No SMA-99-3354). Rockville, MD, U.S. Department of Health and Human Services, 1999b

Swanson AJ, Pantalon MV, Cohen KR: Motivational interviewing and treatment adherence among psychiatric and dually diagnosed patients. J Nerv Ment Dis 187:630–635, 1999

Turner S, Longshore D, Wenzel S, et al: A decade of drug treatment court research. Subst Use Misuse 37:1489–1528, 2002

UKATT Research Team: United Kingdom Alcohol Treatment Trial (UKATT): hypotheses, design, and methods. Alcohol Alcohol 36:11–21, 2001

UKATT Research Team: Effectiveness of treatment for alcohol problems: findings of the randomized UK alcohol treatment trial (UKATT). BMJ 331:541–545, 2005

U.S. Department of Health and Human Services: Ninth Special Report to the U.S. Congress on Alcohol and Health (NIH Publ No 97-4017). Bethesda, MD, National Institutes of Health, 1997

Velasquez MM, Hecht J, Quinn VP, et al: Application of motivational interviewing to prenatal smoking cessation: training and implementation issues. Tob Control 9 (suppl 3):36–40, 2000

Velasquez MM, Maurer GG, Crouch C, et al: Group Treatment for Substance Abuse: A Stage of Change Therapy Manual. New York, Guilford, 2001

Villanueva M, Tonigan JS, Miller WR: Response of Native American clients to three treatment methods for alcohol dependence. J Ethn Subst Abuse 6:41–48, 2007

Volpicelli JR, Pettinati HM, McClellan AT, et al: Combining Medication and Psychosocial Treatments for Addictions: The Brenda Approach. New York, Guilford, 2001

Vuchinich RE, Heather N (eds): Choice, Behavioural Economics, and Addiction. New York, Pergamon, 2003

Wagner CC, Conners W: Motivational interviewing: resources for clinicians, researchers, and trainers. 2007. Available at: http://motivationalinterview.org/clinical/group.html. Accessed February 17, 2010.

Walker DD, Roffman RA, Stephens RS, et al: Motivational enhancement therapy for adolescent marijuana users: a preliminary randomized controlled trial. J Consult Clin Psychol 74:628–632, 2006

West R, Sohal T: "Catastrophic" pathways to smoking cessation: findings from national survey. BMJ 332:458–460, 2006

Wickizer T, Maynard C, Atherly A, et al: Completion rates of clients discharged from drug and alcohol treatment programs in Washington State. Am J Public Health 84:215–221, 1994

Wilk AI, Jensen NM, Havighurst TC: Meta-analysis of randomized control trials addressing brief interventions in heavy alcohol drinkers. J Gen Intern Med 12:274–283, 1997

Winhusen T, Kropp F, Babcock D, et al: Motivational enhancement therapy to improve treatment utilization and outcome in pregnant substance users. J Subst Abuse Treat 35:161–173, 2008

Ziedonis DM, Trudeau K: Motivation to quit using substances among individuals with schizophrenia: implications for a motivation-based treatment model. Schizophr Bull 23:229–238, 1997

Zygmunt A, Olfson M, Boyer CA, et al: Interventions to improve medication adherence in schizophrenia. Am J Psychiatry 159:1653–1664, 2002

6 | Intervention With the Addicted Person

Laurence M. Westreich, M.D.
Eric Leventhal, L.C.S.W.

Intervention is an attempt by those who care about an addicted person to change the addiction's course and promote treatment, by the use of convincing techniques, group support, emotional pressure, and sometimes all three. Although many think of intervention only as the formal group intervention developed by Vernon Johnson (1986) and popularized by television shows such as the A&E Television Network's weekly documentary *Intervention*, true intervention with an addicted person occupies a broad spectrum of convincing and increasingly coercive tactics, ranging from the quiet friendly word to the group intervention to court-mandated treatment.

In this chapter, we discuss the goals of intervention with the addicted person, some general techniques in confronting and then intervening, and some specific intervention models such as Vernon Johnson's seminal intervention, the Community Reinforcement and Family Training (CRAFT) paradigm, and the Pressures to Change protocol. We address strategies involving dually diagnosed patients, medication, legal intervention, and professional interventionists, and therapeutic use of books and videos in the intervention process. The focus throughout is on practical suggestions for helping the addicted person engage in and benefit from addiction treatment.

Goals of Intervention

The goals of intervention with an addicted person are 1) to preserve life and physical well-being, 2) to obtain a full evaluation as soon as possible, and 3) to help the addicted person receive good treatment and to support that treatment over time. Clinicians, family, and friends should focus on these three intervention goals if they want to change the trajectory of the addicted person's behavior. An effective intervention is not a dynamic interpretation that results in a cathectic reaction from the addicted person; instead, it is a focused process of convincing and pushing the addicted person to get into and stay with the appropriate treatment.

First and foremost, any intervention must ensure the addicted person's safety. Obsessing about the addicted person's family dynamics or codependence while he or she uses crack cocaine is a serious mistake. Waiting for the addicted person to "hit bottom" can result in catastrophe, so those who care must sometimes take drastic action such as calling 911 or driving the addicted person to a hospital's emergency department. This sort of dramatic intervention may serve as the basis for an immediate evaluation and ongoing engagement with treatment, and will at the very least render the addicted person as safe as possible in the critical moment.

The second goal of an intervention, whether a dramatic acute intervention or a more relaxed ongoing intervention, is to get the addicted person an in-depth evaluation. By definition, an intervention is only a bridge to a longer evaluation process that can better define any need for detoxification, the effects of the particular substances involved, cues to use that substance, mental health problems, and the most likely effective treatment modalities. For instance, the mother of young children who drinks and drives with her children in the car will not be well served by a quick evaluation by her internist. Rather, an in-depth assessment that can only come from a clinician experienced in addiction treatment will delineate the boundaries of the problem and the best treatment for the addicted mother and her family. The time immediately after an initial evaluation presents an opportunity for the addicted person to slip away from treatment, so the clinician and loved ones must insist on the person's continued engagement with treatment.

After a comprehensive evaluation, which can range from an outpatient clinic assessment to a longer inpatient comprehensive evaluation, the addicted person and those who care about him or her face the difficulties of achieving the third goal of an intervention: actually engaging in the recommended treatment. Research data support the idea that addiction is usually a chronic, relapsing condition (Hser 2008), so the continuing process of intervention should encompass the clinician, family members, and friends continuing to support the addicted person in sticking with treatment.

General Techniques of Intervention

Although some specific intervention techniques have been developed, as we describe below, the skilled and effective clinician uses some common modalities, regardless of the actual protocol or set of protocols being deployed. One of these techniques, *motivational interviewing*, was developed and studied by William Miller and Stephen Rollnick, who organized some commonsense principles into a coherent set of readily usable recommendations for promoting change in the addicted person (Miller and Rollnick 1991). The five general principles of motivational interviewing are to 1) express empathy, 2) develop discrepancy, 3) avoid argumentation, 4) roll with resistance, and 5) support self-efficacy. These five ideas are tied to practical and concretely described procedures for guiding the addicted person toward treatment, engagement with that treatment, and eventual recovery. One important attribute of motivational interviewing is that it adheres to the important and unavoidable principle of all psychotherapy to "start where the client is." Even the addicted person who as yet has no interest in changing can be engaged by using the ideas of motivational interviewing, which engenders hope in both the therapist and the patient.

Another important method for promoting hope and optimism in the addicted person is to make sure that the framework for any intervention establishes that addiction is a disease rather than a moral failing, personal weakness, or sign of possession by the devil. Defining addiction as a disease, with comparisons to other chronic conditions such as diabetes or hypertension, allows the addicted person to avoid the self-flagellation so common in patients with this condition, and defining it in this way sets up the medical or medicalized interventions that may be necessary: detoxification, psychotherapy, and medications. Also, the disease concept promotes the idea that the patient's addiction—like diabetes, for instance—may be chronic and lifelong and may therefore require lifelong vigilance if not lifelong treatment.

In 1960, E.M. Jellinek, an early promoter of this disease model, wrote *The Disease Concept of Alcoholism* (Jellinek 1960), which described the growing evidence for addiction as a medical illness, as seen by researchers, clinicians, and peer-led self-help groups such as Alcoholics Anonymous. The American Medical Association (AMA) agreed, clearly defining alcoholism and drug dependencies as diseases: "The AMA endorses the proposition that drug dependencies, including alcoholism, are diseases and that their treatment is a legitimate part of medical practice" (American Medical Association 2010). Even more important than the views of writers and professional groups, however, is the continuing accretion of scientific evidence (Volkow et al. 2007) that places addiction squarely in the realm of medical illness as opposed to poor choice. These appeals to authority and medical research can be made and discussed with the addicted person as evidence that his or her affliction is not a result of moral badness, but rather an illness with specific treatments in which—and this is most important—the addicted person must engage in order to improve. This requirement is precisely the same as that for many other medical illnesses. For example, the Type II diabetic individual who refuses to manage his diet or take insulin will suffer the consequences of this "resistance" to treatment.

Of course, some may object to the disease concept of addiction, opining that there should be a bright line between biological diseases, such as cancer, and conditions with some apparent volitional component, such as addiction. Although many medical illnesses (including some cancers) have a large element of choice involved in their risk factors and ultimate treatment, this is not a useful debate to have while intervening with the addicted person. It is probably best to simply acknowledge that perspectives can differ on the subject of addiction as disease and move on to the more important task of getting the addicted person into recovery.

In addition to using motivational interviewing techniques and framing the addiction as a disease, those who intervene with an addicted person would be well advised to use a low expressed emotion (low EE) approach. Although this approach was initially promoted as a useful method for working with patients with schizophrenia (Sturgeon et al. 1984), using the low EE approach while intervening with addicted individuals is important because addicted persons are likely to become defensive, angry, and resistant when presented with evidence of the damage they have caused themselves, their families, and those who love them. In the low EE approach, the interveners momentarily suppress their understandably powerful feelings of anger and fear, in the service of getting the addicted person to engage with treatment.

Vernon Johnson Intervention

Among the specific methods for intervention, the intervention protocol developed by Vernon Johnson is the most widely known; it promotes the idea that chemical dependency is a disease one cannot blame on the individual (Johnson 1986). This method challenged the long-held opinion that "nothing could be done with alcoholics until they 'hit bottom' or that only those chemically dependent people who were 'properly motivated' would respond to professionally delivered remedial care" (Johnson 1986, p. iii).

According to Liepman (1993, p. 55), family involvement is an important component of Johnson's method:

> Using family influence to motivate the alcoholic to begin recovery is important in two ways. First, the family, as a significant and meaningful component of the social network, can have substantial influence that seems to enhance the likelihood that the alcoholic will initiate and stick with recovery. Such up-front involvement of the family and significant others assures greater social support for sobriety during and after treatment. Second, the involvement of the family in this initiation phase can provide an opportunity for the therapist to hook family members into the recovery process so that family recovery occurs in tandem with the individual recovery of the alcoholic.

In *Intervention*, Johnson (1986) wrote, "Intervention is a process by which the harmful, progressive, and destructive effects of chemical dependency are interrupted and the chemically dependent person is helped to stop using mood-altering chemicals and to develop new, healthier ways of coping with his or her needs and problems" (p. 61). He also defined an intervention as "presenting reality to a person out of touch with it in a receivable way" (p. 61). He continued, "By 'presenting reality,' we mean presenting specific facts about the person's behavior and the things that have happened because of it. A 'receivable way' is one that the person cannot resist because it is objective, unequivocal, nonjudgmental, and caring" (p. 61).

According to Johnson (1986), "In an intervention, confrontation means compelling the person to face the facts about his or her chemical dependency....It is an attack upon the victim's wall of defenses, not upon the victim as a person" (p. 62). In Johnson's view, such an intervention is based on empathy rather than sympathy. The family member or friend agrees to take part in an intervention out of concern for the chemically dependent person. Johnson stated, "The only 'surprises' during the process should be those the victim experiences when finally met head-on with the realities of his or her disease" (p. 62).

Johnson (1986, p. 103) listed the following principles of intervention:

1. Meaningful persons in the life of the chemically dependent person are involved.
2. All of the meaningful persons write down specific data about the events and behaviors involving the dependent person's chemical use which legitimize their concern.
3. All of the meaningful persons tell the dependent person how they feel about what has been happening in their lives, and they do it in a nonjudgmental way.
4. The victim is offered specific choices—this treatment center, or that hospital.

According to a study performed by Loneck et al. (1996), individuals who underwent a Johnson intervention were more likely to enter treatment than were individuals in four other referral groups. The study also compared the individuals who experienced the Johnson intervention with other referrals to evaluate the role of relapse during treatment. They found that relapse rates across the five types of referrals ranged from 37% to 78%. Those in the Johnson intervention group had the highest rate of relapse (78%), and those who relapsed were less likely to complete treatment. The authors emphasized that the Johnson intervention, "in spite of its high relapse rate, is very effective in retaining those who relapse because it is very effective in retaining all clients, whether they relapse or not" (p. 1). Compared with other groups, "with control variables included in the model, those in the Johnson Intervention group were equally likely to complete treatment as those in the coerced referral group and were more likely to complete it than those in the non-coerced referral, Unrehearsed Intervention, and Unsupervised Intervention groups" (p. 5).

Community Reinforcement and Family Training

Developed by Jane Ellen Smith and Robert J. Meyers, CRAFT is a therapy program for family members or friends of people with substance abuse problems who have been unwilling to accept treatment (Smith and Meyers 2004). CRAFT-trained therapists work with a "concerned significant other" (CSO) and an "identified patient" (IP) to accomplish three major goals: 1) to influence the individual, ultimately, to enter treatment; 2) in the meantime, to reduce that individual's alcohol or drug use; and 3) to help the CSO improve her or his own psychological functioning, whether or not the substance-abusing person enters treatment.

CRAFT is different from other CSO programs because it "promotes active, positive participation in engaging the IP into treatment, as opposed to detachment or confrontation" (Smith and Meyers 2004, p. 33). According to Smith and Meyers, "CSOs are considered ideal collaborators in the treatment engagement process because they have a great deal of knowledge about the IP's behavior and are likely to be successful at influencing it due to their frequent contact with the IP and their high level of personal motivation" (p. 33). Many CSOs are unwilling or unable to step aside and remain uninvolved. The methods of Al-Anon and Nar-Anon, which advocate for "loving detachment" from the drinker or drug user and an acceptance of the CSO's own inability to control the substance-abusing individual's behavior, have met resistance from these families (Smith and Meyers 2004, p. 3). CSOs have also demonstrated discomfort with the highly confrontational role expected of them in the Johnson intervention (Barber and Gilbertson 1997).

CRAFT, based on behavioral principles, uses reinforcement strategies as opposed to confrontational techniques. According to Smith and Meyers (2004), "CSOs receiving the CRAFT treatment in a series of studies were taught how to rearrange contingencies in the IP's environment, such that clean and sober behavior was reinforced and drinking and drug use was effectively discouraged. The CSOs' new skills were geared toward ultimately influencing IPs to enter treatment" (p. 4).

According to Smith and Meyers (2004, pp. 4–5), the following are the major components of CRAFT:

1. *Motivational strategies.* Setting positive expectations by describing the CRAFT program, its success, and the potential benefits for the CSO.
2. *Functional analyses of the IP's substance-using behavior.* Outlining the triggers and consequences of the IP's use and developing CSO intervention strategies based on this information, such that the environmental contingencies to encourage and support clean and sober behavior are rearranged.
3. *Domestic-violence precautions.* Assessing the potential for violence in the CSO-IP relationship, identifying the triggers for IP aggression, and devising prevention and protection plans.
4. *Communication training.* Examining the CSO's current communication style with the IP, providing a rationale for improving communication, teaching positive communication skills, and rehearsing through the use of role playing.
5. *Positive reinforcement training.* Identifying appropriate small rewards for the IP and instructing the CSO in how to use these to reinforce only clean and sober IP behavior.
6. *Discouragement of using behavior.* Showing the CSO how to use "timeouts" from positive reinforcement at IP substance-using times, demonstrating how to allow the natural consequences for using, and teaching a standard problem-solving strategy.
7. *CSO self-reinforcement training.* Exploring the CSO's dissatisfaction in various life areas, developing goals and a plan to address these problems, and assisting the CSO in identifying and "sampling" reinforcers for her- or himself.
8. *Suggestion of treatment to the IP.* Determining the best time and manner for suggesting treatment, preparing the CSO to face a possible refusal, and having arrangements in place at a treatment agency or with a provider to accept the IP for treatment without delay.

CRAFT presents a "menu" approach in that not every component of CRAFT is used with every client (Smith and Meyers 2004). A central effort of the program is to teach new skills and a sense of when best to use them. Clients are trained to state their views calmly but assertively. Some of the skills that the CSOs will learn are geared directly toward influencing the IP's use: "CSOs will be asked to change their behavior in specific ways so that sober behavior is rewarded and substance-using behavior is ignored or discouraged" (pp. 35–36).

According to Smith and Myers (2004), "In a series of studies, CRAFT-trained CSOs were able to influence resistant substance abusers to enter treatment in 64%–86% of their cases" (p. 10). In addition, the CSOs "typically felt better about themselves after treatment regardless of whether or not the IP entered therapy" (p. 10).

A Relational Intervention Sequence of Engagement

A Relational Intervention Sequence for Engagement (ARISE), as developed by Judith Landau and James Garrett in their book *Invitational Intervention: A Step by Step Guide for Clinicians Helping Families Engage Resistant Substance Abusers in Treatment* (Landau and Garrett 2006), "mobilizes family members to motivate Addicted Individuals (AIs) who have been resistant to treatment, or who have relapsed many times, to get into treatment and/or self-help" (p. 1). The method was inspired by the authors' explicit belief in the inherent competence and resilience of families. Landau and Garrett (2006, p. 6) describe the program as follows:

> ARISE is a three-level Invitational Intervention™ method designed to harness the immense energy and driving force behind Family Motivation to Change®; provide encouragement to mobilize the support system, herein referred to as the Intervention Network; and begin the process of an Invitational Intervention with the goal of getting a resistant AI started in treatment.... [The] AI is "invited" into the process, without secrecy or initial confrontation, but with openness, love, and concern. ARISE maximizes the effort of the family (defined for this purpose as the members of the natural support system), while minimizing the need for considerable time and effort on the part of the professional.

Landau and Garrett (2006) detail the first two levels of intervention:

> Level I is set in motion when the First Caller or Concerned Other (CO) reaches out to a treatment agency or individual treatment provider for assistance in getting a resistant, addicted loved one into treatment. The First Caller or CO subsequently becomes the "Family Link"—a person who serves as a bridge between the ARISE Invitational Interventionist and the extended family support system. (pp. 1–2)

> In Level II, between one to five face-to-face sessions are held with the Intervention Network, with or without the AI present. These meetings are

designed to mobilize the group and focus on the goal of treatment engagement. (p. 2)

Landau and Garrett (2006, p. 3) depict Level III, "the formal ARISE Intervention," as follows, while noting that less than 2% of families need to proceed to this level:

> By Level III, the Intervention Network is functioning as a support group for all its members, who are able to implement new boundary setting and consequences with the AI, while continuing to offer consistent support for the individual getting into treatment.

The authors elaborate on the relationship between the family and the trained interventionist (Landau and Garrett 2006, p. 8):

> The ARISE-trained Interventionist shows his/her commitment and trust by believing that the family has inherent strengths and is capable of overcoming its difficulties by accessing these strengths and resources....The collaborative relationship that is formed relies on the implicit notion that the family is the expert on itself and its problems. The ARISE Interventionist is the expert in understanding the interface of addiction and the complexity of family relationships. Thus, the family is trusted to do much of the work on its own with solid guidance, but minimal direct involvement, from the ARISE Interventionist.

Another central concept of the ARISE approach is the Intervention Network (Landau and Garrett (2006, pp. 9–10):

> [The Intervention Network is] an extended support group of family members, friends, neighbors, clergy, and treating professionals who agree to meet with the express purpose of helping the AI enter treatment....The research on ARISE demonstrates a correlation between the size of the Intervention Network and the likelihood that the AI will enter treatment: the larger the network the greater the likelihood of treatment entry.... A large network can serve as a reminder, not only of the particular strengths and resources, but also of the resilience and survival of the intergenerational family across time.

Landau and Garrett (2006, pp. 11–12) summarize their study of ARISE as follows:

> A recent non-randomized clinical trial of the ARISE Invitational Intervention showed that following the family initiating the ARISE method, 83% ($n=91$) of 110 severely addicted and resistant alcoholics and substance abusers enrolled in treatment ($n=86$) or attended self-help meetings ($n=5$). In cumulative terms, 55% entered treatment in Level I; another 26% were engaged in Level II, bringing the total to 81%. Level III added an-

other 2%, completing the final figure of 83%....Half of those who entered treatment did so within one week of the Concerned Other contacting an agency or Interventionist. By the end of two weeks, 76% of those who eventually entered treatment had done so, and 86% had entered by the end of week three....Finally, the study showed that ARISE Interventionists averaged less than an hour and a half of coaching the First Caller and family members to mobilize their network to motivate the AI to enter treatment.

Pressures to Change

In the Pressures to Change approach developed by Barber and Crisp (1995), "the principal question under investigation was whether partner intervention could advance precontemplators toward change (Prochaska 1986). For the purposes of the study, behavior change was operationally defined as the drinker either (a) seeking treatment; (b) ceasing drinking; or (c) reducing drinking to a level acceptable to the partner" (Barber and Crisp 1995, p. 272).

According to Barber and Crisp (1995, pp. 272–273):

[The Pressures to Change approach] involves training partners in how to use five levels of pressure on drinkers to seek help or moderate their drinking. The five levels are arranged in ascending order with the last level (confrontation) being reserved for when all else has failed. Phase I of the treatment is completed in four or five weekly sessions and clients are then given 3 months to employ the strategies before a single follow-up session (Phase I) is arranged. In total, the procedure requires between five and six treatment sessions. Only at Phase II is Level 5 pressure raised as a possibility.

The Level 1 pressure involves *feedback and education.* According to Barber and Crisp (1995, p. 273):

[Level 1 pressure] consists largely in providing the partner [(i.e., the drinker)] with information and feedback on his or her test scores. The objective at this stage is to maximize the client's motivation for change, prepare him or her for frustrations and setbacks, and to explain the principles of the Pressures to Change approach.

The objectives of treatment are explained as being "(a) to help clients cope by being more in control of their reactions; (b) to encourage their partners to reduce their drinking; and/or (c) to entice their partners into treatment" (Barber and Crisp 1995, p. 273). It is explained to clients that drinkers change with pressure from the environment.

The Level 2 pressure involves *incompatible activities.* According to Barber and Crisp (1995, p. 273):

Towards the end of the first session clients are provided with a simple drink diary in which they are asked to record for the week ahead: (a) the situations in which the partner drinks; (b) whether or not the partner becomes intoxicated; (c) the problems caused to clients by their partner's drinking; and (d) the client's responses to the drinking. Clients are taught to identify the drinker's high risk times and to plan incompatible activities (including the cues and consequences of drinking too much) to coincide with these occasions. As far as possible, the incompatible activities chosen seek to address the benefits of alcohol as identified by a functional analysis.

The Level 3 pressure is *responding*. Barber and Crisp (1995, p. 273) state:

Clients draw up a list of reinforcers derived by the drinker from the relationship (for example, conversation, companionship, sex, meals, etc.) and are instructed in how to provide these reinforcers contingently. When drinking becomes unacceptable, partners are instructed to point this out calmly and without anger and then to remove all reinforcers.

The Level 4 pressure is defined as *contracting* between client and drinker (Barber and Crisp 1995, p. 274):

Pressure is increased when clients try to negotiate an explicit drinking contract with the drinker.... [The best contracts] commit drinkers to abstinence or moderation at high risk times. Sometimes these contracts involve a degree of *quid pro quo* in which the partner agrees to exchange some reinforcers for sobriety.... [When a contract is broken,] clients are reminded of the skills learned during Level 3 related to exploiting crises. Moreover, with each acknowledgment of failure to control their drinking, precontemplators must reexamine their assumption that drinking is not a problem for them.

The Level 5 pressure is *confrontation*. Level 5 is used only after Levels 2–4 have been tried and proven to be unsuccessful. According to Barber and Crisp (1995, p. 274):

Clients are introduced to a confrontation technique similar to that developed by Johnson (1973)....Confrontation consists merely in providing feedback about the effects of drinking on those who mean the most to the drinker....These individuals are then taught to write personal testimonials comprised of three parts: (a) a declaration of the author's love for the drinker; (b) feedback about the ways in which drinking is diminishing their relationship; (c) a simple unambiguous plea to change or seek help.

Barber and Crisp (1995, p. 274) state:

Each session begins with clients reporting back on how the strategies have been working. Inevitably, some strategies are more effective than others, and some clients decide to pursue lower level strategies for some time before increasing the pressure. Where strategies have proven ineffective, however, clients are encouraged to move on to the next level. Given that some of the strategies may run counter to familiar patterns of behavior, constant monitoring and rehearsal is necessary. Treatment is terminated when the drinker decides to change or seek treatment, or when the Phase II interview has been completed.

In the authors' study, as reported in their article (Barber and Crisp 1995), 10 of the 16 drinkers who received intervention changed their behavior, and 7 made appointments to discuss treatment options with the researchers—demonstrating that partner interventions can be successful in promoting change in resistant drinkers. As noted in posttest diaries, one drinker gave up drinking by himself and two drinkers cut down to under four standard drinks per day. The authors stated, "In contrast, no drinking partner of the seven clients in the control group sought treatment from any source or modified their drinking in any way over the same period of time" (p. 274). Barber and Crisp added, "The objective of this study was to ascertain whether working through partners was capable of beginning, not necessarily ending, the process of change" (p. 275).

Barber and Crisp (1995) claim that the Pressures to Change procedure has "at least two potential advantages over previous partner interventions. First, it is a relatively brief intervention, requiring no more than five or six sessions in its present form. Secondly, Pressures to Change is a standardized technique that is easy to describe and replicate" (p. 275). The results of the study suggest that "Pressures to Change can be offered on an individual or group basis with equal effect" (p. 275).

Screening, Brief Intervention, and Referral to Treatment

Babor et al. (2007, p. 8) describe Screening, Brief Intervention, and Referral to Treatment (SBIRT) as

> a comprehensive, integrated, public health approach to the delivery of early intervention and treatment services for persons with substance use disorders, as well as those who are at risk of developing them. SBIRT is based on public health principles and procedures, and is designed to reduce the burden of injury, disease, and disability associated with the misuse of psychoactive substances, particularly alcohol, illicit drugs, tobacco products, and prescription medications with high abuse potential.

The core components of SBIRT are screening, brief intervention, brief treatment, and referral to treatment, as described below by Babor et al. (2007, p. 8).

SBIRT begins with the introduction of *systematic screening* into the normal routine at medical facilities and other community settings where persons with substance use disorders are likely to be found. Screening is by definition a preliminary procedure to evaluate the likelihood that an individual has a substance use disorder or is at risk of negative consequences from use of alcohol or other drugs. Whereas screening tests were initially developed to identify active cases of alcohol and drug dependence, in recent years the aim has been expanded to cover the full spectrum ranging from risky substance use to alcohol or drug dependence.

The term *brief intervention* refers to any time-limited effort (e.g., 1–2 conversations or meetings) to provide information or advice, increase motivation to avoid substance use, or to teach behavior change skills that will reduce substance use as well as the chances of negative consequences. Brief interventions are typically delivered to those individuals at low to moderate risk. Among the most cost-effective and time efficient interventions are brief motivational conversations between a health care professional and a substance user.

Brief treatment refers to the delivery of time-limited, structured (or specific) therapy for a substance use disorder by a trained clinician and is typically delivered to those at higher risk or in the early stages of dependence. It generally involves 2–6 sessions of cognitive-behavioral or motivational enhancement therapy with clients who are seeking help. Brief treatment may also include the ongoing management of substance use disorders in primary care settings, especially with the use of new pharmaceutical agents.

Screening often identifies those who already have a substance-related health condition or a suspected substance use disorder that warrants a formal diagnosis and possible *referral to treatment*. The referral process facilitates access to care (including brief treatment) for those individuals who have more serious signs of substance dependence and require a level of care outside the scope of brief services.

A key aspect of SBIRT is the *integration and coordination* of these four components into a system of services linking the specialized treatment programs in a community with a network of early intervention and referral activities that are conducted in medical and social service settings.

Commenting further on the SBIRT approach, Babor and colleagues (2007, p. 10) state:

One important function of SBIRT is to fill the gap between primary prevention efforts and more intensive treatment for persons with serious substance use disorders. From a public health perspective, the goal of SBIRT is to improve the health of a community by reducing the prevalence of adverse consequences of substance misuse, including but not limited to diagnosable abuse or dependence, through the coordination of early intervention and referral to specialized treatment....Perhaps the most significant development in this evidence-based movement to test and disseminate new screening and intervention technologies in the U.S. is the Substance Abuse [and] Mental Health [Services] Administration's SBIRT initiative, which consists of a variety of demonstration programs operating in 11 states.

Based on an extensive review of the literature related to SBIRT, Babor et al. (2007) concluded, "Brief interventions can reduce alcohol use for at least 12 months in non-dependent heavy drinkers. The approach is acceptable to both genders and to adolescents and adults. Cost-effectiveness has been demonstrated in several countries. Brief interventions are effective with smokers and risky drinkers, and there is some evidence that they work well with marijuana users. Brief treatments are effective with persons who are dependent on alcohol, marijuana or other drugs" (p. 25). Babor et al. (2007) added, "There is general agreement on the need to 'broaden the base' of treatment by expanding SBIRT services to less severe cases and populations at risk" (p. 25). According to the federal government's Center for Substance Abuse Treatment, by 2007 more than 536,000 people had been screened using SBIRT in trauma centers, emergency rooms, community clinics, health centers, and school clinics (Substance Abuse and Mental Health Services Administration 2010).

The following case example (provided by L.W.) illustrates the use of an SBIRT protocol.

> **Ellen,** a 16-year-old high school sophomore being raised by her mother, had been seen for her well-child care since infancy in a public hospital pediatrics clinic. Although she had evidenced no serious illnesses throughout her life, as part of an SBIRT protocol, the pediatrics resident treating her asked about alcohol and drug use at her yearly checkup. Ellen readily admitted having tried alcohol several times, and marijuana once. Though not overly concerned, the resident briefly mentioned the dangers of both, including driving while intoxicated and making herself vulnerable while intoxicated. The resident also gave Ellen a brochure about teens and drugs, and scheduled an early follow-up appointment 3 months later.
>
> At the 3-month checkup, Ellen had used substantially more alcohol and told the resident that although she was worried about the alcohol use, she did not want her mother told about it. The resident agreed, provided Ellen spoke with a therapist in the hospital's mental health clinic, to which Ellen gladly agreed. The therapist did not diagnose an addictive disorder but did request that Ellen come in for a weekly session to talk about her development as a young woman and her choices about alcohol. Again, Ellen agreed provided her mother would not be told about the details of the therapy sessions, an arrangement that was acceptable to the mother.
>
> On her graduation from high school 2 years later, Ellen's alcohol use had not progressed and, with encouragement from her therapist, had actually decreased. Using the SBIRT protocol had identified Ellen as at risk for an alcohol problem and—perhaps because of her pediatrics resident's intervention and referral—the alcohol use never rose to the level of abuse or dependence.

Intervention With the Dually Diagnosed

In one study sponsored by the National Institute of Mental Health, an estimated 45% of individuals with an alcohol use disorder and 72% of individuals with a drug use disorder had at least one co-occurring psychiatric disorder (Regier et al. 1990). Brady and Malcolm (2004, p. 530) wrote:

> In general, treatment efforts addressing psychiatric and substance use disorders have developed in parallel. To design treatments specifically tailored for patients with comorbidity, it is necessary to determine the appropriate integration of treatment modalities from both the psychiatric and substance abuse fields. Psychosocial treatments are powerful interventions for both substance use and psychiatric disorders. There are common themes in the psychosocial treatments from both fields, and these themes can be built on to optimize outcome.

According to Brady and Malcolm (2004), "Research in pharmacotherapies for both substance use and psychiatric disorders is progressing rapidly. Integration of information from both the psychiatric and substance abuse fields has led to the testing of strategies targeting individuals with both disorders" (p. 530).

On dual diagnosis, Westreich (2007, pp. 275–276) commented:

> The important thing to remember about a dual diagnosis is that both the diagnosis itself and its eventual treatment will be more complicated than it would be with addiction alone. This is because even after the addictive substance is totally out of the addict's body, he or she will suffer from psychiatric symptoms that have to be treated....Such treatment usually includes a combination of appropriate medications, psychotherapy, group therapy, and peer-led support groups and should be coordinated by a clinician—most likely an addiction psychiatrist—who's familiar with the integrated treatment of addiction and mental illness.

The following case example (provided by L.W.) illustrates issues in assessing and treating a dually diagnosed young adult:

> **Roger,** a 21-year-old college senior, was referred for evaluation because he was skipping classes; had several run-ins with the police; and, according to his parents, smoked "way too much marijuana." At the evaluation session, Roger initially said very little, staring at his feet and hands, while his parents talked about the yearlong decline in his school attendance, social life, and even personal hygiene. The therapist perceived the strong odor of marijuana coming from Roger's clothes and hair and, after the parents had left the room, asked Roger how much he had been smoking. Roger ignored the question and, never making eye contact with the therapist, talked about several classmates who had been harassing him via Facebook

and his cell phone, peering into his window, and even figuring out when he was thinking about them. His paranoia had become so severe that he rarely slept, and he only calmed himself through the use of marijuana.

Further investigation with Roger's parents revealed that Roger's uncle had been hospitalized many times for "nervous breakdowns" and had not held a job in 20 years. Although Roger was reluctant to take medications, he agreed when he was told that, among other things, the medications would help him sleep. The medication, together with weekly relapse prevention therapy sessions, lessened Roger's paranoia and marijuana use. Once he was able to sleep better, he further decreased his marijuana use to essentially nil, and even returned to school on a part-time basis. Although his initial referral had been for an addiction problem, the apparent schizophreniform disorder was so closely linked that only a simultaneous intervention would have proved useful.

Special Situations: Medications, Legal Intervention, and Interventionists

The clinical scenario with some addicted people may necessitate the prescription of medications to enhance the intervention, the use of legal or pseudo-legal procedures to coerce the person into treatment, or the assistance of professional interventionists to manage the entire procedure. Although patients who are dually diagnosed with mental illness and addictive disorders will most likely need medications during the treatment of their various conditions, medications may be of some use in intervening even with individuals who have only an addictive disorder. Given the increasingly large pharmacopoeia available for treating addiction (Westreich and Finklestein 2008), clinicians are well advised to make medication a part of any intervention for disorders for which medications appear to be useful.

Even though medications alone are unlikely to be curative of any addictive disorder, or even the primary agent that brings the addicted person into treatment, medications can still exert a powerful effect on an addiction's course. In an obvious example, relieving an alcohol user's painful withdrawal can be both lifesaving and suggestive to the individual that treatment might have something to offer in terms of decreasing alcohol use and also in terms of just feeling better. The addicted person who reacts negatively to the prescription of medications may be showing evidence of a simple reaction formation, a commonsense desire to avoid more substances, or both. Whatever the psychological underpinnings of the addicted person's reluctance to take a medication, the reaction should be framed by the clinician as a positive thought about substances in general. Nonetheless, the addicted person should be presented with potentially useful medications using a standard risk-benefit analysis, in the same way (the clinician hopes) that the addicted person will view all substance use in the future.

Although the nonmedical side of the addiction treatment field has traditionally been reluctant to support the use of medications in the treatment of addicted people, this attitude is shifting as medications with better efficacy and less addictive potential arrive on the market, and as prescribing psychiatrists better understand the addictive process and the multifaceted approach necessary for its treatment. One study of 1,400 addiction counselors' attitudes toward pharmacotherapy for alcoholism (Abraham et al. 2009) found, predictably, that when counselors were educated about the various medications for treating alcoholism, they were receptive to the use of these medications. Because counselors and nonmedical therapists have such a large role in treating addiction, it is incumbent on the field to provide effective and accurate education about these powerful if imperfect medication strategies.

While most clinicians and families prefer to avoid legal intervention with an addicted person, in fact the legal system can be quite helpful in bringing the addicted person to treatment. Framing a "brush with the law" as a defining moment in a worsening addiction can promote entrance into and engagement with treatments. Dedicated drug courts, family courts, and even general criminal courts are increasingly empowered to mandate addiction treatment, or to allow addiction treatment as a mitigating factor in sentencing. An epidemiological study of adolescents with addiction problems (Substance Abuse and Mental Health Services Administration 2007) found that fully 55% of those in treatment had been referred by the courts. Some states do allow for civil commitment for the treatment of addiction, even if there has been no criminal involvement; using this civil commitment procedure requires the advice of an attorney knowledgeable about the specific state's mental health laws.

In addition to pursuing legal methods for bringing the addicted person to treatment, some families hire professional interventionists to assist in or manage the process. Although most of the modalities mentioned in this chapter would require the assistance of a clinician skilled in the treatment of addiction, the professional interventionist is a breed apart, usually focused entirely on the acute intervention itself and knowledgeable about available treatment facilities, local mental health laws, and various strategies for initiating treatment. Because the title of "interventionist" is self-awarded and has no licensure or education requirements, families should make sure that the person they are hiring does have the training and experience necessary for the work. One proprietary Web site (Intervention Resource Center 2010) recommends that an interventionist have at least 5 years' experience in the addiction field, experience with at least five facilitations, model intervention training, references from three peers, and any relevant licensure or malpractice coverage.

Therapeutic Use of Video and Literature

Books—particularly memoirs—and films have served as sources of support, education, and comfort for people with substance abuse issues and their families. Many family members have noted that hearing other families' stories has made them feel less alone and helped them develop empathy for the addicted person. Additionally, substance abusers and their families have been moved by and derived hope and optimism from hearing stories of people who have successfully learned to stay sober. Artistic renditions of the addictive process, whether fiction or documentary, can be used in the intervention process, specifically to help the family members develop empathy for the addicted person.

Westreich (2007) lists a number of memoirs that have helped families and their addicted relatives, including Augusten Burroughs's *Dry: A Memoir* (2004), Pete Hamill's *A Drinking Life: A Memoir* (1994), Caroline Knapp's *Drinking: A Love Story* (1996), Ann Marlowe's *How to Stop Time: Heroin From A to Z* (1999), George McGovern's *Terry: My Daughter's Life-and-Death Struggle With Alcoholism* (1996), and William Styron's *Darkness Visible: A Memoir of Madness* (1990). We would add the following: David Carr's *Night of the Gun* (2008), Nic Sheff's *Tweak: Growing Up on Methamphetamines* (2007), David Sheff's *Beautiful Boy: A Father's Journey Through His Son's Addiction* (2008), and James Frey's *A Million Little Pieces* (2003). *Sober Siblings: How to Help Your Alcoholic Brother or Sister—and Not Lose Yourself,* by Petros Levounis and Patricia Olsen (2008), describes how alcoholism affects the sibling relationship.

The present authors also recommend several films about addiction, including *Requiem for a Dream* (2000), which is also a novel by Hubert Selby Jr.; *Fear and Loathing in Las Vegas* (1998), which is also a fictionalized memoir by Hunter S. Thompson; *Leaving Las Vegas* (1995); *Clean and Sober* (1988); *Drugstore Cowboy* (1989); *28 Days* (2000); *Rachel Getting Married* (2008); and *Permanent Midnight* (1998).

Conclusion

Intervention, broadly defined, serves as an entry point for the addicted person into, ideally, a lifetime of sobriety. Given the course of most addictions, however, intervention is usually a distinct though oft-repeated reentry into the addiction treatment system. Contrary to much rhetoric in the media, this pattern should not be taken as sad and demoralizing evidence that addiction is untreatable and the addicted person is doomed to a lifetime "revolving door" of constant cycling into and out of various treatment centers and therapists' offices.

Rather, this common pattern of multiple interventions represents hope for the addicted person who stays on top of his or her illness, the clinicians who treat the individual, and those who care about and love the person. The best comparison for the addicted patient who has multiple interventions is the cancer patient who has a relapse but then undergoes successful treatment that brings about a remission. The hope and expectation that the interventions will bring about a permanent remission are realistic, reasonable, and the best possible framework for treatment.

Key Clinical Concepts

- Use motivational interviewing techniques when intervening with an addicted person.

- During any intervention with an addicted person, addiction is best framed as a disease.

- Use a low expressed emotion approach when intervening with an addicted person.

- Medication can be used as an integral part of the treatment plan presented to the addicted person.

- If necessary, legal interventions such as drug courts, pressure from a prosecutor, or civil commitment can be used in intervening with an addicted person.

Suggested Reading

Babor TF, McRee BG, Kassebaum PA, et al: Screening, Brief Intervention, and Referral to Treatment (SBIRT): toward a public health approach to the management of substance abuse. Subst Abuse 28:3–30, 2007

Barber JG, Crisp BR: The Pressures to Change approach to working with the partners of heavy drinkers. Addiction 90:269–276, 1995

Johnson VE: Intervention: How to Help Someone Who Doesn't Want Help. Minneapolis, MN, Johnson Institute Books, 1986

Liepman MR: Using family influence to motivate alcoholics to enter treatment: the Johnson Institute intervention approach, in Treating Alcohol Problems: Marital and Family Interventions. Edited by O'Farrell TJ. New York, Guilford, 1993, pp 54–57

Miller WR, Rollnick S: Motivational Interviewing: Preparing People to Change Addictive Behavior. New York, Guilford, 1991

Smith JE, Meyers RJ: Motivating Substance Abusers to Enter Treatment: Working With Family Members. New York, Guilford, 2004

References

Abraham AJ, Ducharme LJ, Roman PM: Counselor attitudes towards pharmaco-therapies for alcohol dependence. J Stud Alcohol Drugs 70:628–635, 2009

American Medical Association: H-95.983 Drug Dependencies as Diseases. 2010. Available at: http://www.ama-assn.org/ama1/pub/upload/mm/388/alcoholism_treatable.pdf. Accessed February 17, 2010.

Babor TF, McRee BG, Kassebaum PA, et al: Screening, Brief Intervention, and Referral to Treatment (SBIRT): toward a public health approach to the management of substance abuse. Subst Abuse 28:3–30, 2007

Barber JG, Crisp BR: The Pressures to Change approach to working with the partners of heavy drinkers. Addiction 90:269–276, 1995

Barber JG, Gilbertson R: Unilateral interventions for women living with heavy drinkers. Soc Work 42:69–78, 1997

Brady KT, Malcolm RJ: Substance use disorders and co-occurring Axis I psychiatric disorders, in The American Psychiatric Publishing Textbook of Substance Abuse Treatment, 3rd Edition. Edited by Galanter M, Kleber HD. Washington, DC, American Psychiatric Publishing, 2004, pp 529–537

Hser YI, Huang D, Brecht ML, et al: Contrasting trajectories of heroin, cocaine, and methamphetamine use. J Addict Dis 27:13–21, 2008

Intervention Resource Center: Factors in choosing an intervention specialist. 2010. Available at: http://www.interventioninfo.org/referrals/factors.php. Accessed February 17, 2010.

Jellinek EM: The Disease Concept of Alcoholism. New Haven, CT, Hillhouse Press, Yale Center of Alcohol Studies, 1960

Johnson VE: I'll Quit Tomorrow. New York, Harper, 1973 (cited in Barber and Crisp 1995).

Johnson VE: Intervention: How to Help Someone Who Doesn't Want Help. Minneapolis, MN, Johnson Institute Books, 1986

Landau J, Garrett J: Invitational Intervention: A Step by Step Guide for Clinicians Helping Families Engage Resistant Substance Abusers in Treatment. New York, Haworth Press, 2006

Liepman MR: Using family influence to motivate alcoholics to enter treatment: the Johnson Institute intervention approach, in Treating Alcohol Problems: Marital and Family Interventions. Edited by O'Farrell TJ. New York, Guilford, 1993, pp 54–57

Loneck B, Garrett JA, Banks SM: The Johnson Intervention and relapse during outpatient treatment. Am J Drug Alcohol Abuse 22:363–375, 1996

Miller WR, Rollnick S: Motivational Interviewing: Preparing People to Change Addictive Behavior. New York, Guilford, 1991

Prochaska JO: Toward a comprehensive model of change, in Treating Addictive Behaviors: Processes of Change. Edited by Miller WR, Heather N. New York, Plenum, 1986, pp 3–27. Cited in: Barber JG, Crisp BR: The Pressures to Change approach to working with the partners of heavy drinkers. Addiction 90:269–276, 1995

Regier DA, Farmer ME, Rae DS, et al: Comorbidity of mental disorders with alcohol and other drug abuse: results from the Epidemiologic Catchment Area (ECA) study. JAMA 264:2511–2518, 1990

Smith JE, Meyers RJ: Motivating Substance Abusers to Enter Treatment: Working With Family Members. New York, Guilford, 2004

Sturgeon D, Turpin G, Kuipers L, et al: Psychophysiological responses of schizophrenic patients to high and low expressed emotion relatives: a follow-up study. Br J Psychiatry 145:62–69, 1984

Substance Abuse and Mental Health Services Administration: Adolescent treatment admissions by gender: 2005. The Dasis Report, May 24, 2007. Available at: http://www.oas.samhsa.gov/2k7/youthTX/youthTX.pdf. Accessed February 17, 2010.

Substance Abuse and Mental Health Services Administration, Center for Substance Abuse Treatment: Screening, Brief Intervention, and Referral to Treatment. About SBIRT. 2010. Available at: http://sbirt.samhsa.gov/about.htm. Accessed February 18, 2010.

Volkow ND, Fowler JS, Wang GJ, et al: Dopamine in drug abuse and addiction: results of imaging studies and treatment implications. Arch Neurol 64:1575–1579, 2007

Westreich L: Helping the Addict You Love: The New Effective Program for Getting the Addict Into Treatment. New York, Simon & Schuster, 2007

Westreich LM, Finklestein D: New medications for the treatment of substance use disorders. Prim Psychiatry 15:73–80, 2008

7 | Cognitive-Behavioral Therapies

Kathleen M. Carroll, Ph.D.

Cognitive-behavioral treatments are among the most well-defined and rigorously studied psychotherapeutic interventions for substance use disorders. Although the focus of this chapter is primarily on cognitive-behavioral therapy (CBT) approaches, the reader should be aware that CBT shares several features with other empirically supported behavioral approaches. First, cognitive, behavioral, and motivational therapies are applicable across a broad range of substance use disorders; that is, well-controlled trials have supported their efficacy for populations dependent on alcohol, stimulants, marijuana, and opioids. Second, these approaches were developed from well-founded theoretical traditions with established theories and principles of human behavior. Third, these approaches are highly flexible and can be implemented in a wide range of clinical modalities and settings. Moreover, they are compatible with a variety of pharmacotherapies and, in many cases, foster compliance and enhance the effects of pharmacotherapies that include methadone, naltrexone, and disulfiram. Finally, these are relatively brief/short-term and highly focused approaches that emphasize rapid, targeted change in patients with substance use and related problems. As such, they are highly compatible with a health care environment that is increasingly influenced by managed care, best clinical practice models, and professional accountability.

Support was provided by National Institute on Drug Abuse grants P50 DA09241, U10 DA13038, R37 DA15969, and K05 DA00457.

Theoretical Basis

Cognitive-behavioral treatments have their roots in classical behavioral theory and the pioneering work of Ivan Pavlov, John Watson, B.F. Skinner, and Albert Bandura (see reviews by Craighead et al. 1995; Rotgers 1996). Pavlov's work on classical conditioning demonstrated that a previously neutral stimulus could elicit a conditioned response after being paired repeatedly with an unconditioned stimulus. Furthermore, repeated exposure to the conditioned stimulus without the unconditioned stimulus would eventually lead to extinction of the conditioned response. The power of classical conditioning was demonstrated in drug abuse by Wikler (1973), who confirmed that persons addicted to opioids exhibited conditioned withdrawal symptoms upon exposure to drug paraphernalia. Today classical conditioning theory is the basis of several behavioral approaches to substance use treatment, such as cue exposure (Childress et al. 1999; Monti et al. 1993) as an early component of many addiction counseling approaches.

Skinner's work on operant conditioning demonstrated that behaviors that are positively reinforced are likely to be exhibited more frequently. The field of behavioral pharmacology, which has convincingly demonstrated the reinforcing properties of abused substances in both humans and animals, is grounded in operant conditioning theory and principles. Behavior therapies assume that drug use and related behaviors are learned through their association with the positively reinforcing properties of the drugs themselves, as well as their secondary association with other environmental stimuli. CBT attempts to disrupt this learned association between drug-related cues or stimuli and drug craving or use by understanding and changing these behavior patterns. A wide range of behavioral interventions, including those that seek to provide alternative reinforcers to drug use or to reduce reinforcing aspects of abused substances, also are based on operant conditioning theory.

Cognitive-behavioral therapies conceive substance use disorders as complex, multidetermined problems, with a number of influences playing a role in the development or perpetuation of the disorder. These influences may include family history and genetic factors; the presence of comorbid psychopathology; personality traits such as sensation seeking or impulsivity; and a host of environmental factors, including substance availability and lack of countervailing influences and rewards. Although cognitive-behavioral therapies primarily emphasize the reinforcing properties of substances as central to the acquisition and maintenance of substance abuse and dependence, these etiological influences are seen as heightening risk or vulnerability to the development of substance use problems.

For example, some individuals may find substances unusually highly rewarding secondary to genetic vulnerability, comorbid depression, a high need for sensation seeking, and modeling of family and friends who use substances or environments devoid of alternative reinforcers.

Cognitive-behavioral treatments also reflect the pioneering work of Albert Ellis and Aaron Beck, which emphasizes the importance of the person's thoughts and feelings as determinants of behavior. CBT evolved in part from dissatisfaction with the extreme positions of radical behaviorism (e.g., emphasis on overt behaviors) and classical psychoanalysis (emphasis on unconscious conflicts or representations). CBT emphasizes that how the individual perceives and interprets life events is an important determinant of behavior (Meichenbaum 1995). A person's conscious thoughts, feelings, and expectancies mediate the individual's response to the environment. CBT also seeks to help patients become aware of maladaptive cognitions and "teach them how to notice, catch, monitor, and interrupt the cognitive-affective-behavioral chains and to produce more adaptive coping responses" (Meichenbaum 1995, p. 147).

Empirical Support

CBT has been shown to be effective across a wide range of substance use disorders (Carroll 1996; Irvin et al. 1999), including alcohol dependence (Miller and Wilbourne 2002; Morgenstern and Longabaugh 2000), marijuana dependence (Marijuana Treatment Project Research Group 2004; Stephens et al. 2000), cocaine dependence (Carroll et al. 1994a, 1998; McKay et al. 1997; Rohsenow et al. 2000), and nicotine dependence (Fiore et al. 1994; Hall et al. 1998; Patten et al. 1998). CBT has also been shown to be compatible with a number of other treatment approaches, including pharmacotherapy (Anton et al. 1999; O'Malley et al. 1992) and traditional counseling approaches (Morgenstern et al. 2001), and thus can be implemented in a wide range of settings. These findings are consistent with evidence supporting the effectiveness of CBT across a number of other psychiatric disorders as well, including depression, anxiety disorders, and eating disorders.

We have been involved in a programmatic series of studies on the effectiveness of CBT, alone and in combination with pharmacotherapy, for the past 15 years. As our understanding of CBT has deepened over time, this series of studies has been marked by progressively larger effect sizes for CBT over the comparison or control conditions. For example, in our first randomized trial, we conducted a direct comparison of CBT with another active therapy, interpersonal psychotherapy (IPT), adapted for cocaine users. In that trial, CBT was not found to have a main effect over

IPT, but was found to be significantly more effective among the more severely dependent cocaine abusers (Carroll et al. 1991), suggesting that the higher levels of structure and emphasis on skills may have been particularly helpful for the more severely impaired cocaine users.

Severity of cocaine dependence as a moderator of CBT effects was also replicated in our next study (Carroll et al. 1994a). This study used a 2×2 factorial design, in which desipramine was compared with placebo and CBT was compared with supportive clinical management, a supportive psychotherapy control condition. This study was the first in the literature to describe that after the study treatments were terminated, those who had been assigned to CBT continued to reduce the frequency of their cocaine use throughout the 1-year follow-up, a finding termed the "sleeper effect" (Carroll et al. 1994b). Evidence of continued improvement associated with CBT in turn led to increasing interest in mechanisms that might underlie this effect, with skills training and behavioral practice through homework assignments as prime candidates, as described in more detail in the sections below.

Thus, in our next study, which found a significant main effect for CBT over supportive clinical management and which replicated the sleeper effect for CBT over a 1-year follow-up (Carroll et al. 2000a), we also evaluated the acquisition of coping skills in CBT and their relationship to outcome in this population. We developed and validated a role-play task for assessing the acquisition of coping skills in CBT (Carroll et al. 1999). The task involves the patient listening to a series of audiotaped high-risk situations (e.g., "What would you do if you found yourself at a party where you didn't think cocaine would be available, and then noticed a lot of people going in and out of a back room?" "What would you do if you started feeling really intense craving?"). The patient's responses are audiotaped and then rated for quality of response, type of coping response, and number of responses generated using a rating method demonstrated to be highly reliable. In this study, evaluation of the role-play task demonstrated the following: 1) coping skills increased significantly after CBT, 2) patients demonstrated increases in coping skills that were parallel to those taught in the treatment they had been assigned (i.e., differential acquisition of specific behavioral and cognitive coping strategies in CBT with respect to alternative behavioral therapies), and 3) greater acquisition of CBT-specific behavioral and cognitive coping skills was associated with significantly less cocaine use over the 1-year follow-up (Carroll et al. 2000a).

In our most recently completed trial (Carroll et al. 2004b), 121 cocaine-dependent individuals were randomized to one of four conditions in a 2×2 factorial design: disulfiram (250 mg/day) plus CBT, disulfiram plus IPT, placebo plus CBT, or placebo plus IPT. Across outcome measures and for the full intention-to-treat sample (as well as across all subsamples, including treatment initiators and treatment completers), patients assigned to CBT reduced their cocaine use significantly more than those assigned to IPT, and patients assigned to disulfiram reduced their cocaine use significantly more than those assigned to placebo. Effects of CBT plus placebo were comparable to those of CBT plus disulfiram. This was our first trial to identify a significant main effect for CBT over another active behavioral therapy (IPT). Furthermore, although retention was a significant predictor of better drug use outcomes, the CBT by time effect remained statistically significant after controlling for retention.

Thus, this series of trials has demonstrated increasingly strong effects for CBT over time, and our follow-up studies have consistently indicated high durability of CBT compared with other approaches. Similar results have been found by other research groups evaluating CBT across a range of substance use disorders; these have been reviewed in detail elsewhere (Carroll et al. 2004a).

Another particularly exciting development in the field of treatment of drug dependence has been the very strong empirical support for contingency management (CM) approaches, in which participants receive incentives (i.e., vouchers redeemable for goods and services, chances to draw prizes from a bowl) contingent on demonstrating acquisition of treatment goals (e.g., submitting drug-free urine specimens, attending treatment sessions) (Higgins and Silverman 1999; Petry 2000). Given that CM has strong immediate effects but those effects tend to weaken after the contingencies are terminated, whereas CBT tends to have more modest effects initially but is comparatively durable, several investigators have begun to evaluate various combinations of CBT and CM, reasoning that the relative strengths and weaknesses of these approaches may be offset by combining them. For example, Rawson et al. (2002) recently compared group CBT, voucher CM, and a combination of CBT and CM in conjunction with standard methadone maintenance treatment for cocaine-using methadone maintenance patients. During the acute phase of treatment, the group assigned to CM had significantly better cocaine use outcomes. However, during the follow-up period, a CBT sleeper effect emerged, in which the group assigned to CBT essentially caught up to the other groups by the 52-week follow-up (Rawson et al. 2002). Similar results were found for a parallel study conducted among a large sample (N=171) of stimulant-dependent individuals treated as outpatients (Rawson et al. 2006); in this study, CM was associated with better retention and substance use outcomes during treatment, but outcomes for CBT and CM were comparable at 1 year.

Epstein et al. (2003) conducted a similar study, again in the context of intensive methadone maintenance, in which participants were offered CM, group CBT, or a combination, in addition to standard individual counseling. Results were largely parallel to the Rawson et al. (2002) study, in that the investigators reported large initial effects for CM, with drop-off after the termination of the contingencies, and best 1-year outcomes for the CM+CBT combination.

CBT Techniques and Strategies

Specific techniques vary widely with the type of cognitive-behavioral treatment used, and a variety of manuals, protocols, and training programs are available that describe the techniques associated with each approach (Annis and Davis 1989; Carroll 1998; Kadden et al. 1992; Marlatt and Gordon 1985; Monti et al. 1989). Simply put, however, most CBT approaches attempt to help individual patients recognize the situations in which they are most likely to use substances, avoid those situations when appropriate, and cope more effectively with a range of problems and problematic behaviors associated with substance use by implementing a range of cognitive and behavioral coping strategies.

Defining Features of CBT

Two key defining features of most cognitive-behavioral approaches for substance use disorders are 1) an emphasis on functional analysis of drug use—that is, understanding drug use with respect to its antecedents and consequences—and 2) emphasis on skills training.

Cognitive-behavioral approaches include a range of skills to foster or maintain abstinence. These typically include strategies for the following:

1. Understanding the patterns that maintain drug use and developing strategies for changing them. This often involves self-monitoring of thoughts and behaviors that take place before, during, and after high-risk situations or episodes of drug use.
2. Fostering the resolution to stop substance use through exploring positive and negative consequences of continued use (also known as the decisional balance technique).
3. Understanding craving and craving cues and developing skills for coping with craving when it occurs. These include a variety of affect regulation strategies (distraction, talking through a craving, "urge surfing," etc.).
4. Recognizing and challenging the cognitions that accompany and maintain patterns of substance use.

5. Increasing awareness of the consequences of even small decisions (e.g., which route to take home from work), and the identification of "seemingly irrelevant" decisions that can culminate in high-risk situations.
6. Developing problem-solving skills, and practicing application of those skills to substance-related and more general problems.
7. Planning for emergencies and unexpected problems and situations that can lead to high-risk situations.
8. Developing skills for assertively refusing offers of drugs, as well as reducing exposure to drugs and drug-related cues.

These basic skills are useful in their application to helping patients control and stop substance use, but it is essential that therapists also point out how these same skills can be applied to a range of other problems. For example, a functional analysis can be used to understand the determinants of a wide range of behavior patterns, skills used to cope with craving can easily be applied to other aspects of affect control, the principles used in the sessions on seemingly irrelevant decisions can be adapted to understanding a wide range of behavior chains, and substance use refusal skills can be transferred to more effective and assertive responding in a number of situations. When therapists teach coping skills, they should emphasize and demonstrate that the skills can be applied immediately to control substance use, but that they can also be used as general strategies across a wide range of situations and problems the patient may encounter in the future.

Broad-spectrum cognitive-behavioral approaches, such as those described by Monti et al. (1989) and adapted for use in Project MATCH (Matching Alcoholism Treatment to Client Heterogeneity; Kadden et al. 1992), expand to include interventions directed to other problems in the individual's life that are seen as functionally related to substance use. These interventions may include general problem-solving skills, assertiveness training, strategies for coping with negative affect, awareness of anger and anger management, coping with criticism, increasing pleasant activities, enhancing social support networks, and job-seeking skills, among others.

In comparison with many other behavioral approaches, CBT is typically highly structured. That is, CBT is generally brief (12–24 weeks) and organized closely around well-specified treatment goals. Usually, an articulated agenda exists for each session, and the clinical discussion remains focused around issues directly related to substance use. Progress toward treatment goals is monitored closely and often, with frequent monitoring of substance use through urine toxicology screens, and the therapist takes an active stance throughout treatment. Generally, sessions take place within a weekly scheduled therapy "hour." In broad-spectrum cognitive-behavioral approaches, sessions often are organized roughly in thirds (the 20/20/20 rule); the first third of the session is devoted to assessment of the patient's substance use and general functioning in the past week and a report of current concerns and problems, the second third is more didactic and devoted to skills training and practice, and the final third allows time for therapist and patient to plan for the week ahead and to discuss how new skills will be implemented (Carroll 1998). The therapeutic relationship is seen as principally collaborative. Thus, the role of the therapist is one of consultant, educator, and guide, someone who can lead the patient through a functional analysis of his or her substance use, aid in identifying and prioritizing target behaviors, and consult in selecting and implementing strategies to foster the desired behavior changes.

Although structured and didactic, CBT is a highly individualized and flexible treatment. That is, rather than viewing CBT treatment as cookbook "psychoeducation," the therapist carefully matches the content, timing, and nature of presentation of the material to the individual patient. The therapist attempts to provide skills training at the moments the patient is most in need of them. That is, the therapist does not belabor topics such as breaking ties with cocaine suppliers with a patient who is highly motivated and has been abstinent for several weeks. Similarly, the therapist does not race through material in an attempt to "cover" all of it in a few weeks; some patients may require several weeks to master a basic skill.

Extrasession Practice as a Possible Mediator of CBT

In CBT, therapists encourage patients to practice new skills; such practice is a central and essential component of treatment. The degree to which the treatment offers a skills *training* over merely a skills *exposure* approach has to do with the degree to which opportunity is available to practice and implement coping skills, making extrasession practice and homework all the more important. It is critical that patients have an opportunity to try out new skills within the supportive context of treatment. Through first-hand experience, patients can learn what new approaches work or do not work for them, where they have difficulty or problems, and so on. There are many opportunities for practice within CBT, both within sessions and outside of them. Within each session, patients have opportunities to rehearse and review ideas, raise concerns, and get feedback from the therapist.

As noted earlier, interest has been growing in understanding not only what treatments work, but also how they work. Understanding the mechanisms of action of CBT and other empirically validated therapies has heretofore received very little attention in the literature (Kraemer et al. 2002; Morgenstern and Longabaugh 2000; Weisz et al. 2000), but is an area of great importance. Understanding treatment mechanisms not only can advance the development of more effective treatment strategies, but also can result in more powerful, efficient, and ultimately less expensive treatments.

The converging evidence suggesting that CBT is a particularly durable approach has led to increased focus on unique or distinctive aspects of CBT that might account for its durability. Encouraging clients to implement and practice skills outside of sessions via homework assignments is one possible mechanism for this effect. Homework encourages practice of skills outside sessions and possibly generalization of skills to other problems, and the emphasis on extrasession practice assignments is a unique feature of CBT. Moreover, investigators evaluating CBT in non–substance-related psychiatric disorders have noted the importance of homework in CBT's effectiveness.

The relationship of homework compliance, skills acquisition, and outcome in CBT has received very little attention in the substance abuse literature. Thus, we evaluated homework completion in detail, collecting data on what specific type of homework was assigned and how well it was done (e.g., fully, partially, no attempt made) at every session (Carroll et al. 2005). We found strong relationships between homework compliance and outcome. Compared with the participants assigned to CBT who did not do homework or who did it only rarely, the participants who did homework consistently stayed in treatment significantly longer, had more consecutive days of cocaine abstinence (a strong predictor of long-term outcome), and had fewer cocaine-positive urine screens during treatment. Similar effects were found for the subset of participants who completed treatment in this study, suggesting that the effects of homework compliance on better substance use outcomes were not completely accounted for by differential retention. In addition, we found strong relationships between homework compliance and acquisition of coping skills, as well as between homework completion and participants' ratings of their confidence in avoiding use in a variety of high-risk situations. Participants who completed homework had significant increases over time in their self-reported confidence in handling a variety of high-risk situations, whereas self-reported confidence scores for the subgroup that did not do homework did not change over time.

Farabee et al. (2002) evaluated the extent to which cocaine users reported engaging in a series of specific drug-avoidance activities (e.g., avoiding drug-using friends and places where cocaine would be available, exercising, using thought-stopping) after CBT versus alternate treatments (e.g., CM and a control condition). They found that by the end of treatment, participants assigned to CBT reported more frequent engagement in drug-avoidance activities than participants in the comparison treatments. Furthermore, the frequency of drug-avoidance activities was strongly related to better cocaine use outcomes over the 1-year follow-up. Taken together, these studies suggest that CBT interventions that foster the patients' engagement in active behavior change may play a key role in CBT's comparative durability.

> **Peter,** a substance use counselor at an outpatient clinic, had a history of alcohol, cocaine, and marijuana dependence prior to becoming a counselor. Although he had received state certification as a counselor, most of his experience and training was "on the job," and he relied heavily on his experience with the fellowship of Alcoholics Anonymous, which he credited with his own recovery. He had fallen back into occasional drinking during a recent divorce, and ultimately began using marijuana and benzodiazepines fairly regularly to cope with stress and loneliness during this time. He was also referred for weekly individual therapy by his supervisor, as a condition for returning to work after a car accident, and subsequent inpatient hospitalization and detoxification, in addition to naltrexone treatment.
>
> Peter was initially resistant to the idea of CBT, maintaining that he preferred to attend Alcoholics Anonymous meetings. However, after reassurance that CBT was compatible with 12-step approaches and could expand his own clinical repertoire, he became more open. Thus, discussion of CBT concepts took place at multiple levels. First, he learned to apply CBT concepts, such as the functional analysis, to better understand the issues that led to his own relapse and to prevent another one from occurring, with particular emphasis on managing stress and negative cognitions. Second, the clinician took special care to highlight the generalizability of CBT strategies—that is, to connect familiar CBT principles to general concepts and strategies. For instance, she emphasized how a functional analysis could be used to elucidate a range of behavioral problems and patterns, how strategies used to help manage craving could also be used to address affect tolerance, how strategies for refusing offers of drug and alcohol paralleled basic assertive strategies, and particularly how to identify his cognitions associated with negative thinking. This made the treatment "come alive" for Peter and encouraged him to think more broadly about his own problems and his work with clients. He has remained drug-free for several years and has now completed a master's degree in counseling.

This case led to major changes in how we at the Yale Psychotherapy Development Center train clinicians in CBT; rather than simply teaching the elements of CBT as a circumscribed set of strategies to be applied to patients with addictive disorder, we teach them as general concepts and strategies that can be applied to virtually any behavioral problem. This is illustrated by having each trainee apply these principles to a behavioral issue or problem of his or her own that he or she would like to change; this heightens the learn-by-doing aspects of CBT, as well as the need for practice to refine skills.

Training and Competence in CBT

The growing evidence base for CBT and the increased emphasis on incorporating empirically supported therapies into clinical practice have also led to greater focus on training and dissemination. Although standard methods used to train clinicians to use CBT in clinical efficacy trials have generally been associated with high levels of treatment fidelity and comparatively small levels of variation in treatment delivery, these methods (intensive didactic workshop training plus structured feedback on supervised training cases) have not been empirically evaluated, and are not commonly used for training clinicians to use novel approaches (Weissman et al. 2006). Thus, we have initiated a series of studies systematically evaluating different training strategies for clinicians wishing to learn empirically supported therapies, such as CBT, by randomly assigning clinicians working full-time in substance abuse treatment facilities to different training conditions.

In our initial study of CBT training methods (Sholomskas et al. 2005), 78 clinicians were assigned to one of three training conditions: 1) review of the National Institute on Drug Abuse (NIDA) CBT manual only (Carroll 1998); 2) access to a Web-based training site (which included additional frequently asked questions, role-plays, and practice exercises) plus the manual; or 3) a 3-day didactic seminar plus up to three sessions of supervision from a CBT expert trainer based on actual session tapes submitted by the participants. Outcomes focused on clinician behavior and included 1) between-group comparisons of the clinicians' ability to demonstrate key CBT techniques based on structured role-plays administered before and after training and 2) scores on a CBT knowledge quiz. The videotaped role-plays were scored by independent raters, blind to the participants' training condition as well as time (e.g., pretraining vs. posttraining), using adherence/competence ratings of specific CBT techniques from the Yale Adherence and Competence Scale (Carroll et al. 2000b).

Although all groups demonstrated improved adherence and competence scores over time, the only training condition that reached levels of skill consistent with those required of clinicians participating in our CBT efficacy trials was the seminar+supervision condition, with intermediate ratings for the Web condition. The mean effect size for the seminar+

supervision versus manual-only condition comparisons was consistent with a large effect (0.69), whereas the average effect size for the Web versus manual-only condition contrasts was consistent with a medium-size effect (0.30). In addition, as shown in Figure 7–1, significantly more clinicians in the seminar+supervision condition reached criterion levels for adequate fidelity than those assigned to the manual-only condition (54% vs. 15%).

These findings underscore that merely making manuals available to clinicians has little enduring effect on clinicians' ability to implement new treatments. Therefore, the study has important implications for current efforts to disseminate new treatments. Our findings 1) suggest that face-to-face training followed by direct supervision and credentialing may be essential for effective technology transfer and 2) raise questions regarding whether practitioners should feel competent (from an ethical perspective) to administer an empirically supported treatment on the basis of reading a manual alone. Finally, the findings suggest that standard strategies used to train clinicians in clinical trials can be effective for community-based clinicians and may be pursued as a strategy for future dissemination trials and for bridging the gap between research and practice.

Addressing Limitations of CBT

Despite CBT's emerging empirical support, future research is needed to address its limitations. CBT is a relatively complex approach, in that it is comparatively complicated to train clinicians to use this approach or to implement it effectively in clinical practice. As a result, competent delivery of CBT has been shown to be very rare in clinical practice. Independent review of clinician audiotapes from the treatment-as-usual condition in a multisite trial supported by the NIDA Clinical Trials Network indicated that although the clinicians professed using a high level of CBT in their clinical work, interventions associated with CBT (e.g., skills training, focus on cognitions) were extremely rare (Santa Ana et al. 2008).

Another relative weakness of CBT may be the cognitive demands it places on patients, in that they are asked to learn a range of new concepts and skills, including monitoring and remembering cognitions and inner states, implementing new skills while in stressful situations, and so on. Recent data suggest that substance users with higher levels of cognitive impairment may have poorer outcomes in CBT than those who are less impaired (Aharonovich et al. 2006). These findings suggest that clinicians should monitor the cognitive skills of their patients and, in cases where the patients may have memory, attention, or impulse control problems, should adapt the implementation of CBT accordingly, with slower

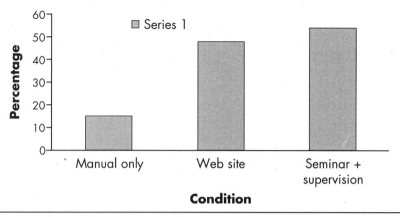

FIGURE 7–1. **Percentage of clinicians trained to criterion, by training condition.**

progression through concepts, frequent repetition of material and checking back with the patient to assess understanding, and more structure provided on extrasession assignments.

Potential strategies for addressing these issues include greater emphasis on understanding CBT's mechanisms of action, so that ineffective components of CBT can be removed and treatment delivery simplified. A more novel strategy is to harness the ability and breadth of technology to standardize CBT and make it more widely available. We have developed a computer-assisted version of CBT, called CBT4CBT, which stands for "computer-based training for cognitive-behavioral therapy." The content of CBT4CBT, which is based closely on the NIDA CBT manual, is delivered in six sessions, or modules, and makes extensive use of the multimedia capabilities of computers to convey CBT principles and illustrate implementation of new cognitive and behavioral strategies (Carroll et al. 2008). Key CBT concepts are taught through short movies, or vignettes, which feature engaging characters in realistic settings confronting a number of challenging situations, as well as a number of interactive games and exercises to teach CBT strategies. Thus, patients are able to see multiple examples of how CBT principles can be implemented, rather than simply hearing sometimes too abstract or incomplete presentations from their therapists.

In a clinical trial in which CBT4CBT was delivered in addition to standard outpatient treatment, exposure to the program was associated with significantly fewer drug-positive urine specimens and longer durations of abstinence during treatment (Carroll et al. 2008). In addition, data from a 6-month follow-up indicated the durability of these effects in that the sleeper effect of CBT appeared to extend to its computer-based version (Carroll et al. 2009). Durability of effects on substance use appeared to have been mediated by significantly higher levels of skill acquisition among those who used the CBT4CBT program (Kiluk et al., in press). Finally, participants' level of neuropsychological functioning did not appear to be associated with outcome in the CBT4CBT program, perhaps because little or no reading of text is required and users can control the rate of speed of material presented, can repeat material as often as they wish, and can select the types of exercises and issues they would like to address, thereby reducing the "cognitive load" of CBT. Although CBT4CBT and other computer-assisted programs have great potential to make empirically supported therapies more widely available and to broaden the base of substance abuse treatment, and some of the early data on their effectiveness is very encouraging, substantially more testing and evaluation are needed before these programs can be widely distributed.

Conclusion

CBT is an empirically supported behavioral approach that has strong theoretical and empirical support with a variety of substance-abusing populations. In recent years, clinical researchers have emphasized moving CBT approaches more broadly into the clinical community, and thus a range of practical resources (e.g., books, videotapes, manuals, training resources and programs) for implementing them effectively in clinical practice is available. Moreover, these approaches can be combined and integrated effectively with a range of other empirically supported behavioral therapies as well as with pharmacotherapies. Therefore, CBT should be a component of all substance abuse clinicians' repertoire.

Key Clinical Concepts

- CBT has strong empirical support across a range of different substance use disorders as well as psychiatric syndromes that frequently co-occur with substance use disorders (e.g., depression, anxiety).

- Key components of virtually all CBT approaches include functional analyses of substance use and individualized skills training, with emphasis on cognitive and behavioral coping.

- Effects of CBT appear to be comparatively durable, with several studies reporting continuing improvement after patients leave treatment. Emphasis on skills training and practice may underlie this effect.

- A variety of manuals, videotapes, and other training materials for CBT may be available. However, specialized coaching and feedback, with structured supervision, may be needed for many clinicians to implement CBT effectively.
- Technology-based models of providing CBT, such as computer-assisted therapies, are showing great promise.

Suggested Reading

Carroll KM, Rounsaville BJ: A vision of the next generation of behavioral therapies research in the addictions. Addiction 102:850–862, 2007

Kazantzis N, Deane FP, Ronan KR, et al (eds): Using Homework Assignments in Cognitive Behavior Therapy. New York, Brunner-Routledge, 2004

Marlatt GA, Donovan D: Relapse Prevention: Maintenance Strategies in the Treatment of Addictions, 2nd Edition. New York, Guilford, 2005

Miller WR, Carroll KM (eds): Rethinking Substance Abuse: What the Science Shows, and What We Should Do About It. New York, Guilford, 2006

Monti PM, Rohsenow DJ, Abrams DB, et al: Treating Alcohol Dependence: A Coping Skills Training Guide in the Treatment of Alcoholism. New York, Guilford, 1989

Wright JH, Basco MR, Thase ME: Learning Cognitive-Behavioral Therapy: An Illustrated Guide. Washington, DC, American Psychiatric Publishing, 2005

References

Aharonovich E, Hasin DS, Brooks AC, et al: Cognitive deficits predict low treatment retention in cocaine dependent patients. Drug Alcohol Depend 81:313–322, 2006

Annis HM, Davis CS: Relapse prevention, in Handbook of Alcoholism Treatment Approaches. Edited by Hester RK, Miller WR. New York, Pergamon, 1989, pp 170–182

Anton RF, Moak DH, Waid LR, et al: Naltrexone and cognitive-behavioral therapy for the treatment of outpatient alcoholics: results of a placebo-controlled trial. Am J Psychiatry 156:1758–1764, 1999

Carroll KM: Relapse prevention as a psychosocial treatment approach: a review of controlled clinical trials. Exp Clin Psychopharmacol 4:46–54, 1996

Carroll KM: A cognitive-behavioral approach: treating cocaine addiction (NIH Publ No 98-4308). Rockville, MD, National Institute on Drug Abuse, 1998

Carroll KM, Rounsaville BJ, Gawin FH: A comparative trial of psychotherapies for ambulatory cocaine abusers: relapse prevention and interpersonal psychotherapy. Am J Drug Alcohol Abuse 17:229–247, 1991

Carroll KM, Rounsaville BJ, Gordon LT, et al: Psychotherapy and pharmacotherapy for ambulatory cocaine abusers. Arch Gen Psychiatry 51:177–197, 1994a

Carroll KM, Rounsaville BJ, Nich C, et al: One-year follow-up of psychotherapy and pharmacotherapy for cocaine dependence: delayed emergence of psychotherapy effects. Arch Gen Psychiatry 51:989–997, 1994b

Carroll KM, Nich C, Ball SA, et al: Treatment of cocaine and alcohol dependence with psychotherapy and disulfiram. Addiction 93:713–728, 1998

Carroll KM, Nich C, Frankforter TL, et al: Do patients change in the way we intend? Treatment-specific skill acquisition in cocaine-dependent patients using the Cocaine Risk Response Test. Psychol Assess 11:77–85, 1999

Carroll KM, Nich C, Ball SA, et al: One year follow-up of disulfiram and psychotherapy for cocaine-alcohol abusers: sustained effects of treatment. Addiction 95:1335–1349, 2000a

Carroll KM, Nich C, Sifry R, et al: A general system for evaluating therapist adherence and competence in psychotherapy research in the addictions. Drug Alcohol Depend 57:225–238, 2000b

Carroll KM, Ball SA, Martino S, et al: Cognitive, behavioral, and motivational therapies, in The American Psychiatric Publishing Textbook of Substance Abuse Treatment, 3rd Edition. Edited by Galanter M, Kleber HD. Washington, DC, American Psychiatric Publishing, 2004a, pp 365–376

Carroll KM, Fenton LR, Ball SA, et al: Efficacy of disulfiram and cognitive-behavioral therapy in cocaine-dependent outpatients: a randomized placebo controlled trial. Arch Gen Psychiatry 64:264–272, 2004b

Carroll KM, Nich C, Ball SA: Practice makes progress: homework assignments and outcome in the treatment of cocaine dependence. J Consult Clin Psychol 73:749–755, 2005

Carroll KM, Ball SA, Martino S, et al: Computer-assisted cognitive-behavioral therapy for addiction: a randomized clinical trial of "CBT4CBT." Am J Psychiatry 165:881–888, 2008

Carroll KM, Ball SA, Martino S, et al: Enduring effects of a computer-assisted training program for cognitive-behavioral therapy: a six-month follow-up of CBT4CBT. Drug Alcohol Depend 100:178–181, 2009

Childress AR, Mozley PD, McElgin W, et al: Limbic activation during cue-induced cocaine craving. Am J Psychiatry 156:11–18, 1999

Craighead WE, Craighead LW, Ilardi SS: Behavioral therapies in historical perspective, in Comprehensive Textbook of Psychotherapy: Theory and Practice. Edited by Bongar BM, Beutler LE. New York, Oxford University Press, 1995, pp 64–83

Epstein DE, Hawkins WE, Covi L, et al: Cognitive behavioral therapy plus contingency management for cocaine use: findings during treatment and across 12-month follow-up. Psychol Addict Behav 17:73–82, 2003

Farabee D, Rawson RA, McCann MJ: Adoption of drug avoidance strategies among patients in contingency management and cognitive-behavioral treatments. J Subst Abuse Treat 23:343–350, 2002

Fiore MC, Smith SS, Jorenberg DE, et al: The effectiveness of the nicotine patch for smoking cessation: a meta-analysis. JAMA 271:1940–1947, 1994

Hall SM, Reus VI, Munoz RF, et al: Nortriptyline and cognitive-behavioral therapy in the treatment of cigarette smoking. Arch Gen Psychiatry 55:683–690, 1998

Higgins ST, Silverman K: Motivating Behavior Change Among Illicit-Drug Abusers. Washington, DC, American Psychological Association, 1999

Irvin JE, Bowers CA, Dunn ME, et al: Efficacy of relapse prevention: a meta-analytic review. J Consult Clin Psychol 67:563–570, 1999

Kadden R, Carroll KM, Donovan D, et al: Cognitive-Behavioral Coping Skills Therapy Manual: a clinical research guide for therapists treating individuals with alcohol abuse and dependence. Project Match Monograph Series, Vol 3 (NIH Publ No 94-3724). Rockville, MD, National Institute on Alcohol Abuse and Alcoholism, 1992

Kiluk BD, Nich C, Babuscio TA, et al: Quantity versus quality: acquisition of coping skills in computer-assisted cognitive behavioral therapy for substance abuse. Addiction (in press)

Kraemer HC, Wilson GT, Fairburn CG, et al: Mediators and moderators of treatment effects in randomized clinical trials. Arch Gen Psychiatry 59:877–883, 2002

Marlatt GA, Gordon JR (eds): Relapse Prevention: Maintenance Strategies in the Treatment of Addictive Behaviors. New York, Guilford, 1985

McKay JR, Alterman AI, Cacciola JS, et al: Group counseling versus individualized relapse prevention aftercare following intensive outpatient treatment for cocaine dependence. J Consult Clin Psychol 65:778–788, 1997

Meichenbaum DH: Cognitive-behavioral therapy in historical perspective, in Comprehensive Textbook of Psychotherapy: Theory and Practice. Edited by Bongar BM, Beutler LE. New York, Oxford University Press, 1995, pp 140–158

Miller WR, Wilbourne PL: Mesa Grande: a methodological analysis of clinical trials of treatments for alcohol use disorders. Addiction 97:265–277, 2002

Monti PM, Rohsenow DJ, Abrams DB, et al: Treating Alcohol Dependence: A Coping Skills Training Guide in the Treatment of Alcoholism. New York, Guilford, 1989

Monti PM, Rohsenow DJ, Rubnis AV, et al: Cue exposure with coping skills treatment for male alcoholics: a preliminary investigation. J Consult Clin Psychol 61:1011–1019, 1993

Morgenstern J, Longabaugh R: Cognitive-behavioral treatment for alcohol dependence: a review of the evidence for its hypothesized mechanisms of action. Addiction 95:1475–1490, 2000

Morgenstern J, Morgan TJ, McCrady BS, et al: Manual-guided cognitive behavioral therapy training: a promising method for disseminating empirically supported substance abuse treatments to the practice community. Psychol Addict Behav 15:83–88, 2001

Marijuana Treatment Project Research Group: Brief treatments for cannabis dependence: findings from a randomized multisite study. J Consult Clin Psychol 72:455–466, 2004

O'Malley SS, Jaffe AJ, Chang G, et al: Naltrexone and coping skills therapy for alcohol dependence: a controlled study. Arch Gen Psychiatry 49:881–887, 1992

Patten CA, Martin JE, Myers MG, et al: Effectiveness of cognitive-behavioral therapy for smokers with histories of alcohol dependence and depression. J Stud Alcohol 59:327–335, 1998

Petry NM: A comprehensive guide to the application of contingency management procedures in clinical settings. Drug Alcohol Depend 58:9–25, 2000

Rawson RA, Huber A, McCann MJ, et al: A comparison of contingency management and cognitive-behavioral approaches during methadone maintenance treatment for cocaine dependence. Arch Gen Psychiatry 59:817–824, 2002

Rawson RA, McCann MJ, Flammino F, et al: Comparison of contingency management and cognitive-behavioral approaches for stimulant-dependent individuals. Addiction 101:267–274, 2006

Rohsenow DJ, Monti PM, Martin RA, et al: Brief coping skills treatment for cocaine abuse: 12-month substance use outcomes. J Consult Clin Psychol 68:515–520, 2000

Rotgers F: Behavioral theory of substance abuse treatment: bringing science to bear on practice, in Treating Substance Abusers: Theory and Technique. Edited by Rotgers F, Keller DS, Morgenstern J. New York, Guilford, 1996, pp 174–201

Santa Ana E, Martino S, Ball SA, et al: What is usual about "treatment-as-usual": data from two multisite effectiveness trials. J Subst Abuse Treat 35:369–379, 2008

Sholomskas D, Syracuse G, Ball SA, et al: We don't train in vain: a dissemination trial of three strategies for training clinicians in cognitive behavioral therapy. J Consult Clin Psychol 73:106–115, 2005

Stephens RS, Roffman RA, Curtin L: Comparison of extended versus brief treatments for marijuana use. J Consult Clin Psychol 68:898–908, 2000

Weissman MM, Verdeli H, Gameroff MJ, et al: National survey of psychotherapy training in psychiatry, psychology, and social work. Arch Gen Psychiatry 63:925–934, 2006

Weisz JR, Hawley KM, Pilkonis PA, et al: Stressing the (other) three Rs in the search for empirically supported treatments: review procedures, research quality, relevance to practice and the public interest. Clinical Psychology: Science and Practice 7:243–258, 2000

Wikler A: Dynamics of drug dependence: implications of a conditioning theory for research and treatment. Arch Gen Psychiatry 28:611–616, 1973

8 | Contingency Management

Stephen T. Higgins, Ph.D.
Kenneth Silverman, Ph.D.
Yukiko Washio, Ph.D.

Contingency management (CM) treatments for substance use disorders (SUDs) have been in the published literature since the 1960s but have achieved a higher profile within the past two decades (see Higgins et al. 2008). CM treatments can vary in many respects, but the central feature common to all of them is the systematic application of reinforcing or punishing consequences to achieve therapeutic goals. With regard to treatment of SUDs, CM most commonly involves the systematic application of positive reinforcement, both to increase abstinence from drug use (an approach referred to as *abstinence reinforcement therapy*) and to facilitate other therapeutic changes, including retention in treatment, attendance at therapy sessions, and compliance with medication regimens. Typically, CM is used as part of a more comprehensive treatment intervention. In this chapter, we outline the scientific rationale underlying this treatment approach, discuss the basic elements of CM, and discuss its treatment efficacy and effectiveness.

Scientific Rationale

CM is a generic behavioral intervention based on the principles of operant conditioning, namely reinforcement and punishment. The idea of using behavioral interventions to treat SUDs is quite rational considering

Preparation of this manuscript was supported by grants DA09378, DA14028, and DA08076 (Higgins) and grants DA13107, DA19386, and DA19497 (Silverman) from the National Institute on Drug Abuse.

the extensive empirical evidence demonstrating that operant conditioning plays an important role in the genesis and maintenance of repeated drug use and dependence (e.g., Higgins et al. 2004a). An extensive basic science literature going back to the 1940s shows that abused drugs function as unconditioned positive reinforcers for laboratory animals in the same way that food, water, and sex do. Laboratory animals readily learn arbitrary operant responses—such as pressing a lever or pulling a chain—when the only consequence for doing so is the receipt of an injection of a prototypical drug of abuse such as amphetamines, barbiturates, cocaine, or morphine. Laboratory animals not only will voluntarily ingest abused drugs, but when given unconstrained access to cocaine and related drugs, they will consume them to the exclusion of basic sustenance and to the point of overdose and death. There is a growing understanding of the neurobiology of these drug-produced reinforcing effects, which appear to depend critically on effects in the mesolimbic dopamine system.

This basic research has also revealed that although drug-produced reinforcement is powerful, it is also malleable and sensitive to environmental context (Higgins et al. 2004a). For example, alterations in the schedule of drug availability, increases in how much the subject has to work to obtain the drug, and increases in the availability of alternatives to drug use can all produce orderly reductions in drug consumption. That is true with both laboratory animals and drug-dependent human research subjects. In fact, a highly regarded series of studies conducted in the 1970s demonstrated this point with individuals with severe alcoholism (e.g., Bigelow et al. 1975). In these studies, alcoholic subjects resided on a hospital unit where they were permitted to purchase and consume alcohol under medically supervised conditions. Abstinence from voluntary drinking increased when 1) access to an alternative reinforcer (i.e., an enriched ward environment) was made available contingent on abstinence, 2) monetary reinforcement was provided contingent on abstinence, 3) the cost of drinking in the form of the amount of work required to purchase the alcohol was increased, and 4) brief periods of social isolation were imposed contingent on drinking. Each of these outcomes followed from predictions based on alcohol use being a form of operant responding, which by definition is sensitive to environmental consequences. More recent studies conducted with cocaine and opioid abusers, marijuana abusers, and cigarette smokers have similarly conformed to predictions based on operant conditioning and demonstrated sensitivity of these different forms of drug use to systematically arranged environmental consequences (Higgins et al. 2004a).

An obvious question is, if drug use is so sensitive to environmental consequences, why do individuals continue abusing drugs despite the many horrific adverse consequences that they experience? There are many answers to that question, but here are three important ones to consider. First, many individuals do respond to adverse consequences; that is, the majority of those who experiment with drug use, including the use of highly addictive drugs like cocaine, do not go on to become dependent, and many of those who do become dependent resolve their problem later without professional treatment. Also, those drug-dependent individuals who seek treatment often do so following some untoward health or social consequences related to their drug abuse. A safe assumption is that naturalistic reinforcement and punishment contingencies are operative in these scenarios.

Second, the reinforcing effects of drugs are relatively immediate and reliable, whereas associated adverse consequences are typically more delayed and intermittent. Temporal delays and inconsistent delivery weaken the effect of behavioral consequences. These features would favor a greater influence by the reinforcing effects of abused drugs than by their adverse effects.

Third, research has revealed potentially important individual differences with regard to sensitivity to temporal delays and frontal lobe executive functions that may be involved in vulnerability to drug dependence (see Bechara 2005; Bickel et al. 2007). A normal aspect of the human biological makeup is a preference for more immediate over delayed reinforcement, all else being equal. Such a bias would have had obvious survival advantage in evolutionary history. However, as with most everything biological, there is variability in this characteristic, and accumulating evidence indicates that individuals with SUDs discount the value of delayed consequences and may have deficiencies in behavioral regulatory abilities, either preexisting or resulting from chronic drug use, that increase vulnerability to addiction to a significantly greater extent than in nonabuser matched controls (Bickel et al. 2007). For example, individuals with SUDs are more biased toward immediate reinforcement than delayed reinforcement compared with healthy control subjects, even when the more immediate option is of less value. Such a bias can be expected to work against recovery from SUDs, because the benefits of quitting drug use in terms of improved health, marriage, or vocation are going to be delayed in time relative to the immediate reinforcing effects that will follow in short order from a return to drug abuse. Indeed, in one of the first studies to look into this matter, greater discounting of delayed monetary reinforcement assessed at treatment entry predicted postpartum relapse to smoking among women who quit smoking during pregnancy (Yoon et al. 2007). This relationship held even though the antepartum baseline assessment of delayed discounting was conducted almost 1 year prior to the 6-month postpartum assessment, when most relapse to smoking was noted.

Overall, when considered together, the extensive data supporting an important role of operant conditioning in drug use, the sensitivity of drug use to systematically delivered environmental consequences, and a possible bias of drug-dependent individuals toward immediate rather than delayed reinforcement suggest that CM should be quite useful in the treatment of SUDs. To drive recovery, CM interventions use the same reinforcement process that drives repeated drug use. As we discuss in the following section, CM programs are designed to produce frequent, relatively immediate positive reinforcement for abstaining from drug use, rather than relying exclusively on more delayed naturalistic reinforcing consequences of recovery. This can be thought of as tailoring treatment to the known characteristics of the patient population. As outlined below, the extant evidence on the efficacy of CM interventions for improving treatment outcomes across a wide range of different types of SUDs, populations, and settings suggests that the reinforcement process has as important a role to play in recovery as it does in the genesis and maintenance of drug abuse (Lussier et al. 2006).

Basic Elements of Contingency Management

Before we turn to the literature on the efficacy of CM interventions for SUDs, some discussion of the basic elements of these interventions is warranted. A brief discussion is sufficient because these basic elements have been outlined elsewhere (e.g., Higgins et al. 2008). Briefly, CM interventions promote behavioral change through the use of one of the following generic types of contingencies administered alone or in combination:

- *Positive reinforcement.* The delivery of a reinforcing consequence (e.g., a monetary voucher) contingent on meeting a therapeutic goal (e.g., abstinence from recent drug use).
- *Negative reinforcement.* The removal or a reduction in the intensity of an aversive event (e.g., job suspension) contingent on meeting a therapeutic goal (e.g., successful completion of treatment).
- *Positive punishment.* The delivery of an aversive event (e.g., social reprimand) contingent on evidence of the occurrence of a therapeutically undesirable response (e.g., failure to attend therapy sessions).
- *Negative punishment.* The removal of a positive condition (e.g., forfeiture of clinic privileges) contingent on the occurrence of an undesirable response (e.g., resumption of drug use).

Reinforcement and punishment interventions are effective with SUDs, but the latter are disliked by patients and staff and can inadvertently increase treatment dropout. The evidence suggests that CM interventions composed largely of high rates of positive reinforcement along with judicious use of occasional negative punishment can be very effective at retaining patients in treatment, reducing drug use, and improving other therapeutic outcomes (Lussier et al. 2006).

To be effective, CM interventions need to be carefully designed and implemented; with CM, the details matter. Below are 10 points to consider when designing an effective CM intervention.

1. *Use a written contract.* A written contract is recommended.
2. *Operationally define the therapeutic target.* For example, for a CM intervention used to reinforce cocaine abstinence, the target would be abstinence from recent cocaine use as defined by a cocaine-negative urine toxicology result.
3. *Stipulate the schedule on which progress will be monitored.* The schedule for monitoring progress should be well specified. Staying with the example of a CM intervention for cocaine abstinence, the schedule might be a three-times-a-week (Monday, Wednesday, Friday) assessment of recent cocaine use.
4. *Schedule frequent opportunities for patients to experience the programmed consequences.* CM interventions are designed to promote new behavior while decreasing the frequency of well-learned behavior. As in any learning experience, repetition is important. The thrice-weekly schedule mentioned above has been effective in reinforcing abstinence from cocaine and opioids. When designing the frequency of monitoring, the clinician should consider practical issues, such as the half-life of the abused drug.
5. *Objectively verify that the target response occurred.* The methods for verifying that the target response occurred must be specified and should be objective; reliance on patient self-reports is not adequate for these purposes. Furthermore, because family, friends, and employers may have lost confidence in the individual's veracity by the time he or she enters treatment, objective monitoring of abstinence has the added benefit of providing an effective means to reduce suspicion about progress in treatment and to rebuild respect among significant others. For CM interventions to be effective, they must be precise, and that is only possible when there is precision in determining whether the target response occurred. In applications with SUDs, objective and precise verification typically entails some form of testing for biological markers of recent drug use—for example, urine toxicology

testing with specimen collection observed by a same-sex staff member would be conducted at the thrice-weekly assessments.

6. *When feasible, target single rather than multiple responses.* CM interventions that focus on a single target (e.g., cocaine abstinence) produce larger treatment effects on average than those that have multiple targets (e.g., abstinence from multiple substances) (Lussier et al. 2006). This appears to be simply a matter of trying to have a reasonable balance between the behavioral change that is being targeted and the magnitude of the consequence being delivered.

7. *Specify what consequences will follow when the target response occurs and when it does not occur.* The consequences that will follow success and failure to emit the target behavior need to be made clear. For example, cocaine-negative urine toxicology results would earn a voucher with a specified monetary value that can be used to purchase retail items in the community. A cocaine-positive urine toxicology report would result in no voucher and a recommendation for the patient to meet with his or her counselor as soon as possible. The exact schedule of voucher earnings over the course of the intervention would be specified.

8. *Specify the duration of the contract.* For example, the voucher program would be operative from weeks 1 through 12 of treatment.

9. *Minimize delays in delivering consequences following verification.* Delays weaken behavioral consequences. Delivering the consequence on the same day that occurrence of the target response is verified produces larger treatment effects than delivering the consequence on the next day or later (Lussier et al. 2006). Treatment outcome studies have not shown whether differences in response occur as a function of still further delays. Human laboratory studies suggest that the size of the treatment effect would progressively decrease as the length of the delay increased, until a delay was reached beyond which efficacy would disappear (see Higgins et al. 2004a).

10. *Use a consequence of sufficient magnitude or intensity to function as an effective reinforcer or punisher.* On average, larger-value incentives produce larger treatment effects (Lussier et al. 2006).

With respect to the last point in the list above, it is important to note that the magnitude of reinforcement or punishment necessary to change behavior will depend on the nature of the behavioral change involved, the patient population, and the larger economic context, among other things. Empirically, it has been shown that on average, larger-value reinforcement results in larger treatment effects, with effect size varying in a graded manner across daily incentive values of less than $5, $5–$10.99,

$11–$16, and greater than $16 (Lussier et al. 2006). Direction in choosing appropriate incentive magnitudes for the various populations and types of therapeutic targets with which one may be working is best obtained by consulting previously published studies involving those populations and therapeutic targets (or at least close approximations of them). The CM literature is sufficiently large at this time that a clinician should be able to find a relevant study or two that provides at least some initial guidance in selecting appropriate parameters. Thereafter, some initial pilot testing of the new intervention with the targeted clinical population is essential to working out unforeseen problems and fine-tuning the parameters. Importantly, the clinician should not assume that incentive values used in interventions implemented in developed countries will be necessary to promote healthy behavior change for patients in developing countries. Indeed, large-scale antipoverty programs are being implemented throughout Latin America and other regions that utilize basic contingency management principles, or what is being called conditional cash transfers, to promote healthy behavior change (Higgins 2009; Lagarde et al. 2007). The incentive values used in these programs are appropriately based on local economics. The principles that cut across economies are those relating to effective use of contingent reinforcement.

In the CM literature on the treatment of SUDs, the effects of varying the intensity of punishment have not been assessed in any systematic manner because of the sparse use of all but minimal punishment interventions. The basic operant literature would suggest that effect size can be expected to vary as a function of the intensity of the punishment, and if the research calls for a higher-intensity punishment, it is best to implement it early in the intervention rather than gradually escalating intensity, which fosters habituation.

Evolution of a Treatment Approach: Treatment Outcome Studies on Contingency Management and Substance Use Disorders

Early Contingency Management Applications

As is typical of treatment development, early reports on the use of CM to treat SUDs first appeared in the form of uncontrolled case studies in which, for example, smokers earned back portions of a monetary deposit contingent on remaining abstinent from smoking, amphetamine abusers earned retail items donated by community businesses contingent on drug abstinence, and individuals with chronic alcohol dependence earned coupon booklets contingent on submitting alcohol-negative breath specimens. A particularly impressive seminal controlled study in this area was reported by Miller (1975). In this study, 20 homeless men with severe alcohol dependence were randomly assigned to a control condition or to a CM intervention. Those in the control condition received the usual social services in the form of food, clothing, and housing, whereas those in the CM condition received those same services as long as they sustained abstinence, verified through breath alcohol testing and observation for signs of gross intoxication. Evidence of drinking resulted in a 5-day suspension from such services. Results showed that arrests for public drunkenness decreased and days of employment increased among those in the contingent condition compared with those in the control condition.

These impressive findings were not followed up in the published literature in any systematic manner, but CM began to be pursued as a treatment for other types of SUDs. Several controlled studies in the 1980s reported that abstinence levels increased when cigarette smokers had to submit monetary deposits that they earned back in portions contingent on remaining abstinent (e.g., Bowers et al. 1987). Other investigators reported controlled studies demonstrating that contingent cash payments increased abstinence from cigarette smoking (e.g., Stitzer and Bigelow 1982). Large-scale workplace and community incentive-based interventions for smoking cessation appeared in the 1980s; however, results from those interventions were not encouraging, most likely because of a failure by investigators to adhere to the points listed in the numbered list earlier in this chapter, especially the points regarding reinforcement magnitude and frequency in the monitoring of abstinence. (For a more detailed examination of CM and smoking, see a review by Sigmon et al. 2008.)

A particularly influential and programmatic series of controlled experimental studies was conducted with patients enrolled in methadone treatment for opiate dependence (see Stitzer et al. 1984). These studies firmly established the efficacy of using contingent positive reinforcement, such as access to clinic privileges (e.g., methadone take-home privileges), cash payments, and adjustments in methadone dose, for increasing abstinence from illicit drug use. For example, 10 patients who were receiving methadone maintenance treatment and who had consistently positive urine toxicology results for benzodiazepine use participated in a study using a within-subject reversal design (Stitzer et al. 1982). During a 12-week intervention period, patients earned 2 days of medication take-home privileges, a cash payment ($15), or a 20-mg methadone dose adjustment contingent on submitting benzodiazepine-negative urine toxicology results. Reinforcers were not available during the baseline periods that preceded and followed the intervention period. During the intervention period, 43% of specimens were benzodiazepine negative, compared with only 3.6% and 7.9% in the initial and final baseline periods.

These controlled studies from the 1980s provided a strong empirical foundation and clear proof-of-concept evidence for the development of CM as a formal treatment for SUDs. Other uncontrolled studies conducted with health care workers during this same period suggested that CM may be efficacious in treating cocaine dependence (e.g., Crowley 1985–1986), which was an important observation considering that cocaine dependence was emerging as a major public health concern in the United States when these studies were conducted. The cocaine epidemic caught drug abuse experts unprepared and created a strong need for effective treatments; however, many of the treatments that were examined, both behavioral and pharmacological, were ineffective. An exception was a CM intervention that has come to be known as voucher-based reinforcement therapy (VBRT).

Voucher-Based Reinforcement Therapy

Cocaine and Opiate Abuse

With VBRT, patients earn vouchers that are exchangeable for retail items, contingent on biochemically verified abstinence from recent drug use or meeting some other therapeutic target. The initial trials with VBRT integrated it with an intensive behavioral therapy known as the community reinforcement approach (CRA) and thus did not allow for inferences regarding what contributions VBRT was making to the positive outcomes obtained with the CRA plus VBRT intervention (Higgins et al. 1991). Nevertheless, the positive outcomes obtained with the CRA plus VBRT intervention were in such contrast with the many negative outcomes that were being reported in efforts to treat cocaine dependence that the combined intervention garnered a large amount of attention.

Inferences about the contributions of VBRT to research outcomes were made possible through a series of experiments in which 40 cocaine-dependent outpatients were randomly assigned to 24 weeks of CRA treatment, with half of the patients also receiving VBRT during weeks 1–12 (Higgins et al. 1994). Seventy-five percent of patients assigned to the VBRT condition were retained in treatment for the recommended 24 weeks, compared with only 40% in the condition without VBRT. Those who received VBRT achieved an average of 11.5+2.0 weeks of continuous cocaine abstinence, compared with only 6.0+1.5 weeks of abstinence by those not receiving VBRT. This trial demonstrated that VBRT increased treatment retention and cocaine abstinence among cocaine-dependent outpatients, a group for whom there were no reliably efficacious treatments. Subsequent randomized clinical trials conducted in this same clinic demonstrated the reliability of the treatment effects and showed that the positive effects of VBRT on cocaine abstinence remained discernible throughout the 2 years following treatment entry (e.g., Higgins et al. 2007).

Because the basic voucher schedule arrangement used in those original studies by Higgins et al. (1994) with cocaine-dependent outpatients became the prototype on which most subsequent VBRT interventions were based, we describe it in detail here. Urine specimens were collected during treatment weeks 1–12 and tested for benzoylecgonine, a cocaine metabolite. Specimens that tested negative for cocaine earned points that were recorded on vouchers, which were given to subjects. Each point was worth the equivalent of $0.25. The first specimen to test negative for cocaine per subject earned 10 points, or $2.50. The value of each subsequent consecutive cocaine-negative specimen increased by 5 points. The equivalent of a $10 bonus was provided for each three consecutive cocaine-negative specimens. The intent of the escalating magnitude of reinforcement and bonuses was to reinforce continuous cocaine abstinence. Cocaine-positive specimens or failure to submit a scheduled specimen reset the value of vouchers back to the initial $2.50 value. This feature was designed to punish relapse back to cocaine use following a period of sustained abstinence, with the intensity of the punishment tied directly to the length of sustained abstinence that would be broken. To provide patients with a reason to continue abstaining from use following a reset, submission of five consecutive cocaine-negative specimens following a cocaine-positive specimen returned the value of points to where it was prior to the reset. Points could not be lost once earned. Use of vouchers had to be approved by staff, who recommended patients use them to support the healthy lifestyle changes that were being encouraged as part of the CRA therapy they received. Of course, all purchases had to be legal and not involve alcohol, cigarettes, or firearms. Testing positive for drug use other than cocaine did not affect the voucher program or have any other programmed consequence.

Key to the successful development of VBRT was demonstrating that it was efficacious when used by other investigators and, even more important, demonstrating that it had efficacy with an inner-city population of cocaine abusers. The VBRT studies by Higgins and colleagues were conducted in Burlington, Vermont, a small metropolitan area in a largely rural state with an almost exclusively white population (Higgins et al. 1991, 1994). That patient population included a large proportion of intranasal cocaine users (such users generally have a better prognosis). The seminal study extending VBRT to the large, inner-city setting was a randomized, controlled trial conducted with 37 intravenous cocaine abusers enrolled in methadone maintenance treatment for opiate dependence (Silverman et al. 1996). The schedule arrangement in the experimental condition was largely the same as in the studies by Higgins et al. (1991, 1994), with patients assigned to 12 weeks of VBRT in which earning vouchers was contingent on cocaine abstinence. Those assigned to a noncontingent control condition earned vouchers in an amount and pattern that was yoked to the experimental condition but delivered independent of cocaine use. Those assigned to the abstinence-contingent voucher condition achieved significantly greater cocaine abstinence compared with those assigned to the control condition; for example, 47% of patients assigned to abstinence-contingent vouchers achieved between 7 and 12 weeks of continuous abstinence, compared with 0% in the noncontingent voucher control condition. Only one patient (6%) assigned to the noncontingent control condition achieved greater than 2 weeks of continuous cocaine abstinence. The results of this study provide compelling evidence supporting the generalizability of earlier findings about VBRT to inner-city populations and methadone patients. Other VBRT trials investigated the efficacy of VBRT in promoting abstinence from illicit opioid abuse (Silverman et al. 1996), demonstrated that the use of opioids sometimes decreased along with cocaine use when CM explicitly targeted only cocaine abstinence (Silverman et al. 1998), and supported the efficacy of increasing the magnitude of VBRT in order to promote a treatment response in recalcitrant cocaine abusers (e.g., Silverman et al. 1999).

Interest in and research on VBRT as a treatment for SUDs grew considerably after the first publication on that form of CM, extending use of the intervention to a wide range of different substances, populations, and settings. A meta-analysis by Lussier et al. (2006) on VBRT identified more than 60 reports of controlled studies published in peer-reviewed journals examining VBRT as a treatment for SUDs, with robust evidence supporting its efficacy. Figure 8–1 shows average effect sizes for VBRT across different drugs targeted by the intervention as well as potential moderator variables. No significant differences were noted across the different types of drug abuse targeted, although a clear trend toward smaller effect sizes when targeting multiple substances is discernible. The only drug for which the 95% confidence intervals overlapped with zero (suggesting no significant treatment effect) was alcohol, on which there was only a single study and thus larger variance. Analyses of potential moderator variables indicated that greater monetary value of potential daily earnings and immediate (same-day) versus delayed delivery of the voucher were associated with larger treatment effects.

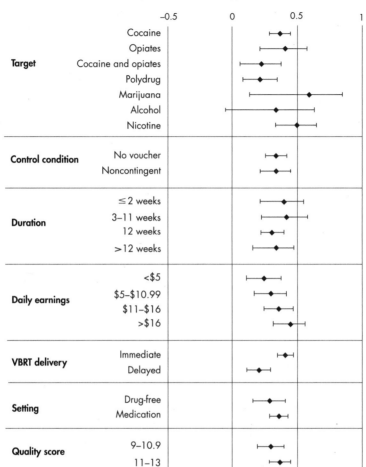

FIGURE 8–1. Estimated effect size (r) and 95% confidence intervals for voucher-based reinforcement therapy (VBRT) across variables.

Weighted average effect sizes and 95% confidence intervals for subsets of studies as a function of the moderator variables: target, control condition, duration, daily earnings, VBRT delivery immediacy, setting, and study quality. All studies targeted abstinence ($N=30$). Weighted average effect sizes are represented by closed diamonds and 95% confidence intervals by solid lines. Where confidence intervals do not overlap, differences between subsets of studies are significantly different at the 0.05 level.

Source. Reprinted from Lussier JP, Heil SH, Mongeon JA, et al.: "A Meta-Analysis of Voucher-Based Reinforcement Therapy for Substance Use Disorders." *Addiction* 101:192–203, 2006. Used with permission.

Building on the success of VBRT in reducing cocaine abuse among cocaine-dependent methadone patients, other studies were conducted demonstrating efficacy in reducing illicit opiate abuse in this population. In one such study, 120 methadone patients who continued to abuse heroin were randomly assigned to receive a methadone dose increase, abstinence-contingent vouchers (maximum earnings of $554 in 8 weeks), a combination of the methadone dose increase with abstinence-contingent vouchers, or continued treatment with a standard intervention technique. Contingent vouchers increased opiate abstinence significantly above the standard intervention, whereas the methadone dose increase did not. The combination treatment was equal to the vouchers-only condition, suggesting that it was the vouchers that produced the increases in abstinence (Preston et al. 2000).

Other Drugs of Abuse

As illustrated in Figure 8–1, VBRT has been extended to a broad range of different SUDs. For illustration purposes, we discuss here the extension to marijuana use disorders. Some thought CM would not be feasible in treating marijuana abuse because of the long half-life of tetrahydrocannabinol, which might be expected to result in too long a delay in being able to deliver contingent reinforcement for abstinence. Such concerns notwithstanding, VBRT has been successfully extended to outpatient treatment of marijuana dependence. For example, a study examining the addition of VBRT to a treatment of motivational enhancement and coping skills therapy increased end-of-treatment abstinence more than threefold compared with the motivational enhancement therapy alone or motivational therapy plus coping skills (Budney et al. 2000).

Fishbowl Procedure

Petry et al. (2000) developed a variation of VBRT designed to lower cost without losing efficacy. In this procedure, rather than having each occurrence of the target response reinforced, patients earned the opportunity to draw from a fishbowl that contained vouchers of varying value, including many that were of zero value but offered verbal praise, some that were of relatively low monetary value (e.g., $1), still fewer of moderate value ($20), and a very few of high monetary value ($100). Instead of exchanging these vouchers for the opportunity to make retail purchases in the community, patients chose among prize items already available at the clinic. Importantly, this modified arrangement has been demonstrated to be efficacious for increasing cocaine and opioid abstinence in drug-free and methadone community clinics; however, there is no evidence that this more complex schedule arrangement results in better outcomes than the more conventional voucher program that uses vouchers of lower value. In the only direct comparison of the fishbowl and conventional voucher programs offered at comparable values, both methods improved outcomes above a control condition, and no significant difference was found between the fishbowl and conventional voucher programs (Petry et al. 2005a).

The important contributions of the development of the fishbowl procedure are that it is less costly than the original VBRT intervention and it is efficacious, giving it a better likelihood than more expensive arrangements of being adopted by community clinics, in which cost concerns are an important priority. The likelihood of its increased use seems certain given the results obtained in two multisite trials conducted in community clinics as part of the National Institute on Drug Abuse Clinical Trials Network, in which the procedure was shown to improve outcomes of stimulant abusers enrolled in drug-free (Petry et al. 2005b) and methadone (Peirce et al. 2006) clinics. There is no evidence that lowering costs with this fishbowl arrangement gets around the relationship between treatment effect size and reinforcement magnitude in VBRT interventions. Indeed, as expected, effect sizes obtained with the fishbowl intervention appear to be smaller than those achieved with more expensive VBRT interventions in comparable populations (Lussier et al. 2006).

Treating Special Populations

Identifying effective treatments for special populations of individuals with SUDs is an important challenge, and another important development of VBRT is its extension to the treatment of such populations (for a review, see Higgins et al. 2008). The application of VBRT in treating pregnant smokers provides an excellent example of this extension of VBRT. Maternal cigarette smoking is a leading preventable cause of poor pregnancy outcome and pediatric morbidity. Effective interventions for promoting smoking cessation among pregnant women are available, but only about 15% of women who receive them actually quit smoking. Controlled trials indicated that VBRT could increase quit rates to more than 30%. In one of these trials, VBRT was studied with 58 women who were still smoking upon entering prenatal care and were assigned to either contingent or noncontingent voucher conditions (Higgins et al. 2004b). In the contingent condition, vouchers were earned for biochemically verified smoking abstinence; in the noncontingent condition, vouchers were earned independent of smoking status. Contingent vouchers significantly increased abstinence over noncontingent vouchers at the end-of-pregnancy (37%

vs. 9%) and at 12-week postpartum (33% vs. 0%) assessments. The effect of contingent vouchers remained significant at the 24-week postpartum assessment (27% vs. 0%), which was 12 weeks after discontinuation of the voucher program. The magnitude of these treatment effects exceeds levels typically observed with pregnant and postpartum smokers. These promising results were replicated in a randomized clinical trial comparing these same treatment conditions, as well as sonographic estimates of fetal growth (Heil et al. 2008). Smoking abstinence rates were again several orders of magnitude greater in the contingent than in the noncontingent condition, and estimated fetal weight gain, femur length, and abdominal circumference were significantly greater in the contingent than in the noncontingent condition as well. The following case vignette illustrates this intervention involving a woman treated in the contingent condition.

> **Vicki** was a 38-year-old white woman who was still smoking upon entering prenatal care in a community obstetrics clinic. She was conscientious and entered prenatal care at approximately 8 weeks gestation. Upon learning that she was a current smoker, study staff invited her to participate in a study on behavioral interventions to assist pregnant women to quit smoking. She accepted and was assigned to the contingent condition. Vicki was particularly concerned about her smoking because she had been a regular cigarette smoker since age 13 years, had smoked throughout her one prior pregnancy, and was still smoking approximately 20 cigarettes daily since learning of the current pregnancy several weeks earlier. In the way of sociodemographics, she was divorced, had completed 14 years of education, and was currently employed but without private health insurance. Smoking status was verified using breath carbon monoxide level during the initial week of the cessation effort and urine cotinine thereafter.
>
> Vicki had an excellent outcome. She was continuously abstinent throughout the remainder of her pregnancy and sustained abstinence through the last follow-up assessment conducted at 6 months postpartum, 3 months after the incentive program was discontinued. No women with a comparable level of heavy smoking quit in the noncontingent condition. Regarding birth outcomes, Vicki's baby was delivered at 39.2 weeks gestational age and weighed 3,910 g, both well beyond the risk for preterm delivery (<37 weeks) and low birth weight (<2,500 g) associated with smoking during pregnancy. The birth outcomes also exceeded levels observed among mothers treated in the control condition, in which the vast majority (90%) of mothers smoked throughout the pregnancy, with mean gestational age at delivery of 38.3±0.3 weeks and birth weight of 3,086±70.6 g. Despite a prior history of smoking while pregnant and a relatively high rate of daily smoking after learning of the pregnancy, Vicki successfully quit smoking, delivered a healthy baby, and looked to be on her way to sustaining longer-term abstinence.

Another example of extending this treatment approach to special populations is a study in which Krishnan-Sarin et al. (2008) used VBRT to promote smoking cessation among adolescents. Twenty-eight adolescent smokers participated in a 1-month, school-based smoking cessation program in which they were randomly assigned to receive either cognitive-behavioral therapy (CBT) alone or CM combined with weekly CBT. In the CM plus CBT group, biochemical verification of abstinence was obtained twice daily during the first 2 weeks, followed by daily appointments during the third week and appointments once every other day during the fourth week. Participants earned monetary reinforcement contingent on abstinence. At the end of weeks 1 and 4 , abstinence verified using quantitative urine cotinine levels was higher in participants in the CM plus CBT group (week 1: 76.7%; week 4: 53.0%) compared with those receiving CBT alone (week 1: 7.2%; week 4: 0%).

Improving CM Interventions: Initial Treatment Response and Longer-Term Outcomes

Although the treatment effects obtained with CM are impressive, often 50% or more of treated patients do not have positive outcomes. The 10-point list provided earlier in this chapter, under "Basic Elements of Contingency Management," represents what is known about how to increase treatment response. Using a higher magnitude of reinforcement, minimizing delay in reinforcement delivery, targeting one response rather than multiple responses, and monitoring abstinence more frequently are all associated with larger treatment effects (Lussier et al. 2006). The parameter for which there is the greatest amount of evidence, including experimental evidence and results from meta-analyses, is reinforcement magnitude (e.g., Higgins et al. 2007; Silverman et al. 1999).

Regarding longer-term outcomes, several studies have shown that VBRT effects on abstinence sometimes last for as long as 21 months following discontinuation of the intervention (e.g., Higgins et al. 2007). However, many patients exposed to VBRT or other CM interventions resume drug use following discontinuation of the intervention. Identifying ways to sustain treatment effects over time is a priority with CM just as it is with virtually all treatments for SUDs. A number of trials have investigated combining VBRT with relapse prevention therapy, but there is no evidence that this combination extends treatment effects beyond those obtained with VBRT alone (Rawson et al. 2002).

Another avenue being pursued is use of VBRT to increase the proportion of patients who achieve a sustained period of abstinence during treatment. This approach grew out of observations in studies in which

VBRT effects that were sustained during posttreatment follow-up were compared with effects of control treatments. In those studies, the probability of posttreatment abstinence during follow-up increased as a function of the duration of continuous abstinence achieved during treatment to a comparable extent in the VBRT and control treatments (e.g., Higgins et al. 2007).

Knowing that greater reinforcement magnitude produces larger effects during the treatment period, Higgins et al. (2007) conducted a randomized clinical trial to see if posttreatment outcomes could be increased as well by increasing reinforcement magnitude. In this study, 100 cocaine-dependent adults were randomly assigned to receive treatment based on either CRA plus VBRT set at a relatively high monetary value (maximal value=$1,995/12 weeks) or CRA plus VBRT set at a relatively low monetary value (maximal value=$499/12 weeks). The high-value vouchers were used to test the concept and not with the idea that they would have direct practical application. Earning vouchers was contingent on cocaine-negative urinalysis results during the initial 12 weeks of the 24-week outpatient treatment. Results indicated that increasing the voucher value significantly increased the duration of continuous cocaine abstinence achieved during treatment, and, as hypothesized, point prevalence cocaine abstinence assessed every 3 months throughout an 18-month posttreatment follow-up period was greater in the high-value than in the low-value voucher condition (Figure 8–2). As in prior studies, the duration of abstinence achieved during treatment predicted posttreatment abstinence, although that relationship weakened over time. Overall, increasing the value of abstinence-contingent incentives during the initial 12 weeks of treatment represented an effective method for increasing during-treatment and longer-term cocaine abstinence, although the positive association of during-treatment abstinence with longer-term outcome dissipated over time. This is a research avenue that will continue to be evaluated.

Dawn was a 33-year-old community resident who presented for treatment at an outpatient research clinic for cocaine dependence after testing positive for drug use when applying for a new job and consequently being turned down for the position. She was currently residing with a live-in boyfriend and her 14-year-old daughter. She reported that the boyfriend encouraged treatment following the aforementioned incident. Dawn had a long-standing history of cocaine and alcohol dependence, being a regular cocaine user since age 17 and a regular drinker since age 16. She primarily used the intranasal route of cocaine administration, using about 1 g per episode of use, and always concurrent with alcohol. She has an extensive family history of substance abuse, and the family, including the

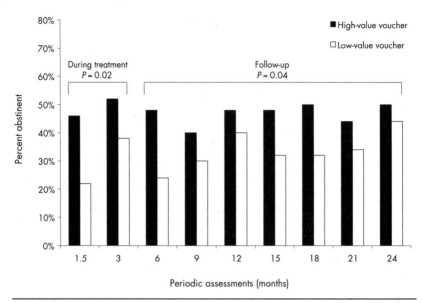

FIGURE 8–2. **Periodic abstinence assessments.**

Percentages of participants abstinent at each of the periodic assessments conducted with subjects retained in treatment as well as dropouts. Data points represent point prevalence abstinence at the respective assessments. Abstinence was defined as a self-report of no cocaine use in the past 30 days and cocaine-negative urinalysis results. In categorical modeling, abstinence levels were significantly higher in the high-value than low-value voucher conditions, based on assessments during treatment (1.5 and 3.0 months, $P=0.02$) and follow-up (6- through 24-month assessments, $P=0.04$).

Source. Reprinted from Higgins ST, Heil SH, Dantona R, et al.: "Effects of Varying the Monetary Value of Voucher-Based Incentives on Abstinence Achieved During and Following Treatment Among Cocaine-Dependent Outpatients." *Addiction* 102:271–281, 2007. Used with permission.

patient, has owned and worked in bar settings. She reported using cocaine eight times in the 30 days prior to treatment entry. In her one prior treatment experience in this same clinic, 8 years earlier, she received the same treatment but with the usual voucher value ($997.50 maximum earnings across 12 weeks) and had a relatively poor outcome (maximum of 4 weeks of continuous abstinence).

With the higher voucher value, Dawn had an excellent response to treatment, which was sustained through 2 years of posttreatment follow-up. She was continuously abstinent from cocaine throughout the 24 weeks of treatment, during which time she also was compliant with disulfiram therapy for alcohol dependence and abstained from drinking as well. She regularly attended self-help meetings, developed new friendships with healthy people, reinitiated contact with healthy family members, developed new recreational activities, and worked regularly as a cosmetologist. At a final assessment conducted 2 years after treatment entry, she was still cocaine abstinent and showing substantial improvement from baseline in almost all areas of functioning. Comparing her intake to follow-up composite scores on the Addiction Severity Index captures that sustained improvement quite nicely: Drug, 0.22 to 0.02; Alcohol, 0.59 to 0.06; Employment, 0.21 to 0.13; Medical, 0.92 to 0.00; Family/Social, 0.69 to 0.20; and Psychiatric, 0.47 to 0.14. She had no legal problems at any assessment. This profile shows a broad and stable improvement in Dawn's cocaine and alcohol dependence and related areas of functioning.

Silverman et al. (2004) conducted a seminal study examining the use of VBRT as a maintenance intervention. This study examined whether long-term abstinence reinforcement could maintain cocaine abstinence throughout a 1-year period. Patients who injected drugs and used cocaine during methadone treatment (N=78) were randomly assigned to one of two abstinence-reinforcement groups or to a usual-care control group. Participants in the two abstinence-reinforcement groups could earn take-home methadone doses for providing opiate- and cocaine-free urine samples; the participants in one of those groups could also earn $5,800 in vouchers for providing cocaine-free urine samples over 52 weeks. Both abstinence-reinforcement interventions increased cocaine abstinence, but the addition of the voucher intervention resulted in the largest and most sustained abstinence (Figure 8–3). Indeed, those patients in the condition with take-home doses and VBRT who achieved a period of continuous cocaine abstinence often sustained it through the duration of the voucher program and beyond. Patients in the other treatment conditions rarely achieved comparable levels of sustained abstinence. The study provided proof of the concept that VBRT could be a highly effective maintenance intervention for cocaine abstinence in methadone-treated patients.

Dissemination: Community Drug Abuse Treatment Programs

Cost is an important obstacle when considering dissemination of CM into community substance abuse treatment clinics, and there have been encouraging developments in this area. The positive outcomes obtained in the multisite trials using the fishbowl procedure are quite promising and are likely to facilitate successful dissemination (Peirce et al. 2006; Petry et al. 2005b). The New York City Health and Hospitals Corporation, the largest provider of public treatment for substance abuse in New York City, launched low-cost CM programs in five of its community substance abuse treatment clinics that were supported through public funds (Kellogg et al. 2005). In an initiative that received broad media coverage (e.g., Ornstein 2005), the San Francisco Department of Public Health

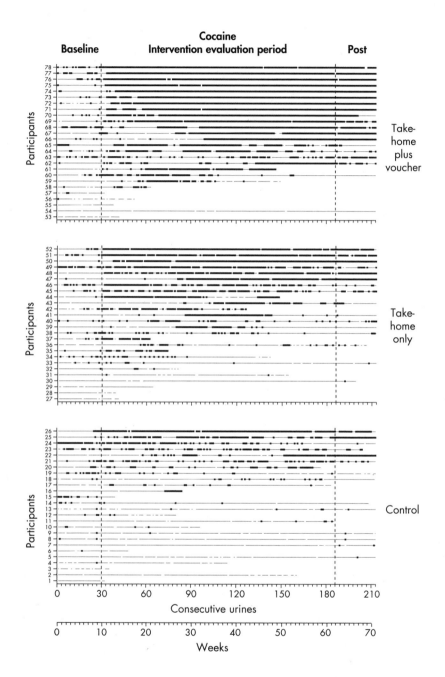

FIGURE 8–3. **Cocaine urinalysis results across consecutive urine samples for individual participants in each of the three experimental conditions *(opposite page).***

Top, middle, and bottom panels represent data for the take-home plus voucher, take-home only, and usual-care control conditions, respectively. The vertical dashed lines divide each panel into three periods, the baseline (left), the intervention (center), and the postintervention (right) periods. Within each panel, horizontal lines represent the cocaine urinalysis results for individual participants across the consecutive scheduled urine collections of the study. The heavy portion of each line represents cocaine-negative urinalysis results, the thin portions of each line represent cocaine-positive urinalysis results, and the blank portions represent missing urine samples. Within each panel, participants are arranged from those showing the least abstinence (fewest cocaine-negative urine samples) on the bottom of the panel to participants with the most abstinence on the top. The numerals on the ordinates represent participant identification numbers.

Source. Reprinted from Silverman K, Robles E, Mudric T, et al.: "A Randomized Trial of Long-Term Reinforcement of Cocaine Abstinence in Methadone-Maintained Patients Who Inject Drugs." *Journal of Consulting and Clinical Psychology* 72:839–854, 2004. Used with permission.

established a VBRT program for gay and bisexual methamphetamine abusers, demonstrating how acute public health need can sometimes surmount cost concerns.

Another strategy is to integrate existing community services into CM arrangements. Two programs offer exciting examples of how this can be done effectively. In one program for patients with SUDs and serious mental illness, the CM program is built around patients' Social Security disability benefits (Ries et al. 2004). The clinic serves as the designated payee, and patients gain progressively greater control over the use of those benefits contingent on verified abstinence from drug use.

Another exciting program is being conducted as part of the U.S. Department of Veterans Affairs Compensated Work Therapy program, which provides veterans who have chronic employment problems access to paid training and supported paid employment. Perhaps not surprisingly, SUDs are an important problem in these programs. Drebing et al. (2007) demonstrated how VBRT can be used to increase abstinence as well as job-seeking and job placement activities in that setting. As we mentioned above, in what is without question the largest-scale contingency management effort ever, contingent cash incentives are being used to promote healthy behavior change in antipoverty programs involving many millions of families across the globe (Lagarde et al. 2007).

Workplaces offer important opportunities to arrange abstinence reinforcement opportunities because of the resources that they control in the form of wages and benefits. Silverman et al. (2002) developed a model referred to as the *therapeutic workplace* that is designed to treat chronically unemployed adults. This program has been evaluated with pregnant and recently postpartum women who were continuing to abuse cocaine and heroin despite being enrolled in methadone treatment. Forty women were randomly assigned either to the therapeutic workplace or to usual care. For those assigned to the therapeutic workplace, daily entry into the work setting was contingent on verified abstinence from cocaine and opiate use, and once in the program they earned vouchers contingent on job performance. The intervention was in place for several years, with significantly more women in the therapeutic workplace abstinent from cocaine and opiates than those in usual care (30% vs. 5%) during year 3 (Silverman et al. 2002). More recent adaptations of the therapeutic workplace have included both genders (Silverman et al. 2007). Volpp et al. (2009) successfully implemented an impressive CM-based smoking-cessation intervention in a large corporate setting.

The emergence of the U.S. drug court system holds tremendous promise for the successful dissemination of CM into mainstream rehabilitation for SUDs (see Marlowe and Wong 2008). Drug courts are themselves an explicit CM program wherein reinforcers and punishers, termed *incentives* and *sanctions* within the drug court literature, are used to systematically leverage nonviolent criminals with SUDs to obtain the treatment they need. It is difficult to imagine a better setting in which to successfully disseminate CM practices. In the United Kingdom, feasibility studies are being undertaken to investigate nationwide implementation of voucher-based CM for treatment of SUDs in community substance abuse treatment clinics (Pilling et al. 2007).

Conclusion

CM treatments have developed in many exciting directions during the past two decades and represent an important part of evidence-based treatments for SUDs. The varied CM applications outlined in this chapter demonstrate the relevance of basic principles of behavioral science to the treatment of SUDs, the striking effectiveness and versatility of CM interventions, and the feasibility of disseminating these interventions in society, both through community treatment clinics and through other settings, such as workplaces, the Veterans Affairs hospital system, and drug courts. Despite the promise of CM interventions suggested in this extensive body of research, the research reviewed in this chapter also shows that more work is needed to find ways to increase the effectiveness of the interventions so that they will succeed with even more patients, to develop methods that will ensure longer-term maintenance of beneficial effects over time, and to continue to develop and refine practical applications that will be used widely in society. Thus, we have outlined in this chapter the impressive effectiveness and promise of CM interventions, as well as the areas in which additional research and more development are needed.

As is amply shown in the research reviewed in this chapter, CM interventions are not a bag of arbitrary tricks but rather an orderly set of procedures that are based on fundamental principles of behavioral science. Further improvement and development of these procedures can be guided by the basic scientific principles on which the interventions are based. The broad success the field has achieved to date in applying these basic principles to treat SUDs across populations, drugs, and settings should give great confidence that CM interventions can continue to be developed and improved to address the costly and devastating consequences of SUDs.

Key Clinical Concepts

- Contingency management (CM) is based on an extensive basic science literature that demonstrates an important role for operant conditioning in the genesis and maintenance of drug use.

- CM is an efficacious intervention for a wide range of different types of substance use disorders and populations.

- CM has some basic features, outlined in the section "Basic Elements of Contingency Management," that are important to effective implementation.

Suggested Reading

Higgins ST, Silverman K, Heil SH (eds): Contingency Management in the Treatment of Substance Use Disorders. New York, Guilford, 2008

References

Bechara A: Decision making, impulse control, and loss of willpower to resist drugs: a neurocognitive perspective. Nat Neurosci 8:1458–1463, 2005

Bickel WK, Miller ML, Yi R, et al: Behavioral and neuroeconomics of drug addiction: competing neural systems and temporal discounting processes. Drug Alcohol Depend 90 (suppl 1):S85–S91, 2007

Bigelow G, Griffiths R, Liebson I: Experimental models for the modification of human drug self-administration: methodological developments in the study of ethanol self-administration by alcoholics. Fed Proc 34:1785–1792, 1975

Bowers TG, Winett RA, Frederiksen LW: Nicotine fading, behavioral contracting, and extended treatment: effects on smoking cessation. Addict Behav 12:181–184, 1987

Budney A, Higgins ST, Radonovich KJ, et al: Adding voucher-based incentives to coping skills and motivational enhancement improves outcomes during treatment for marijuana dependence. J Consult Clin Psychol 68:1051–1061, 2000

Crowley TJ: Doctors' drug abuse reduced during contingency-contracting treatment. Alcohol Drug Res 6:299–307, 1985–1986

Drebing CE, Van Ormer EA, Mueller L, et al: Adding contingency management intervention to vocational rehabilitation: outcomes for dually diagnosed veterans. J Rehabil Res Dev 44:851–865, 2007

Heil SH, Higgins ST, Bernstein IM, et al: Effects of voucher-based incentives on abstinence from cigarette smoking and fetal growth among pregnant women. Addiction 103:1009–1018, 2008

Higgins ST: Comments on contingency management and conditional cash transfers. Health Econ Aug 7, 2009 [Epub ahead of print]

Higgins ST, Delaney DD, Budney AJ, et al: A behavioral approach to achieving initial cocaine abstinence. Am J Psychiatry 148:1218–1224, 1991

Higgins ST, Budney AJ, Bickel WK, et al: Incentives improve outcome in outpatient behavioral treatment of cocaine dependence. Arch Gen Psychiatry 51:568–576, 1994

Higgins ST, Heil SH, Lussier JP: Clinical implications of reinforcement as a determinant of substance use disorders. Annu Rev Psychol 55:431–461, 2004a

Higgins ST, Heil SH, Solomon LJ, et al: A pilot study on voucher-based incentives to promote abstinence from cigarette smoking during pregnancy and postpartum. Nicotine Tob Res 6:1015–1020, 2004b

Higgins ST, Heil SH, Dantona R, et al: Effects of varying the monetary value of voucher-based incentives on abstinence achieved during and following treatment among cocaine-dependent outpatients. Addiction 102:271–281, 2007

Higgins ST, Heil SH, Rogers RE, et al: Cocaine, in Contingency Management in the Treatment of Substance Use Disorders. Edited by Higgins ST, Silverman K, Heil SH. New York, Guilford, 2008, pp 19–41

Kellogg SH, Burns M, Coleman P, et al: Something of value: the introduction of contingency management interventions into the New York City Health and Hospital Addiction Treatment Service. J Subst Abuse Treat 28:57–65, 2005

Krishnan-Sarin S, Duhig A, Cavallo D: Adolescents, in Contingency Management in the Treatment of Substance Use Disorders. Edited by Higgins ST, Silverman K, Heil SH. New York, Guilford, 2008, pp 222–240

Lagarde M, Haines A, Palmer N: Conditional cash transfers for improving uptake of health interventions in low- and middle-income countries: a systematic review. JAMA 298:1900–1910, 2007

Lussier JP, Heil SH, Mongeon JA, et al: A meta-analysis of voucher-based reinforcement therapy for substance use disorders. Addiction 101:192–203, 2006

Marlowe DB, Wong CJ: Contingency management in the adult criminal drug courts, in Contingency Management in the Treatment of Substance Use Disorders. Edited by Higgins ST, Silverman K, Heil SH. New York, Guilford, 2008, pp 298–333

Miller PM: A behavioral intervention program for chronic public drunkenness offenders. Arch Gen Psychiatry 32:915–918, 1975

Ornstein C: Quitting meth pays off. Los Angeles Times, November 14, 2005. Available at: http://articles.latimes.com/2005/nov/14/local/me-meth14. Accessed March 3, 2010.

Peirce JM, Petry NM, Stitzer ML, et al: Effects of lower-cost incentives on stimulant abstinence in methadone maintenance treatment: a National Drug Abuse Treatment Clinical Trials Network study. Arch Gen Psychiatry 63:201–208, 2006

Petry NM, Martin B, Cooney JL, et al: Give them prizes, and they will come: contingency management for treatment of alcohol dependence. J Consult Clin Psychol 68:250–257, 2000

Petry NM, Alessi SM, Marx J, et al: Vouchers versus prizes: contingency management treatment of substance abusers in community settings. J Consult Clin Psychol 73:1005–1014, 2005a

Petry NM, Peirce JM, Stitzer ML, et al: Effect of prize-based incentives on outcomes in stimulant abusers in outpatient psychosocial treatment programs: a National Drug Abuse Treatment Clinical Trials Network study. Arch Gen Psychiatry 62:1148–1156, 2005b

Pilling S, Strang J, Gerada C: Psychosocial interventions and opioid detoxification for drug misuse: summary of NICE guidance. BMJ 335:203–205, 2007

Preston KL, Umbricht A, Epstein DH: Methadone dose increase and abstinence reinforcement for treatment of continued heroin use during methadone maintenance. Arch Gen Psychiatry 57:395–404, 2000

Rawson RA, Huber A, McCann M, et al: A comparison of contingency management and cognitive-behavioral approaches during methadone maintenance treatment for cocaine dependence. Arch Gen Psychiatry 59:817–824, 2002

Ries RK, Dyck DG, Short R, et al: Outcomes of managing disability benefits among patients with substance dependence and severe mental illness. Psychiatr Serv 55:445–447, 2004

Sigmon SC, Lamb R, Dallery J: Tobacco, in Contingency Management in the Treatment of Substance Use Disorders. Edited by Higgins ST, Silverman K, Heil SH. New York, Guilford, 2008, pp 99–119

Silverman K, Higgins ST, Brooner RK, et al: Sustained cocaine abstinence in methadone maintenance patients through voucher-based reinforcement therapy. Arch Gen Psychiatry 53:409–415, 1996

Silverman K, Wong CJ, Umbricht-Schneiter A, et al: Broad beneficial effects of cocaine abstinence reinforcement among methadone patients. J Consult Clin Psychol 66:811–824, 1998

Silverman K, Chutuape MA, Bigelow GE, et al: Voucher-based reinforcement of cocaine abstinence in treatment-resistant methadone patients: effects of reinforcement magnitude. Psychopharmacology (Berl) 146:128–138, 1999

Silverman K, Svikis D, Wong CJ, et al: A reinforcement-based therapeutic workplace for the treatment of drug abuse: three-year abstinence outcomes. Exp Clin Psychopharmacol 10:228–240, 2002

Silverman K, Robles E, Mudric T, et al: A randomized trial of long-term reinforcement of cocaine abstinence in methadone-maintained patients who inject drugs. J Consult Clin Psychol 72:839–854, 2004

Silverman K, Wong CJ, Needham M, et al: A randomized trial of employment-based reinforcement of cocaine abstinence in injection drug users. J Appl Behav Anal 40:387–410, 2007

Stitzer ML, Bigelow GE: Contingent reinforcement for reduced carbon monoxide levels in cigarette smokers. Addict Behav 7:403–412, 1982

Stitzer ML, Bigelow GE, Liebson IA, et al: Contingent reinforcement for benzodiazepine-free urines: evaluation of a drug abuse treatment intervention. J Appl Behav Anal 15:493–503, 1982

Stitzer ML, Bigelow GE, Liebson IA, et al: Contingency management of supplemental drug use during methadone maintenance treatment. NIDA Res Monogr 46:84–103, 1984

Volpp KG, Troxel AB, Pauly MV, et al: A randomized, controlled trial of financial incentives for smoking cessation. N Engl J Med 360:699–709, 2009

Yoon JH, Higgins ST, Heil SH, et al: Delay discounting predicts postpartum relapse to cigarette smoking among pregnant women. Exp Clin Psychopharmacol 15:176–186, 2007

9 | Psychodynamic Psychotherapy

Hallie A. Lightdale, M.D.
Avram H. Mack, M.D.
Richard J. Frances, M.D.

Psychoanalytic and psychodynamic theories are fundamental to modern psychiatric practice, including addiction treatment. Although some investigators have argued that psychodynamic treatment has only a minor role in the treatment of substance abuse (Vaillant 2005), others have shown how psychodynamic understanding can add depth to work with individuals and groups, further the rehabilitation process (Dodes and Khantzian 2004; Frances et al. 1989; Khantzian and Albanese 2008), and increase the usefulness of 12-step programs (Dodes 1988). For many patients, self-medication with addictive substances plays a part in the move to dependence. Relapsing patients understand better what affects they are seeking, but alternative approaches to relief from suffering are of help to patients. In a transtheoretical integrated treatment model, understanding of psychodynamic principles can be used by the therapist to help the addicted patient recognize that he or she has a problem and then to identify what might provide effective motivation for that individual to change. This approach helps patients in actualizing their wish to change by helping them move along the continuum from contemplation of a problem, such as smoking, to contemplation of the need for change, to taking action and then maintaining abstinence. In addition, memory and transference from past relationships into the current therapeutic interaction are an inevitable part of the treatment process, and understanding one's resistance to treatment is a tool for change.

Neurobiological approaches, including pharmacotherapy, can be fruitfully combined with psychodynamic approaches. Psychodynamics integrated with neurobiological models of addiction provide a deeper understanding of the patient and the factors that might help a particular patient to change. From a neurobiological perspective, psychotherapy can be understood as a controlled form of learning that occurs in the context of a therapeutic relationship (Etkin et al. 2005) and that may produce alterations of gene expression and thereby alter neurobiology. Studies of basal brain metabolism and blood flow as well as studies of stimulus-response imaging have demonstrated that psychotherapy produces changes in the brains of patients who have been diagnosed with anxiety and mood disorders; some of these changes may be shared with those induced by pharmacotherapy, and others may be modality specific (Etkin et al. 2005). This is one avenue by which psychodynamic and neurobiological issues can be explored in tandem.

The following case illustrates how important it is for the clinician to have the capacity to approach substance misuse from a psychodynamic perspective.

> **Sabrina** was a 25-year-old graduate student who presented with anxiety after failing a major exam. She had been abusing cannabis daily for years, and she drank alcohol daily, with multiple binges per month (often with blackouts). She felt that anxiety had prevented her from studying for and passing the exam. She described a strong family history of alcohol dependence. Initially, she denied substance use was problematic and refused urine drug testing, stating that a positive test could damage her career.
>
> From the first meeting, it was clear that Sabrina had in mind a secondary gain: the opportunity to retake her exam required the provision of special educational accommodations. Getting the psychiatrist to support her request for accommodations was the main initial reason that she engaged in psychotherapy and helped her to remain in therapy as the initial sessions focused on confrontation of her substance abuse problem. The focus of the first six sessions was on taking a thorough history, and on reframing Sabrina's substance abuse (rather than anxiety) as her primary problem. She reflected on how her father's alcohol dependence had affected her, and she began to speak about her ambivalence toward her father. In a following session, she made a connection between this ambivalence and her current relationship with her boyfriend, who was her cannabis source. She observed that she always used alcohol with her father or family and cannabis with her boyfriend, and that the substance was a focal point of gatherings with both. After identifying these connections, Sabrina was able to agree to a trial of abstinence from cannabis for 1 week; she failed the trial, and was able to discuss how frightened that failure made her.
>
> Over the next 2 months, Sabrina reduced her cannabis and alcohol abuse to a controlled-use pattern and began to negotiate with the goal of abstinence. After retaking and passing the exam, she was able to recognize that she habitually used other people for secondary gain, and that she had difficulty with intimacy and trust in relationships. Working

through this issue helped her form a solid therapeutic alliance and increased her motivation for change.

Our approach, as highlighted in Sabrina's case, is that psychodynamic principles are a set of skills, knowledge, and attitudes that may be used in selected dimensions of the care of individuals who misuse substances, regardless of the actual psychotherapeutic modality. In this chapter, we review some basics of the psychodynamic approach in general and then specific to substance misuse. This is followed by a guide to the application of psychodynamic concepts in addiction treatment, including indications and contraindications, and a discussion of how psychoanalytic theory can be used to enhance standard treatment techniques and deepen understanding of addiction treatment.

Review of Psychodynamics and Addiction

Classical and Early Psychoanalysis

Psychodynamic treatment is based on Sigmund Freud's work in discovering the importance of unconscious phenomena; on his development of a theory of the relationship between id, ego, and superego, with an emphasis on resistance, defenses, and conflict; and on his use of techniques such as free association, clarification, and interpretation. Childhood experience, dreams, memory, and other aspects of development are important to understanding emotional problems in dynamic theory. Freud (1905/1953), Abraham (1908/1960), and Radó (1933/1984) each posited trauma-related developmental issues—including orality, regression toward infantile fixations, defenses against homosexuality, sexual and social inferiority, emotional immaturity, depressive tendencies, and insecurity—as psychopathological pathways leading to substance abuse (Lorand 1948). Freud (1930/1964) also connected the elation of intoxication, which he believed relaxed superego repression, to manic states. Glover (1932/1956) noted the important role of aggressive drives in substance abuse.

Modern Psychoanalysis and Psychodynamics

As the focus of psychoanalytic theory has moved from drives to developmental and structural deficits and affective experience, psychoanalytic approaches to addictions have been redrawn as well. A number of theorists have contributed important ideas on the role of ego defenses, defense deficit, and affective experience in drug abuse and alcoholism. Although each authority may have focused his or her work on a particular facet of psychodynamic theory, the modern clinician integrates these ideas as they best apply to individual patients. In the following subsections, we review many of these positions.

Alexithymia and Affective Dysregulation

Affective regulation has been a major area of interest among those studying the psychodynamics of addiction. Krystal (1982–1983) emphasized a defective stimulus barrier, resulting from early psychic trauma, and the attempt to use substances to fortify against the onslaught of overwhelming affects. He described the inability of patients to label affects, which he called *alexithymia*, and the inability of addicted individuals to verbalize affective states. McDougall (1984) focused on drug use as a dispersion of affects into action. Lewis (1987) highlighted pathological shame, affecting one's core sense of self, as an affect associated with substance abuse. Dodes and Khantzian (2004) emphasized the addicted individual's sense of helplessness and powerlessness, often in the face of intolerable affects, and the drive to restore through drug use a sense of power and control to which the individual feels entitled. In this perspective, the goal of substance use is pharmacological control or change of one's affective state.

Psychosexual Development

Addictions have also been explained in terms of fixation or delay of psychosexual development. Krystal (1982–1983) described an inability in addicted individuals to take over the internal maternal functions associated with care of the self. Bean-Bayog (1988) described the addiction itself and the resultant loss of control as a sort of severe psychic trauma that leads to characteristic defensive patterns. Wurmser (1984) and Meissner (1986) emphasized narcissistic collapse as a cause of substance use: individuals use substances to compensate for a punctured grandiose or idealized self. According to Wurmser (1984), feelings of emptiness, boredom, rage, shame, depression, and guilt are symptoms of narcissistic wounds and superego regression, which prompt substance use. He further characterized addiction as self-medication for claustrophobia, a feeling of being trapped, with substance use becoming a means of escape. These authors stressed the severity of psychopathology underlying drug dependence. Silber (1974) emphasized the alcoholic individual's pathological identification with destructive or psychotic parents.

Object Relations and Self Psychology

Both object relations and self psychology perspectives have been applied to addictions. Some authors have attempted to analyze the substance itself, framing alcohol as a fetish object (Keller 1992), or have described alcohol abuse in terms of falling in love with the reward state of intoxication (DuPont 1998). Kohut and Wolf (1978) considered substance problems as narcissistic behavior disorders, in that the drugs serve as substitute idealized selfobjects for selfobjects missing developmentally in addicted individuals. Kernberg (1991) described addictive behavior as a reunion with a forgiving parent, an activation of "all good" selfobject images, and a gratification of instinctual needs. Kernberg (1991) identified subsets of addicted individuals with malignant narcissism, which is associated with strong antisocial features.

Self-Medication Hypothesis

Although the questions of primary and secondary effects of alcoholism were originally raised by Hippocrates more than 2,000 years ago, they were raised again in 1911, when Bleuler (1911/1921) hypothesized that drinking was often the cause of neurotic disturbances and that clinicians should not be taken in by the "stupid excuses" of heavy drinkers. Ferenczi (1912/1916) and Freud and Ferenczi (1908–1914/1993), on the other hand, viewed alcoholism as an "escape into narcosis" from underlying psychodynamic causes. The self-medication hypothesis originated from this theory.

The self-medication hypothesis evolved starting in the 1970s and is based on observations of patients with dual diagnoses. Theorists such as Wieder and Kaplan (1969), Milkman and Frosch (1973), and Khantzian (1997) have discussed the importance of the specific effects of particular drugs on affect and the choice of a particular substance on the basis of specific sought-after effects. Khantzian (1997) highlighted this self-medication hypothesis in describing the use of opioids to assuage end-point feelings of rage and aggression and the use of cocaine to counter feelings of depressive anergic restlessness or to augment grandiosity. Alcohol has been related to deep-seated fears of closeness, dependence, and intimacy, with the effects of alcohol promoting the tolerance of loving or aggressive feelings.

Moving the self-medication hypothesis beyond strict psychiatric diagnoses and toward underlying psychological states, Khantzian (1997) emphasized affect regulation, tolerance, self-regulation of affect, self-esteem, need satisfaction, relationships, and self-care. He also related psychodynamic concepts to the total care of addicted patients, providing a better understanding of how 12-step programs are helpful. He described substance-abusing individuals as lacking an internal, comforting sense of self-validation. These individuals also have difficulty obtaining nurturance and validation from others in a consistent, mature way. Self-care relates to the individual's developmental inability to anticipate danger or to worry about or consider the consequences of his or her actions, resulting in self-defeating and self-destructive behavior. Galanter (2002) emphasized the value of self-help groups and religious and social networks in providing a calming, soothing release of anxiety and a support for failing functions of the individual's ego and superego.

Interpersonal Relationships

Luborsky (1984) and Klerman et al. (1984) stressed the importance of clarifying the impact of drugs on the addicted individual's interpersonal relationships. Empirical research (using structured instruments) has failed to demonstrate high levels of dissociation among previously traumatized adults with substance use disorders, and the theory has been promoted that alcohol subsumes the expected dissociation (Langeland et al. 2002).

Application of Psychodynamics to Treatment

Applied psychodynamic theory must be distinguished from psychoanalysis. Whereas psychoanalysis is a specific form of therapy, psychodynamic principles can be used to inform individual and group therapies, rehabilitation, and other aspects of addiction treatment. Psychoanalysis as a treatment involves seeing an analyst four or five times per week, with the analyst providing relatively little feedback, being quite neutral, and providing little reassurance in order to allow the patient to experience frustration and have regressive fantasies. The patient lies on a couch to facilitate regression, and the therapist interprets the fantasies as they relate to the patient's childhood experiences. Psychoanalysis is not appropriate for most recovering addicted patients.

Psychodynamic psychotherapy (also referred to as insight-oriented psychotherapy) is a modified form of such treatment: individual sessions usually occur one or two times per week, possibly in addition to other modalities, and the patient sits up, facing the therapist. (Use of a couch is generally avoided because it facilitates regression.) Abstinence from the addictive substance is essential for successful treatment. Vigilant efforts at relapse prevention and helping patients get back on track after relapse are very much part of psychodynamic psychotherapy with addicted patients. Psychodynamic psychotherapy and 12-step self-help programs are compatible approaches for the maintenance of long-term abstinence.

Today, rather than dwelling on childhood experiences, psychodynamic approaches tend to focus on current conflicts and the therapeutic relationship as they relate to the past. Psychodynamic understanding takes into account the patient's childhood history; temperament; existing conflicts at the oral, anal, phallic, or genital levels; development of defenses;

and ego and superego development, including object relations and relationships with parents, siblings, and friends and ways they affect the doctor-patient relationship (Khantzian and Albanese 2008). With these insights, the therapist can help the patient to identify what motivates him or her for change. The therapist, aware of the patient's characteristic defenses and particular ego weaknesses and strengths, provides empathic interpretations and takes an active and supportive role. The therapist-patient relationship is discussed openly to work through resistance, and no effort is made to foster further regression. Psychodynamic techniques aimed at increased self-awareness, growth, and the working through of conflicts can be combined with cognitive approaches, case finding, relapse prevention, motivational techniques, suggestions, education, and provision of support and reassurance as indicated. Utilizing a transtheoretical treatment model, the therapist can help a particular patient to move along through the stages of change and recovery. Therapists skilled in these techniques use depth psychology in both listening and talking to patients, and this furthers empathy and mindfulness. Some authors use techniques such as mentalization to describe an empathic awareness of self and others.

A real danger in the history of psychoanalysis has been a reductionism in which attempts are made to apply one theory or approach to every situation. A broad and flexible use of psychodynamic thinking takes into account the total range of structural issues, including id, ego, and superego; developmental factors; conflict theory; self psychology; affect regulation; and cognitive deficits. Perry et al. (1987) clarified how three psychodynamic theoretical models—self psychology; object relations; and classical ego, id, and superego conflict theory—can be used to fit the metaphor that is most useful to a particular patient or psychodynamic history.

Psychodynamics in Differential Therapeutics

Clinical Indications and Rationale for Psychodynamic Psychotherapy

Psychodynamic principles are applicable throughout the various forms of psychotherapy and are relevant to addiction treatment. Insight-oriented therapy may be especially sought out by individuals for whom this kind of approach represents a particularly good fit. Individual psychodynamic psychotherapy may be the sole treatment or may be combined with group, family, psychopharmacological, self-help, or cognitive-behavioral therapy, as well as other treatment approaches. Individual psychodynamic psychotherapy may be reserved for treatment-resistant cases, or it may be the treatment of choice because of patient factors. Some patients refuse to participate in group or self-help programs and seek out individual psychodynamic therapy because of a wish for privacy, confidentiality, and insight. Patients with certain characteristics may especially seek out psychodynamic psychotherapy. Positive characteristics of such patients may include high intelligence, interest, and insight; psychological mindedness; a wish to understand or find meaning in behavior; a capacity for intimacy; identification with a therapist; ample time; ample funds; and a wish to change aspects of self that are not acceptable. As with most forms of psychotherapy, positive prognostic indicators are higher socioeconomic status, marital stability, less severe psychopathology, and minimal sociopathy (Woody et al. 1986). Some relatively negative characteristics associated with other treatments are social phobia, avoidance, and fears, which make attendance at Alcoholics Anonymous (AA) and Narcotics Anonymous (NA) meetings difficult for some patients. Factors that may lead some individuals to consider psychodynamic psychotherapy instead of other treatments include initial reactions of distaste toward spirituality, as may occur in some atheists; strong negative reactions to groups in general; unwillingness to take medication when indicated; and a lack of a rational approach to the world (patients with such a deficit might also benefit from cognitive-behavioral treatment). Some aspects that are nonspecific to treatment philosophy include the building of trust, empathy, openness, being nonjudgmental, honesty, and being supportive.

For adolescents and young adults sorting out identity issues, problems regarding individuation, and a need for independence, an insight-oriented approach may be beneficial. For patients in whom denial, projection, splitting, and projective identifications are prominent defenses, consistent interpretation of defenses may be needed to form a working alliance that can be used to achieve sobriety and growth. Patients who continue to be anxious, depressed, and troubled after detoxification are more likely to seek out additional psychotherapy. In many ways, patients who benefit from psychodynamic psychotherapy and have abused substances are similar to those who benefit from such therapy and have not abused substances. At the same time, however, many patients who failed to respond to psychodynamic psychotherapy when they were drinking find that they do benefit from this form of treatment when they are sober. Insight-oriented psychotherapy may be used to achieve or maintain the benefits of abstinence and to prevent relapse.

Those affected by traumatic disasters often turn to substances for relief of painful affects, and psychotherapy might prevent addiction or relapse in vulnerable individuals. Alcohol and substance use can increase vulnerability to posttraumatic stress disorder, and the disorder itself can increase alcohol and drug problems. In one study, alcohol use was decreased among victims of the Oklahoma City bombing, and alcohol did not alleviate symptoms but in fact increased functional impairment in these individuals (Pfefferbaum and Doughty 2001).

Recovering addicted patients are often members of families with heavy addiction, and the danger of relapse is greater among patients who have conflicts about enjoying and enhancing their success at abstinence. These patients may fear being more successful in this regard than an addicted parent or sibling, and insight into the sources of self-defeating behavior can be essential to preventing relapse. In the case of patients for whom self-care, self-destructiveness, suicidality, and masochism are major issues, an awareness of unconscious forces of self-destructive behavior can be useful to both patient and therapist. Many patients are not aware that their alcoholism may be what Menninger (1938) called "a slow form of suicide." Awareness of risk-taking aspects of behavior may lead the patient to take greater caution. Addiction and suicide are long-term solutions to what are often short-term problems, and the therapist's job is to help the patient realize this.

The rationale for using psychodynamic principles is frequently based on an in-depth clinical understanding of a particular patient's life situation. The study of temperament is leading to intriguing implications for psychiatric treatment, including treatment of addictions (Cloninger 1987). Psychodynamics are used to deepen the patient's understanding of the rehabilitation process and group psychotherapy, and to help him or her understand how self-help groups work (Frances et al. 1989). Awareness of the importance of an unconscious wish to return to drinking, especially during periods of stress, is used in treatment. When unconscious factors have repeatedly led to relapse, exploratory psychotherapy may be particularly useful (Dodes and Khantzian 2004). For example, a patient's association of a "lost weekend," a drunk dream, or a planned vacation to a location where relapses frequently occurred in the past may be a warning sign of a possible relapse and can be used to help the patient to recognize that a craving still exists and should be addressed.

An awareness of reasons not to drink and the strengthening of that side of the patient's internal conflict may help, along with increased insight into the sources of the internal struggle. The greatest focus of attention has been on how substances may be used to self-medicate for other psychiatric disorders or to self-regulate affect, and how their use may be a symptom of an underlying problem (Khantzian and Albanese 2008). Abused substances may be used to push painful thoughts from one's consciousness and to numb feelings associated with painful knowledge, or they may be used to gain access to unconscious material and to facilitate the experience or expression of anger and other feelings that may be avoided during sobriety.

For patients for whom affect regulation is an issue, psychodynamic psychotherapy may be especially valuable. A patient with an underlying dysthymia, depression, or affective disorder may need to understand how he or she has used substances to cope with unmanageable feelings. Given that alcohol or drugs invariably cause additional life difficulties, psychodynamic approaches may help the patient deal with the psychosocial effects associated with the toxic metabolic complications of substance use. The application of psychodynamic theory to the treatment of comorbid psychiatric problems, such as Axis II personality disorders (including borderline, narcissistic, and avoidant personality disorders), is important, especially because alcoholism and drug abuse are overrepresented in these patients. The literature on comorbidity of Axis I and Axis II disorders is extensive, and a presentation of findings is beyond the scope of this chapter (for further discussion, see Kessler et al. 1997). It may be especially hard to identify the boundaries of temperament, acute substance-induced personality change, other Axis I disorders, secondary personality features, and independent personality disorders. Exploratory psychotherapy with patients with borderline personality disorder who have a history of addiction must be informed by a good knowledge of addiction psychiatry and an emphasis on structure and limit setting in treatment, including the vital parameter of abstinence.

Kernberg (1991) discussed the deception and projection often seen in the initial therapeutic alliance with patients with borderline or narcissistic personality disorder, as well as the need to confront distorted views of reality in the therapeutic relationship. The use of insight in interpreting negative transference and acting out may deepen a positive transference and ultimately foster open expression. As a patient develops a clearer picture of his or her life through exploratory psychotherapy, the value of openness and honesty becomes apparent, and the tie to the therapist is cemented. Frequently, addicted patients have lied to themselves and others and are tired of feeling false and phony. The therapist's healthy ability to tolerate being conned by highly skilled, manipulative patients may minimize damaging countertransference reactions. If the therapist finds himself or herself doing something with a patient (either positive or negative) that is out of the ordinary, some examination of countertransference is always warranted.

It may be hard to tell whether a personality change that occurs early in treatment is attributable to a gradual return to better function due to physical, social, and psychological recovery from addiction effects; is best accounted for by an incorrect initial diagnosis of personality disorder; or is the result of psychodynamic therapy and/or a 12-step program. Some patients experience a "rebound high" in terms of improved functioning overall (analogous to the "practicing" subphase of development in the second year of life, when there is a burst of autonomous development [Mahler et al. 1975]).

Many addicted patients who have narcissistic traits or personality disorder, and in whom the toxic effects of addiction heighten narcissism, feel a sense of specialness and entitlement, have no empathy for others, are unable to allow themselves gratification of dependence needs, and experience loneliness. For these patients, rehabilitation often involves acceptance of vulnerability and of being ordinary and similar to others with the same problem; a reaching out for help; and encouragement to develop a new humility. Whether this rehabilitation is achieved through 12-step programs, application of Beck's cognitive therapy (A.T. Beck et al. 1993; J.S. Beck et al. 2004), or psychodynamic exploration of the narcissistic vulnerability, or a combination of the above, these issues should be dealt with in this substantial subpopulation.

Dodes (1996) suggested that addictions are in the same category as compulsions, and because compulsions have been seen as treatable with traditional psychodynamic psychotherapy, addictions should also be treatable by similar approaches. Evidence indicates that alcohol problems can either cause or result from anxiety disorders and that more often than not, agoraphobia, social phobia, and obsessive-compulsive disorder precede rather than follow an alcohol problem (Kushner et al. 1990). Although cognitive-behavioral and pharmacological approaches may be first-line treatments for panic disorder, agoraphobia, and social phobia, psychodynamic approaches are often used with patients whose conditions have been resistant to, or have only partially responded to, other psychotherapies and medications (Frances and Borg 1993).

Contraindications for Psychodynamic Psychotherapy

Contraindications for psychodynamic psychotherapy include active use of substances, severe organicity, psychosis, and, for the most part, antisocial personality disorder. Some patients who regress too readily in individual therapy, who develop psychotic transferences, or who develop negative therapeutic reactions benefit from the diffusion of transference that takes place in group therapy. If the principal problem is marital, family therapy is the treatment of choice.

Utilizing Treatment Outcome Research

The state of the art in addiction treatment involves being aware of the results of treatment outcome studies but also selecting a combination of treatments that takes into account current knowledge and patient characteristics. Treatment recommendations depend on a wide range of considerations, and trial results are only one factor. The American Psychiatric Association (2006) developed practice guidelines for the treatment of substance use disorders based on reviews of the literature on treatment and outcomes. These guidelines recommend individualizing treatment planning and include treatment of comorbid conditions.

Woody et al. (1986) showed meaningful differences in efficacy between supportive-expressive psychotherapy and drug counseling in patients receiving methadone maintenance treatment. Carroll et al. (1994) pointed out that there is a delayed emergence of effects of psychotherapy after cessation of short-term treatments in cocaine-dependent patients. O'Malley et al. (1996) compared psychotherapy with or without naltrexone therapy in alcoholic patients and found that the combined treatment had favorable results.

With managed care entering the arena of health care, studies of cost-effectiveness and outcomes are becoming increasingly important. Humphreys and Moos (1996) found reduced substance-related health care costs in a study involving veterans participating in AA. O'Brien (1997a) found favorable efficacy when comparing specific treatment approaches for addictive disorders with specific treatments for other chronic disorders such as diabetes and asthma. O'Brien (1997b) also pointed to studies that have shown a cost saving of $4–$12 for every dollar spent on substance abuse treatment.

It is too early in addiction outcome research to make hard-and-fast recommendations regarding treatments to be used. Treatment guidelines and the treatment outcome studies discussed in this book provide useful information but not definitive instructions to clinicians. Although clinicians agree on some points (e.g., the usefulness of abstinence as a goal, pharmacological treatment of comorbid disorders such as panic attacks, the value of adding education and cognitive-behavioral approaches), the value of 12-step programs and psychodynamic psychotherapy has not been strongly proved in controlled studies, although each treatment has a commonsense rationale. Where definite answers are still lacking, clinicians need to be aware of a growing literature of outcome study findings, of the methodological problems involved in conducting good studies, and of the problems in reliability and validity in applying these results. Uncertainties about the exact value of psychodynamic and combined treatments should not deter clinicians from using what has seemed useful, especially with patients who have specific favorable characteristics, such as motivation and capacity for insight, and who have destructive patterns amenable to interpretation. When definitive conclusions about the effectiveness of treatment components have been drawn, targeting of treatment will improve.

Engaging in Psychodynamic Psychotherapy

Initiation of Treatment

Some authors recommend waiting 6–12 months before beginning psychodynamic psychotherapy with a patient (Bean-Bayog 1988). We believe that psychodynamic treatment can be initiated early; however, timing should be tailored to the patient. The greatest opportunity to develop a treatment alliance is often early, while the patient is in crisis. Supportive elements, such as confrontation, clarification, support of defenses, and building on ego strengths, may be more prominent early in treatment. The therapist should also take into account state-related problems of organicity, physical illness, and affective vulnerability, all of which can lead to an inability to utilize interpretations. In their work on initiating treatment, Prochaska et al. (1992) discussed the stages in which patients develop awareness of their addiction problems. Focusing on motivational aspects of treatment and confronting denial of a need for help are essential elements in initiating treatment. Promoting identification as a recovering person can boost self-esteem and provide stability.

The psychodynamic psychotherapist needs to consider the effects of intoxication and withdrawal, as well as the chronic organic effects of alcohol. However, during intoxication or withdrawal, there are patients for whom psychodynamic interpretations are indicated from the very outset of treatment, regardless of the stage of addiction. Interpretations may help the patient work through resistances to accepting help. They may also provide a meaningful explanation for destructive patterns, one that can inspire a wish for change.

Timing of interpretations is crucial. A patient who may need to project blame and responsibility for his or her actions onto substances early in recovery may later be able to accept responsibility for those actions. For example, one patient admitted later in treatment that having an affair, embezzling money, and being abusive were things he wanted to do anyway and that he used alcohol and cocaine abuse as an excuse. The individual may not be ready to take full responsibility for his or her actions early in abstinence, but over time, these issues can be explored and pointed out, denial can be worked through, and acceptance of responsibility can be achieved. Defenses may need to be supported at first, including denial of affect related to some of the losses. Interpreting those defenses may be most effective when the patient is facing life challenges that offer a particular motivation for change. For example, a 67-year-old successful professional with alcohol dependence used the defenses of denial and displacement to avoid the grief he felt at how he had sabotaged his relationship with his children throughout their lives. When presented with the opportunity for a relationship with his grandchildren, he was more able to face his desperate wish to win back respect and love from his family. His wish to not be remembered as "that old drunk" motivated him to take steps toward recovery.

Confrontation should concentrate initially on denial surrounding addictive behaviors. Clarification, confrontation, and interpretation of denial, lying, splitting, and projective defenses in other areas ultimately need to be expanded. However, in selected cases, with repeated treatment failure, an initial intervention may require active, across-the-board confrontation and interpretation of inconsistencies and denial in order to help the patient accept a need for change. In a patient with alexithymia or constricted affect, interpretations are aimed at increasing the patient's awareness of feeling states and helping him or her connect thoughts and feelings without the use of substances.

Session Frequency, Setting, and Goals

Psychodynamic psychotherapy with alcoholic patients is usually conducted one to two times per week, is often combined with group psychotherapy, and includes a parameter of abstinence and a long-term goal of sobriety. It can be done during an inpatient stay or in an organized outpatient or office practice, and it can be time limited and focused or long-term. It is foolhardy for psychotherapists to promise that once underlying causes of a "symptom of drinking" are dealt with, the patient will be able to return to controlled drinking. Similarly, it is unwise to promise that once a patient is fully treated with psychoanalytically oriented psychotherapy, he or she will never need additional help through 12-step programs or additional psychotherapy. A treatment model that integrates multiple modalities is most likely to facilitate real change. For most alcoholics, shifting from dependence on a chemical such as alcohol to dependence on a therapist, group, or spiritual belief or involvement with anything human is a major step in the direction of growth. Although issues of dependence may be worked through partially, an ongoing positive identification with a therapist, a sponsor, and/or recovering friends may be a major positive outcome of treatment. Active dialogue with the patient and an attitude of empathic concern and sharing on the part of the therapist are optimal. Issues of interruption or termination of individual therapy or graduation from phases of treatment may bring earlier conflicts back to the surface and trigger relapse. The goal of psychodynamic treatment for addicted patients is to help them maintain abstinence, provide them with a richer understanding of and control of their inner lives, and reduce psychological triggers for relapse. Achieving this goal helps improve patient self-esteem, self-care, and affect regulation (Khantzian and Albanese 2008).

General Technical Aspects of Treatment

Advances in object relations theory, ego psychology, and modern psychodynamic understanding of conflicts and affect regulation can be applied to addiction treatment. Psychodynamic principles are applied in conjunction with an understanding of the clinical exigencies of addiction treatment. The therapist needs to modify techniques, especially those related to attaining and sustaining abstinence, and carefully monitor the effects of regression. However, well-established techniques and principles of brief and long-term psychodynamic treatment are generally maintained. The therapist listens for themes relating to the patient's intrapsychic conflicts, developmental impairments, and defenses, paying special attention to how they may relate to substance abuse and relapse potential.

The therapist has some important objectives: to obtain a careful developmental history of the patient, with attention to achievement of milestones of ego development; to evaluate temperament in the patient and significant caretakers; to examine the patient's capacity to identify with and to separate from important figures of identification, including parents, siblings, and admired peers; and to explore the patient's affect regulation, especially in relation to substance use. The therapist's tools include free association, "slips," and dreams, which are examined to find meaning in the unconscious derivatives of behavior (e.g., an unconscious wish to drink, expressed in a dream about being drunk). For example, a 45-year-old male patient described an ambivalent relationship with his father, who had failed in business and was devalued by the patient's overbearing mother. The patient expressed loving and sad feelings for his father. He had developed a pattern of sabotaging his own potential for success with alcoholic relapses. During an extended period of sobriety, he began to dream that he had killed his father and was drinking at his father's funeral. The interpretation of this dream helped the patient to begin to examine his unconscious need to fail so that he would not surpass his father, as well as suppressed rage at his father for his helplessness.

Treatment Parameters

Treatment parameters for patients with addictions, such as structure, clear boundaries, and abstinence, are similar to those used effectively in treating borderline personality disorder. Structure and boundaries help the patient reestablish control and self-regulation and help him or her express feelings verbally rather than by acting them out. The conventional practice of psychodynamic psychotherapy with limit setting is generally helpful, although on rare occasions a more active approach may be needed. For example, a therapist may need to mobilize a family to bring a suicidal alcoholic patient to the emergency room or to the physician's office after a relapse.

While working through the patient's resistance and defenses, the therapist should be aware of how alcohol provides the patient with an escape, can numb or facilitate expression, and can itself alter defensive operations, especially in terms of heightening denial. The therapist should watch closely the interplay of ego function, feeling states, and chemical effects in the patient.

Most therapists in the addiction field believe that abstinence is necessary for psychotherapy to be effective. Many think it is best to first develop a solid relationship with the patient and then aim for gradual achievement of abstinence (Dodes and Khantzian 2004). We believe that although flexibility is often needed for patients with severe psychiatric illness, psychiatric problems for the most part must be treated in synchrony with the addiction disorder, and abstinence is vital to this approach. Unfortunately, sometimes continuation of psychodynamic psychotherapy can enable the addicted patient to continue substance use. Psychodynamic psychotherapy can also raise conflicts that may lead to worsening of the addiction, and thus the treatment can be contraindicated. The following vignette illustrates such a situation:

> A 37-year-old successful journalist was in psychoanalysis 5 days per week for a severe alcohol addiction. He frequently arrived at sessions intoxicated or missed them altogether. During years of analysis, his addiction to alcohol progressed. His family tried to persuade him to see an addiction psychiatrist. He protested that he had a good relationship with his analyst, thought that he was being helped, and used this as a rationale to avoid effective treatment. A divorce, job loss, and health problems followed, none of which were addressed by the therapist.

This patient achieved poor results in treatment because his psychoanalyst was not knowledgeable about addictions and was adhering to a technique that was wrong for the patient. The issue of abstinence was crucial here, but it was ignored. The therapist is more likely to be successful in treating addiction by using the telephone sometimes and occasionally may even need to make a home visit in these situations. Home visits may be more common in nondynamic treatment of addictions, and such an interaction poses significant challenges to a psychodynamically oriented psychotherapy and needs to be handled carefully, with attention to boundaries, trust, and control.

Other Treatment Tools

A combination of psychodynamic approaches, such as clarification, inter-pretation, and genetic reconstruction, may be used along with directive approaches, such as assertiveness training, social skills training, self-efficacy groups, modeling, positive reinforcement, increasing cognitive awareness, and suggestion. A sophisticated familiarity with typical problems that occur in alcohol- or drug-abusing individuals and their families and the use of psychoeducation about these issues help the therapist establish a positive alliance with his or her patient. The literature on adult children of alcoholic patients can aid the therapist's understanding and be used in educating patients and their families.

The following case illustrates the use of combined approaches:

> **Janis,** a 42-year-old recovering alcoholic woman with panic attacks and ag-oraphobia had special problems when flying. Psychodynamic psycho-therapy was useful when added to desensitization, relaxation therapy, exposure to flying, and closely monitored medication for panic attacks (paroxetine and benzodiazepines taken 2 hours before airplane trips). The anxiety persisted at a significant level, frequently interfering with the patient's plans. Her fears of flying were related to childhood conflicts about having to take planes to visit her father after her parents divorced. Janis was "the apple of her father's eye" and had clearly won out over her mother, although she had considerable guilt over her especially favored position. Her oedipal guilt persisted, contributing to difficulty in reach-ing orgasm with her husband and feelings of guilt about enjoying her sex-uality. At the time of treatment, the flights she feared most were those related to visits with her father and those involved in pleasure trips with her husband. Although none of the treatments totally allayed her fears, Janis was able to travel without drinking and was better able to understand and cope with her fears of flying, having gained enhanced insight into the roots of her fears. Use of a selective serotonin reuptake inhibitor helped block her panic attacks. She was increasingly allowing herself to enjoy gradual steps toward success without relapsing.

Initial Focus and Phases of Treatment

The phases of intervention include initial screening, evaluation and inter-vention, rehabilitation, and aftercare. The initial focus is often on conflicts related to the acceptance of addiction as a problem, the patient's reluc-tance to acknowledge dependence and need for treatment, and conflicts resulting from complications of alcoholism (including the loss of relation-ships, health, and jobs) and from missing alcohol itself. As emphasized above in "Treatment Parameters," the first goal is abstinence. More often than is usually the case in insight-oriented psychotherapy, the patient may initially be forced into the consultation by an employer, probation officer, family member, or physician. Especially when coercion has occurred, the therapist must make a considerable effort to develop trust and a working alliance with the patient. The alliance is achieved along with a careful review of the patient's history and the ways in which addiction has interfered with work, family relationships, and other relationships or has caused legal problems, all of which have contributed to pain and the need to escape it. The therapist's integrity, adherence to confidentiality, and ability to be helpful all contribute to the establishment of trust.

The patient is helped to accept a diagnosis and to accept the need for help, which may lead to positive transference. These steps are similar to the first two AA steps, in which patients admit their powerlessness over alcohol and accept their need for help or acknowledge their own dependence needs, which in AA is called "accepting a higher power" and has spiritual overtones. A psychodynamic perspective may aid in the confrontation of denial and other defenses, and through interpretations patients achieve a deeper understanding of certain destructive patterns that have led to the present problem. It is especially challenging to help the patient acknowledge dependence needs that have been channeled into the addiction.

Therapy is a process in which a need for substances is shifted into a need for people, including the therapist. Patients who abuse drugs often refuse to take medications because of fears of using them in compulsive ways, becoming dependent on drugs for relief, and becoming dependent on the therapist to obtain the medications. For example, a 23-year-old alcoholic male with opioid abuse refused to take naltrexone because "I don't like taking pills." The paradox of not wanting to accept medication when also abusing substances represents a resistance that requires exploration, clarification, and confrontation.

From early in treatment of patients with substance use disorders, issues of trust, dependence, separation, loss, disappointment, and truthfulness are frequent themes. In the later stages, the focus of exploratory psychotherapy should not be imposed from the outside—that is, it should not be based on purely theoretical considerations. Rather, the focus should be on the most pressing issue of the moment that may relate to the patient's drinking: a particular conflict; a relationship with a family member or an employer; a problem with self-esteem, self-destructiveness, or self-medication for panic; or other painful affects.

Other major themes include specific conflicts over assertiveness, handling of aggression, and issues of control and inhibition. The disinhibiting role of addiction, leading to risk-taking behavior (including increased sexual activity), may be an issue. Alternatively, alcohol may play a role in distancing the individual from sexual life, or substance use may substitute for sexual activity.

An Approach to Relapse

Patients should be observed carefully for drinking or drug use behavior. Laboratory tests may be useful, and meeting with family and other sources of collateral information may be essential, to get a true picture before confronting patients who dissimulate. Making patients aware that relapse can be facilitated by using any abusable substance is important. As mentioned earlier in "Clinical Indications and Rationale for Psychodynamic Psychotherapy," psychodynamic therapy can help in relapse prevention. Consider the following case:

> A 47-year-old pediatric surgical nurse frequently relapsed in her addiction to diazepam on the evenings after she had had to deal with families of children with disastrous surgical results. As a child, she had been traumatized by a younger sister's postoperative death due to a brain tumor. Her parents had tried to protect her by never discussing her sister's death, and she had always found this to be strange. Her relapses were triggered by unresolved conflicts and grief regarding her dead sister, whom she envied, loved, and, at self-destructive moments, wished to join in death. Her initial treatment plan involved detoxification, support, and an aim of abstinence. However, the effectiveness of relapse prevention was enhanced by psychodynamic treatment that helped her mourn her sister, deal with her guilt as a survivor, and eliminate an important trigger for relapse.

Acceptance of Self in Recovery

An important part of recovery is a change in self-awareness and self-perception. An enormous shift occurs when the patient accepts a diagnosis of alcoholism or substance dependence as an illness. This change entails not only shifting from a moral model (in which the patient sees himself or herself as weak, shameful, and bad for being alcoholic) but also being aware that a problem exists about which a great deal is known, that the problem is treatable, and that it does not have to lead to hopelessness and despair. Sometimes this awareness leads to reaction formation, in which the patient feels grateful for being an alcoholic and turns a disability into an advantage. There may have been real advantages in terms of broadening experience, overcoming a vulnerability, and developing pride, as can occur in any group that finds a way to overcome a stigma. The patient's feeling of relief after he or she is no longer experiencing the consequences of alcoholism and addiction often leads to a rebound after initial abstinence—a rebound that can approach euphoria. This euphoria is often followed by a letdown that accompanies awareness of the multitude of problems that the addiction caused. The shift in moral focus involves no longer feeling guilty about having the illness of addiction but instead feeling responsible for accepting treatment and preventing relapses.

An Ego Psychological Model of Rehabilitation

Assessment of ego function needs to include a search for strengths, talents, and positive qualities that can be used to help the patient. All too often, therapists miss opportunities to enhance self-esteem in patients whose self-criticism leads them to overlook real and potential opportunities for growth. One way to combine positive insight with support is to help patients recall periods in which their values were in place and to give them hope for a return to a higher level of function.

Self-efficacy is a quality that is a good prognostic sign and that needs to be supported at every step of the way. We tell patients, "If you are 100% motivated, you will achieve 100% success."

Even very damaged, impaired individuals from deprived and disadvantaged backgrounds have dreams in their lives that they have buried. Rekindled dreams can foster renewed hope and improve self-esteem. The stigma of the illness can also be lessened by discussing positive role models, such as Betty Ford, who have struggled with the same illness and have worked hard at recovery. An ego psychological model can be applied to the biopsychosocial effects of addiction and to rehabilitation. Chemicals and psychosocial consequences have effects and may lead to regression and impairment of defenses, object relatedness, judgment, reality testing, and superego. It may take time and practice for good ego and superego function to return. The following case demonstrates recovery of function:

> A 47-year-old narcissistic man who had drunk heavily for 25 years had disuse atrophy of ego functions, particularly in his inability to relate to others, and was pushed to function better as part of rehabilitation. He thought of his wife only in terms of what she could do for him, as a part object or a need-satisfying object, and only with practice and with time sober could he relate to her in a more complex way as having needs of her own. He would idealize or devalue everyone and everything, and it took him a long time to relate to others as having both good and bad qualities. To develop friendships and break isolation, he had to practice relatedness in individual therapy, couples therapy, group therapy, and self-help groups.

In this case, the patient's superego had been dissolved in chemicals for years, and it took external structure and parameters to gradually awaken the sleeping policeman within—that is, for the superego to start working again. The program requirements and the external norms of the groups helped him regain structure. His superego was initially inconsistent and vacillated from a lack of restraint and self-indulgence to a primitive punitive masochistic rigidity. Cognitive impairment, especially in the nondominant hemisphere functions of spatial and temporal relationships, was present and improved over time with abstinence.

The defenses initially encountered in treatment are usually the most primitive and include denial, rationalization, splitting, projection, and projective identification. With time and treatment, higher-level defenses such as intellectualization, reaction formation, repression, and sublimation may be more in the forefront. For example, instead of denying alcoholism and projecting poor self-esteem, a patient may feel grateful to have alcoholism and honored to be part of a group that initially was perceived as stigmatizing. Denial of alcohol's harmful effects on the liver, which can be addressed through psychoeducation, can be replaced with curiosity and intellectualization about how liver damage occurs. Use of reaction formation may also lead to noncompliance with psychiatric and other prescribed medications, with the rationale that they could have unknown negative effects on liver and other organ functions. Denial of losses related to addiction may be replaced with repression over time, after grieving over the losses has occurred.

Applications of Psychodynamics to Groups and Self-Help

The addition of group psychotherapy, AA, or NA is especially needed when individual therapy alone is not helping the patient maintain abstinence. Group treatments help diffuse some of the powerful negative transference that may be impossible to overcome early in treatment. Groups can focus on self-care, self-esteem, affect regulation, sharing, and exposure to feared social situations. They can provide social support and models for identification and coping skills, and they can help patients work through family problems. Groups can be targeted to specific additional diagnoses, such as anxiety disorders, or to specific subpopulations, such as persons with chronic mental illness, those with medical complications, women, or adolescents. Groups can be homogeneous (e.g., recovering physicians with anxiety disorders) or heterogeneous (e.g., all patients in a detoxification unit). Khantzian (1997) described a model of modified psychodynamic group therapy for substance-abusing patients involving self-care, self-esteem, and affect regulation. Together, the patient and the individual therapist can look at how the patient projects feelings toward other AA, NA, or group members who, for example, remind the patient of his or her alcoholic relatives. Character flaws can be actively worked on, with immediate and multiple feedback from group members. If the individual therapist is also the group therapist, the individual work may be used to encourage the patient to try a new behavior in the group; conversely, conflicts observed in the group can be worked on individually.

Aspects of 12-step programs may readily lend themselves to integration with psychodynamic treatment. These aspects include accepting a diagnosis, accepting dependence needs, being aware that one cannot control drinking alone, taking a personal inventory (often discussed in terms of a higher power), working at change, dealing with sobriety one day at a time, accepting the structure of a treatment program, and enhancing self-esteem by helping others with the problem, thus living up to an ego ideal. The 12-step programs provide education, auxiliary ego and superego support, and powerful role models for positive identification. Steps in AA that involve taking a personal inventory and making amends can be used in conjunction with the psychotherapeutic process of self-exploration and insight aimed at behavioral change. The addition of AA is especially helpful during periods of relapse and during periods when the therapist is unavailable because either the patient or the therapist is away. Because alcoholism and drug abuse are often chronic relapsing illnesses, both the patient and the therapist must be prepared for the possibility of a relapse. The therapist should be both nonjudgmental and unafraid of confrontation.

The Patient-Therapist Relationship

Many problems related to working with addicted patients concern the challenge of establishing a positive therapeutic relationship between the patient and the therapist. Frequently, errors in treatment occur because of negative feelings and attitudes that therapists have toward addicted patients. Typical therapist mistakes include providing inadequate empathy or overly identifying with patients. A major source of countertransference is the uncritical acceptance by a clinician of roles projected onto him or her in the patient's transference. In many cases, an understanding of the patient's specific transference that may either evoke countertransference problems or prevent compliance with treatment may be essential for good management and a successful alliance with the patient. Typical transference resistance may result from growing up in a household in which the parents were addicted, inconsistent, and either overly harsh or indulgent. Children of alcoholic parents frequently have authority problems and will often trust siblings, peers, and other alcoholic individuals more readily than they will trust teachers, nurses, doctors, or police. When a patient describes a therapist as cold, neglectful, uninvolved, or detached, this may be transference to a parent who fits this description and may lead the therapist to unconsciously behave in this way. It is helpful for the therapist to be able to interpret negative transference and to know how to manage and appropriately use therapist countertransference. The following is an example of projective identification in the therapeutic situation:

> A sadomasochistic homosexual Wall Street accountant addicted to co-caine and cannabis presented with a hostile devaluing transference and would frequently relapse, seemingly to provoke his therapist into feeling hopeless about him, as the patient felt about himself. In addition to a de-pressive disorder and a depressive personality, he also had substance-induced depression, amotivation, and posttraumatic stress disorder fol-lowing his witnessing of the 9/11 terror attacks. He had been the victim of physical and emotional abuse from a sadistic, mentally ill, and substance-using mother throughout his childhood. Unconsciously he tried to re-create that relationship in the therapeutic situation, and it took periodic interpretation of what was happening to help him allow himself to work on staying sober and developing healthier relationships with others.

Alcoholic patients frequently try to evoke feelings of fear, anger, and despair in their therapists and to reenact relationships with alcoholic par-ents, siblings, and spouses through the transference. They may project critical attitudes onto the therapist and keep secrets out of fear that the therapist will respond like a parent. When the patient feels that the ther-apist is like a parent, sibling, or friend, this feeling may have been evoked for specific reasons. The greater the therapist's awareness of what is hap-pening, the more this issue can be brought into the treatment in a con-structive way.

A second major source of countertransference in treating addicted pa-tients is a therapist's weak knowledge base about addiction and its treat-ment. The more knowledgeable the therapist is about addiction psychiatry and about the patient, the less likely the therapist is to project his or her own problems onto the patient. Attitudinal problems on the part of the therapist can be reduced by good training and the experience of having worked through issues related to stigma. The more the therapist is in com-mand of a treatment armamentarium, the less frightened he or she is in the face of what can be a dreadful disease. Ultimately, patients are the best teachers. By listening carefully, the therapist can learn about the addictive experience, addictive practices, and the street language of addiction.

A third source of countertransference is based on a therapist's mostly unconscious transference related to his or her past or present problems. Transference may relate to the therapist's attitudes about substances; present or past problems with addiction; or experience with a parent, spouse, or child with a substance use problem. The therapist's own envy, fear, hopes, and needs can adversely affect his or her prescribing prac-tices and lead to overinvolvement, avoidance, hopelessness, jealousy, and burnout. Some clinicians who have chosen to work in the addiction field because of their wish to overcome personal problems related to addictions may have special difficulty dealing with patients' problems if they have not worked out their own. Frequent mistakes include excessive self-revelation of personal problems and a tendency not to see the specifics of patients' problems clearly because of a need to see everyone as similar to the self. A recovering clinician might consider a patient's problem minor compared with his or her own. Alternatively, some clinicians see every problem only in relation to addictive problems, which results in misdiagnosis and overdiagnosis. One extreme of overinvolvement is sexual or aggressive acting out with a vulnerable substance-abusing patient; this has disastrous consequences for both patient and therapist.

Seeking out second opinions from or supervision by experienced practitioners is advisable when working with difficult patients. Thorough self-exploration by the therapist in personal therapy also helps. Clinicians with maturity, a good support system, and a secure personal life are better protected against countertransference problems. Additional protection is given by working in a team: team members can point out one another's blind spots and assist in improving one another's technique. Feedback from patients and their families can be another means of supervision for the clinician who listens carefully. A wise clinician admits his or her mistakes, learns from them, and tries to avoid future mistakes (Committee on Alcoholism and Addictions 1998).

Myths and Pitfalls to Avoid in Psychodynamic Psychotherapy

Clinical experience suggests that there are common misperceptions (myths) about the role of psychotherapy in treating addictions, misperceptions that can negatively affect treatment planning. There are also avoidable problems (pitfalls) that may arise in psychotherapies by even the most seasoned and well-meaning therapists. The following lists cannot be comprehensive, but they address some of the most frequent and relevant myths and pitfalls in psychodynamic psychotherapies with patients who have addictions.

Myths

- One can first develop a therapeutic relationship and then gradually wean the patient off substances.
- Substance use will disappear with understanding.
- Once conflicts have been resolved, the patient can safely return to drinking.

- If the problem is narcotic addiction, alcohol is safer and legal.
- Addiction is always a symptom, not a primary problem.
- Use of motivational interviewing, cognitive-behavioral techniques, group therapy, and 12-step programs cannot be integrated with insight-oriented therapy.

Pitfalls

- The therapist believes the patient's explanation for drinking, without awareness of rationalization and a patient's need to justify his or her behavior.
- The therapist does not check out the patient's story.
- The therapist conducts treatment as if psychodynamic interpretations were "golden" and other interventions less valuable. Treatment approaches and sequence should be selected on the basis of the patient's needs.
- The therapist does not have a healthy respect for the patient's dependence needs and has overly high expectations for resolving these needs. It is better for the patient to depend on therapists or on AA than on substances, and an endless relationship with AA is a desirable goal—not a compromise of a therapist's goal of self-reliance on the patient's part.
- The therapist is overinvolved or overly distant. Therapists in recovery themselves sometimes have blind spots or may share with the patient more than the patient needs to know.
- The therapist has a bias toward one or another form of treatment and lacks theoretical and practical flexibility. Even moderate biases of this type can be a disservice to the patient.

Conclusion

Psychodynamic theory can play an important role in enriching and informing substance abuse treatment and improving the therapeutic relationship. However, rigid application of psychoanalytic technique is inappropriate in substance abuse treatment and can be counterproductive. Application of psychodynamic understanding—including attending to the unconscious, child development, ego function, affect regulation, and efforts to enhance self-esteem and deal with shame and other narcissistic vulnerability—widens the range of patients who can be treated.

Key Clinical Concepts

- A sophisticated, dynamic understanding of his or her own conflicts can help motivate a patient to accept the presence of a problem and a need for change, can aid in treatment, and can be used to maintain progress.

- Psychodynamic understanding can be integrated with cognitive, behavioral, and pharmacological approaches to enhance treatment.

- Psychodynamic understanding of the substance-using patient requires specific considerations and emphases in different phases of the therapy.

- More research needs to be done on how influencing the mind can affect brain function, including addictive behavior.

Suggested Reading

Khantzian EJ, Albanese MJ: Understanding Addiction as Self Medication: Finding Hope Behind the Pain. Lanham, MD, Rowman & Littlefield, 2008

Prochaska JO, DiClemente CC, Norcross JC: In search of how people change: applications to addictive behaviors. Am Psychol 47:1102–1114, 1992

Vaillant GE: The Natural History of Alcoholism Revisited. Cambridge, MA, Harvard University Press, 1995, pp 362–373

References

Abraham K: The psychological relation between sexuality and alcoholism (1908), in Selected Papers of Karl Abraham. New York, Basic Books, 1960, pp 80–89

American Psychiatric Association: Practice Guideline for the Treatment of Patients With Substance Use Disorders: Alcohol, Cocaine, Opioids, 2nd Edition. Arlington, VA, American Psychiatric Association, 2006. Available at: http://www.psychiatryonline.com/pracGuide/pracGuideTopic_5.aspx. Accessed May 13, 2010.

Bean-Bayog M: Alcoholism as a cause of psychopathology. Hosp Community Psychiatry 39:352–354, 1988

Beck AT, Wright FD, Newman CF, et al: Cognitive Therapy of Substance Abuse. New York, Guilford, 1993

Beck JS, Liese BS, Najavits LM: Cognitive therapy, in Clinical Textbook of Addictive Disorders, 3rd Edition. Edited by Frances RJ, Miller SI, Mack AH. New York, Guilford, 2004, pp 474–501

Bleuler E: Alcohol and the neuroses (1911), in Jahrbuch für psychoanalytische und psychopathologische Forschungen, Jahrbuch der Psychoanalyse 3:848. Abstracted by Blungart L. Psychoanal Rev 8:443–444, 1921

Carroll KM, Rounsaville BJ, Nich C, et al: One-year follow-up of psychotherapy and pharmacotherapy for cocaine dependence: delayed emergence of psychotherapy effects. Arch Gen Psychiatry 51:989–997, 1994

Cloninger CR: A systematic method for clinical description and classification of personality variants: a proposal. Arch Gen Psychiatry 44:573–588, 1987

Committee on Alcoholism and Addictions, Group for the Advancement of Psychiatry: Addiction Treatment: Avoiding Pitfalls—A Case Approach, Vol 142. Washington, DC, American Psychiatric Press, 1998

Dodes LM: The psychology of combining dynamic psychotherapy and Alcoholics Anonymous. Bull Menninger Clin 52:283–293, 1988

Dodes LM: Compulsion and addiction. J Am Psychoanal Assoc 44:815–835, 1996

Dodes LM, Khantzian EJ: Individual psychodynamic psychotherapy, in Clinical Textbook of Addictive Disorders, 3rd Edition. Edited by Frances RJ, Miller SI, Mack AH. New York, Guilford, 2004, pp 457–473

DuPont RL: Addiction: a new paradigm. Bull Menninger Clin 62:231–242, 1998

Etkin A, Pittenger C, Polan HJ, et al: Toward a neurobiology of psychotherapy: basic science and clinical applications. J Neuropsychiatry Clin Neurosci 17:145–158, 2005

Ferenczi S: On the part played by homosexuality in the pathogenesis of paranoia (1912), in First Contributions to Psycho-Analysis. Boston, MA, Richard G Badger, 1916, pp 154–184

Frances RJ, Borg L: The treatment of anxiety in patients with alcoholism. J Clin Psychiatry 54(suppl):37–43, 1993

Frances RJ, Khantzian EJ, Tamerin JS: Psychodynamic psychotherapy, in Treatments of Psychiatric Disorders: A Task Force Report of the American Psychiatric Association, Vol 2. Washington, DC, American Psychiatric Association, 1989, pp 1103–1111

Freud S: Three essays on the theory of sexuality (1905), in The Standard Edition of the Complete Psychological Works of Sigmund Freud, Vol 7. Translated and edited by Strachey J. London, Hogarth Press, 1953, pp 125–245

Freud S: Civilization and Its Discontents (1930). New York, WW Norton, 1964

Freud S, Ferenczi S: The Correspondence of Sigmund Freud and Sandor Ferenczi, Vol 1: 1908–1914. Translated by Hoffer PT. Edited by Brabant E, Falzeder E, Giampieri-Deutsch P. Cambridge, MA, Belknap Press of Harvard University Press, 1993

Galanter M: Healing through social and spiritual affiliation. Psychiatr Serv 53:1072–1074, 2002

Glover E: On the etiology of drug addiction (1932), in Selected Papers on Psycho-Analysis, Vol 1: On the Early Development of Mind. New York, International Universities Press, 1956, pp 187–215

Humphreys K, Moos RH: Reduced substance-abuse-related health care costs among voluntary participants in Alcoholics Anonymous. Psychiatr Serv 47:709–713, 1996

Keller LE: Addiction as a form of perversion. Bull Menninger Clin 56:221–231, 1992

Kernberg OF: Transference regression and psychoanalytic technique with infantile personalities. Int J Psychoanal 72:189–200, 1991

Kessler RC, Crum RM, Warner LA, et al: Lifetime co-occurrence of DSM-III-R alcohol abuse and dependence with other psychiatric disorders in the National Comorbidity Survey. Arch Gen Psychiatry 54:313–321, 1997

Khantzian EJ: The self-medication hypothesis of substance use disorders: a reconsideration and recent applications. Harv Rev Psychiatry 4:231–244, 1997

Khantzian EJ, Albanese MJ: Understanding Addiction as Self Medication: Finding Hope Behind the Pain. Lanham, MD, Rowman & Littlefield, 2008

Klerman GL, Weissman MM, Rounsaville BH, et al: The Theory and Practice of Interpersonal Psychotherapy for Depression. New York, Basic Books, 1984

Kohut H, Wolf ES: The disorders of the self and their treatment: an outline. Int J Psychoanal 59:413–425, 1978

Krystal H: Alexithymia and the effectiveness of psychoanalytic treatment. Int J Psychoanal Psychother 9:353–378, 1982–1983

Kushner MA, Sher KJ, Bertman BD: The relation between alcohol problems and anxiety disorders. Am J Psychiatry 147:685–695, 1990

Langeland W, Draijer N, van den Brink W: Trauma and dissociation in treatment-seeking alcoholics: towards a resolution of inconsistent findings. Compr Psychiatry 43:195–203, 2002

Lewis HB: Shame and the narcissistic personality, in The Many Faces of Shame. Edited by Nathanson DL. New York, Guilford, 1987, pp 93–132

Lorand J: A summary of psychoanalytic literature on problems of alcoholism. Yearbook of Psychoanalysis 1:359–378, 1948

Luborsky L: Principles of Psychoanalytic Psychotherapy: A Manual for Supportive-Expressive Treatment. New York, Basic Books, 1984

Mahler M, Pine R, Bergman A: The Psychological Birth of the Human Infant: Symbiosis and Individuation. New York, Basic Books, 1975

McDougall J: The "dis-affected" patient: reflections on affect pathology. Psychoanal Q 53:386–409, 1984

Meissner WW: Psychotherapy and the Paranoid Process. New York, Jason Aronson, 1986

Menninger KA: Man Against Himself. New York, Harcourt Brace, 1938

Milkman H, Frosch WA: On the preferential abuse of heroin and amphetamine. J Nerv Ment Dis 156:242–248, 1973

O'Brien CP: Progress in the science of addiction. Am J Psychiatry 154:1195–1197, 1997a

O'Brien CP: A range of research-based pharmacotherapies for addiction. Science 278:66–69, 1997b

O'Malley SS, Jaffe AJ, Chang G, et al: Six-month follow-up of naltrexone and psychotherapy for alcohol dependence. Arch Gen Psychiatry 53:217–224, 1996

Perry S, Cooper A, Michels R: The psychodynamic formulation: its purpose, structure, and clinical application. Am J Psychiatry 144:543–550, 1987

Pfefferbaum B, Doughty DE: Increased alcohol use in a treatment sample of Oklahoma City bombing victims. Psychiatry 64:296–303, 2001

Prochaska JO, DiClemente CC, Norcross JC: In search of how people change: applications to addictive behaviors. Am Psychol 47:1102–1114, 1992

Radó S: Classics revisited: the psychoanalysis of pharmacothymia (drug addiction) by Sandor Radó. The Psychoanalytic Quarterly 1933. J Subst Abuse Treat 1:59–68, 1984

Silber A: Rationale for the technique of psychotherapy with alcoholics. Int J Psychoanal Psychother 3:28–47, 1974

Vaillant GE: Conversation with George Vaillant. Addiction 100:274–280, 2005

Wieder H, Kaplan EH: Drug use in adolescents: psychodynamic meaning and pharmacogenic effect. Psychoanal Study Child 24:399–431, 1969

Woody GE, McLellan AT, Luborsky L, et al: Psychotherapy for substance abuse. Psychiatr Clin North Am 9:547–562, 1986

Wurmser L: The role of superego conflicts in substance abuse and their treatment. Int J Psychoanal Psychother 10:227–258, 1984

10 | Network Therapy

Marc Galanter, M.D.
Helen Dermatis, Ph.D.

In recent years, considerable progress has been made in developing psychosocial modalities specific to the treatment of addiction. Indeed, the situation is quite different from when Alcoholics Anonymous (AA) emerged in the 1930s in a climate of inadequate physician attention to the rehabilitation of alcoholic individuals. Professionals in the addiction field now have access to a variety of therapeutic techniques. These include variants of cognitive-behavioral therapy (CBT), motivational enhancement, and family and group therapy modalities that are all tailored to the needs of the patient with alcohol or drug use disorder.

The clinician in office practice, however, often is uncertain as to how to integrate these approaches to meet the needs of a given patient. On the face of it, there is no obvious relationship, for example, between the use of cognitively oriented approaches such as relapse prevention, and the engagement of family support to secure improved motivation. To address this broader issue, in this chapter we examine network therapy (Galanter 1993a, 1993b, 1999), a multimodal approach that has been disseminated to practitioners and has been standardized and studied in the clinical research setting.

The integrated approach that we discuss is called network therapy because it draws on the support of a group of family and peers who are introduced into individual therapy sessions. This approach is allied to the work of Speck and Attneave (1974), who used a large support group drawn from the patient's family and social network as a tool for psychiatric management. These networks were used for both psychological and practical aid in addressing acute psychiatric illness, so as to avert a hospi-

---

See also pp. xix–xxi and the accompanying DVD illustrative of network therapy.

talization until the patient's acute symptoms remitted. Once mobilized, the network became available to aid in ambulatory rehabilitation as well. Network therapy, as discussed here, developed a decade later, integrating many approaches that were later formalized.

A Perspective on the Problem

To understand what the network therapy approach must accomplish, one needs first to consider some unique characteristics of the substance dependence syndrome. For many clinicians, the problems of relapse and loss of control, embodied in the criteria for substance dependence in DSM-IV-TR (American Psychiatric Association 2000), epitomize the pitfalls inherent in addiction treatment. Because addicted patients typically experience pressure to relapse and ingest alcohol or drugs, they are seen as poor candidates for stable treatment. The concept of loss of control has been used to describe addicts' inability to reliably limit consumption once an initial dose is taken. This clinical phenomenon is generally described anecdotally but can be explained mechanistically as well, by recourse to the model of conditioned withdrawal. Wikler (1973), an early investigator of addiction pharmacology, developed this model to explain the spontaneous appearance of drug craving and relapse. He pointed out that drugs of dependence typically produce compensatory responses in the central nervous system at the same time that their direct pharmacological effects are felt, and these compensatory effects partly counter the drug's direct action. Thus, when an opiate antagonist is administered to addicts maintained with morphine, latent withdrawal phenomena are unmasked. Similar compensatory effects were observed in alcoholics maintained with alcohol, who evidenced evoked-potential response patterns characteristic of withdrawal while still clinically intoxicated (Begleiter and Porjesz 1979). A potential addict who has begun to drink or use another drug heavily may be repeatedly exposed to an external stimulus (e.g., a certain mood state) while drinking. Subsequent exposure to these cues may thereby produce conditioned withdrawal symptoms, subjectively experienced as craving.

More dramatic is the phenomenon of affect regression (Wurmser 1977) observed among addicted patients who were studied in a psychoanalytic context. When addicted subjects sustain narcissistic injury, they are prone to a precipitous collapse of ego defenses, followed by intense and unmanageable affective flooding. In the face of such vulnerability, these subjects handle stress poorly and may turn to drugs for relief. This vulnerability can be considered in light of the model of conditioned withdrawal, whereby drug seeking can become an immediate reflexive response to stress, undermining the stability and effectiveness of a patient's coping mechanisms. Drug seeking can occur quite suddenly in patients who have long associated drug use with their attempts to cope with stress.

This discussion helps to explain why relapse is such a frequent and unanticipated aspect of addiction treatment. Exposure to conditioned cues, ones that were repeatedly associated with drug use, can precipitate reflexive drug craving during the course of therapy, and such cue exposure can also initiate a sequence of conditioned behaviors that lead addicted individuals to relapse unwittingly into drug use.

Cognitive-Behavioral Therapy and Social Support

Cognitive-Behavioral Therapy

CBT has been shown to be effective for a wide variety of substance use disorders, including dependence on alcohol (Morgenstern and Longabaugh 2000), marijuana (Stephens et al. 2002), and cocaine (Carroll 1998). The CBT approach is goal oriented and focuses on current circumstances in the patient's life. In network therapy, reference can be made to salient past experiences, both in individual and conjoint sessions. CBT sessions are typically structured, so, for example, patients begin each network session with a recounting of recent events directly relevant to their addiction and recovery. This is followed by active participation and interaction of therapist, patient, and network members in response to the patient's report. CBT emphasizes psychoeducation in the context of relapse prevention, so that circumstances, thoughts, and interpersonal situations that have historically precipitated substance use are identified, and the patient and his or her network members are taught to anticipate where such triggers can precipitate substance use.

The process of guided recall is particularly important because it allows the therapist to use both individual sessions, with the patient alone, and network sessions, with the patient and network members, to guide the patient to recognize a sequence of conditioned stimuli (triggers) that play a role in drug seeking. Such triggers may not initially be apparent to the patient or network members, but through encouragement and prompting, the triggers can emerge over the course of an exploration of the circumstances that have led, either in the past or in a recent "slip," to substance use.

Social Support

Social support has been studied in a variety of data sets in relation to recovery from substance use disorders. For example, in the federal Project

MATCH (Matching Alcoholism Treatment to Client Heterogeneity), three modalities—12-step facilitation, motivational enhancement, and cognitive-behavioral approaches—were compared. In a secondary analysis of findings from this multisite study, Zywiak and Wirtz (2002) found that certain aspects of social support were most predictive of abstinence outcomes. Two social network characteristics that had a positive effect on outcome were the size of the supportive social network in the person's life and the number of members who were abstainers (or recovering alcoholics). In network therapy, network participants without substance-related problems are important to a patient's long-term clinical outcome. In fact, a large number of network members, when their participation is effectively maintained over time, can counter a variety of circumstances that may undermine a patient's abstinence. Additionally, they can provide varied aspects of support relative to the patient's experience in recovery. Of interest in this context, Beckman and Amaro (1986) reported that men are more typically encouraged by their wives to seek help, whereas women are more often encouraged by mothers, siblings, and children.

Community Reinforcement

Family involvement in a patient's substance abuse treatment has long been shown to be effective in improving outcome. Numerous approaches make use of social network involvement in treatment, including behavioral couples therapy (Fals-Stewart et al. 2000), marital therapy (O'Farrell 1986), and the community reinforcement approach (Azrin et al. 1982; Meyers et al. 2003).

More specifically, the Community Reinforcement and Family Training (CRAFT) program includes many aspects of treatment that are employed in network therapy. The CRAFT approach was developed to encourage drinkers to enter therapy and reduce drinking, in part by eliciting support of concerned others, as well as to enhance satisfaction with life among members of the patient's social network who were concerned about the patient's drinking (Smith and Meyers 2004). As in network therapy, the CRAFT program includes a functional analysis of the patient's substance use, with the goal of understanding the substance use with respect to its antecedents and consequences. Like network therapy, the program also serves to minimize reciprocal blaming and defensiveness among the concerned significant others, and to promote a patient's sobriety-oriented activities.

In one large trial in which concerned significant others were randomly assigned to one of three conditions, Miller et al. (1999) compared Al-Anon-facilitated therapy; an approach similar to the Johnson Institute interventions; and the CRAFT model. (For more information on these approaches, see Chapter 6 of this volume.) The CRAFT intervention was found to be most effective in engaging treatment-refusing alcoholic subjects. Similar positive findings were obtained in studies on CRAFT with illicit drug users (Kirby et al. 1999; Meyers et al. 2002). In another study, however, concerned significant others were successfully trained to apply a modified Johnson intervention technique in the absence of a therapist, and this approach was found to be successful in itself (Landau et al. 2004).

Treatment Technique

Selection of Patients

Network therapy is appropriate for individuals who cannot reliably control their intake of alcohol or drugs once they have taken their first dose; those who have tried to stop and relapsed; and those who have not been willing or able to stop. Individuals whose problems are too severe for the network approach in ambulatory care include those who cannot stop their drug use even for a day or who cannot comply with outpatient detoxification. On the other hand, individuals who can be treated with conventional therapy and without a network include those who have demonstrated the ability to moderate their consumption without problems.

The Network's Membership

Networks generally consist of three or four members. Once the patient has come for an appointment, establishment of a network is undertaken with active collaboration between the patient and the therapist. The two, aided by those who join the network initially, must search for the right balance of members. The therapist, however, must carefully promote the choice of appropriate network members. The network will be crucial in determining the balance of the therapy. This process is not without problems, and the therapist must think strategically of the interactions that may occur among network members. The following case illustrates the nature of the therapist's task:

> **John,** a 25-year-old graduate student, had been abusing drugs since high school, in part drawing on funds from his affluent family, who lived in a remote city. At two points in the process of establishing his support network, the reactions of his live-in girlfriend were particularly important. They both agreed to bring in his 19-year-old sister, a freshman at a nearby college. He then mentioned a "friend" of his, a woman whom he had apparently found attractive, even though there was no history of an overt

romantic involvement. The expression on his girlfriend's face suggested that she was uncomfortable with this option. The therapist temporarily put aside the idea of the friend and moved on to evaluating the patient's uncle. Initially, the patient was reluctant to include him in the network because he perceived the uncle as a potentially disapproving representative of the parental generation. The therapist and the girlfriend nonetheless encouraged him to accept the uncle as a network member to round out the range of relationships within the group. The uncle was caring and supportive, particularly after he was helped to understand the nature of the addictive process.

The Network's Task

The therapist's relationship to the network is one of a task-oriented team leader rather than of a family therapist oriented toward restructuring relationships. The network is established to implement a straightforward task, that of aiding the therapist to sustain the patient's abstinence. The network must be directed with the same clarity of purpose with which a task force is directed in any effective organization. Competing and alternative goals must be implicitly suppressed or at least prevented from interfering with the primary task, but the atmosphere must be kept supportive.

Unlike family members involved in traditional family therapy, network members are not led to expect symptom relief or self-realization for themselves. This approach prevents development of competing goals for the network's meetings. It also protects members from having their own motives scrutinized and thereby supports their continuing involvement without the threat of an assault on their psychological defenses. Because network members have kindly volunteered to participate, their motives must not be impugned. Their constructive behavior should be commended. Network members should be acknowledged for the contribution they are making to the therapy. They often have a counterproductive tendency to minimize the value of their contribution. The network must therefore be structured as an effective working group with good morale. This approach is illustrated below:

> **Joan,** 45-year-old single woman served as an executive in a large family-held business, except when her alcohol problem led her into protracted binges. Her father, brother, and sister were prepared to banish her from the business but decided first to seek consultation. The father was a domineering figure who intruded in all aspects of the business, evoking angry outbursts from his children. The children typically reacted with petulance, provoking him in return. The situation came to a head 2 months into treatment, when the patient's siblings angrily petitioned the therapist to exclude the father from the network. This presented a problem because the father's control over the business made his involvement

important in securing the patient's compliance. Relapse by Joan was still a real possibility. The father implied that he might compromise his son's role in the family business. The father's potentially coercive role, however, was an issue that the group could not deal with easily. The therapist supported the father's membership in the group, pointing out the constructive role he had played in getting the therapy started. It was clear to the therapist that the father could not deal with a situation in which he was not accorded sufficient respect and that there was no place in this network for addressing the father's character pathology directly. The children became less provocative as the group responded to the therapist's pleas for civil behavior.

Couples

A cohabiting couple will provide the first example of how natural affiliative ties can be used to develop a secure basis for rehabilitation. Couples therapy for addiction has been described in both ambulatory and inpatient settings, and good marital adjustment has been found to be associated with a diminished likelihood of dropping out and a positive overall outcome (McCrady et al. 1991). However, a spouse must be involved in an appropriate way. Constructive engagement should be distinguished from a codependent relationship or overly involved interaction, which is thought to be a problem in recovery. Indeed, couples managed with a behavioral orientation showed greater improvement in alcoholism than those treated with interactional therapy, where attempts were made to engage them in relational change (McCrady et al. 1991). Thus, we consider here a simple, behaviorally oriented device for making use of the marital relationship: namely, working with a couple to enhance the effectiveness of disulfiram therapy.

The use of disulfiram has yielded relatively little benefit overall in controlled trials when patients are responsible for taking their doses on their own (Fuller et al. 1986). This is largely because this agent is effective only when it is ingested as instructed, typically on a daily basis. Alcoholics who forget to take required doses likely will resume drinking in time. Indeed, such forgetting often reflects the initiation of a sequence of conditioned drug-seeking behaviors.

The involvement of a spouse, however, in observing the patient's consumption of disulfiram has been shown to yield a considerable improvement in outcome (Azrin et al. 1982; Fuller et al. 1986). Patients alerted to taking disulfiram each morning by this external reminder are less likely to experience conditioned drug seeking when exposed to addictive cues and are more likely to comply on subsequent days with the dosing regimen.

The technique also helps in clearly defining the roles in therapy of both the alcoholic and the spouse (typically the wife, as alcoholism is

more prevalent in men), by avoiding the spouse's need to monitor drinking behaviors she cannot control. The spouse does not actively remind
the alcoholic to take each disulfiram dose. She merely notifies the therapist if she does not observe the pill being ingested on a given day. Decisions about managing compliance are then shifted to the therapist, and
the couple does not become entangled in a dispute over the patient's attitude and the possibility of secret drinking. By means of this technique,
a majority of alcoholics in one clinical trial (Galanter 1993c) experienced
marked improvement and sustained abstinence over the period of treatment. The format used in Figure 10–1 can be applied in this context.

A variety of other behavioral devices shown to improve outcome can
be incorporated into this couples format. For example, Stark et al. (1990)
found that scheduling the first appointment for as soon as possible after
the initial telephone contact improves outcome by diminishing the possibility of an early loss of motivation. Spouses also can be engaged in history taking at the outset of treatment to minimize the introduction of
denial into the patient's representation of the illness (Liepman et al.
1989). The initiation of treatment with such a technique is illustrated in
the following case.

> A 39-year-old alcoholic man was referred for treatment. Both the patient
> and his wife were initially engaged by the psychiatrist in a telephone ex-
> change so that all three could plan for the patient to remain abstinent on
> the day of the first session. They agreed that the wife would meet the pa-
> tient at his office at the end of the workday on the way to the appoint-
> ment. This would ensure that cues presented by his friends who were
> going out for a drink after work would not lead him to drink. In the ses-
> sion, an initial history was taken from the spouse as well as the patient, al-
> lowing the wife to expand on the negative consequences of the patient's
> drinking, thereby avoiding his minimizing of the problem. A review of the
> patient's medical status revealed no evidence of relevant organ damage,
> and the option of initiating his treatment with disulfiram was discussed.
> The patient, with the encouragement of his wife, agreed to take his first
> dose that day, continue under her observation, and then be evaluated by
> his internist within a few days. Subsequent sessions with the couple were
> dedicated to dealing with implementation of this plan, and concurrent
> individual therapy was initiated as well.

Patients who take disulfiram in this manner have acquired a cognitive
label (i.e., a specific thing to remind them) to help them avoid a sudden
and unanticipated relapse. The potential efficacy of this approach is illustrated by the reaction of a patient who experiences a precipitous collapse
of psychological defenses and potentially relapses. If he has been taking
disulfiram as described above, his knowledge of a potential disulfiram

Month:

Date/day	Time taken	Therapist checkoff	Date/day	Time taken	Therapist checkoff
1.			17.		
2.			18.		
3.			19.		
4.			20.		
5.			21.		
6.			22.		
7.			23.		
8.			24.		
9.			25.		
10.			26.		
11.			27.		
12.			28.		
13.			29.		
14.			30.		
15.			31.		
16.					

FIGURE 10–1.   **Format for a network member's observation of pill ingestion by the patient.**

reaction can alert him to avoid going out to get a drink. Patients who are maintained with disulfiram, as described, for an initial year of recovery thus have the opportunity to deal in therapy with the issues that precipitate craving, without exposing themselves unduly to the threat of relapse.

It is important to clarify certain aspects of engaging a network member in the treatment, particularly a spouse. Long-standing conflicts between members of a couple should not be allowed to interfere with the disulfiram monitoring of the alcoholic member. For example, the spouse should not be placed in a role in which she must demand compliance. This is why the patient is vested with the responsibility of ingesting the disulfiram so that he is clearly seen by his spouse; her role is only to notify the therapist in a telephone message if she does not see him taking his pill on a given morning. Discussions of compliance per se are therefore initiated by the therapist and not by the spouse. In this way, the role of the spouse as enforcer is eliminated.

Typical Networks

The therapist's intervening with family and friends to start treatment was introduced by Johnson (1986) as one of the early ambulatory techniques in the addiction field. More broadly, the availability of greater social support to patients has been shown to be an important predictor of positive outcome in addiction. In light of the issue of support, it is important to consider what would serve as a useful paradigm for using family and social supports in office treatment. This can be used as well to enhance the stability of the technique for disulfiram observation, as previously described.

There are two options for stabilizing abstinence: the ecological and the problem-solving family treatment. The ecological approach emphasizes the engagement of resources from the patient's family and social environment. It presumes that the pathology is embedded in the broader social context and acknowledges that this context must be used to effect recovery. Many approaches to treatment, from community reinforcement to social service–based models, employ this approach in one form or another. Problem-solving family therapy, originally developed by Haley (1977) and others, relies on an initial assessment of the principal presenting symptom, and subsequent treatment is directed at the problem itself, rather than primarily at restructuring the family relations. By means of these approaches, the therapist can develop an option that parallels the community reinforcement behavioral approach used in multimodality clinics.

> Friends of a 46-year-old alcohol-dependent man sought out consultation to secure his abstinence. At the psychiatrist's suggestion, they brought him along with them to a conjoint session, where he stated that he could

stop drinking on his own. An agreement was made among the network members, the patient, and the psychiatrist that they would maintain contact so that they could act together in case the patient's suggested approach did not succeed. Two months later, after the patient had required brief hospitalization for detoxification following a relapse into drinking, members of the network prevailed on him to pursue treatment. The patient and network members then agreed that he would participate in individual therapy and would meet with the network and psychiatrist at regular intervals. The patient suffered a relapse 6 months later; one of the network members consulted the psychiatrist and stayed with the patient in his home for a day to ensure that he would not drink. He and other network members then accompanied the patient to the psychiatrist's office to reestablish a plan for abstinence.

The previous case illustrates how members of a network can help to counter the patient's inclination to deny his or her drinking problem in the initial stages of engagement and during relapse as well. It shows the value of the network in providing the psychiatrist with the means of communicating with a relapsing patient and of assisting in reestablishment of abstinence. As illustrated in the following case vignette, an effective intervention does not need to involve more than the network members' providing advice in the therapy session. The weight of the patient's relationship with his or her own chosen network members and the patient's ability to respond to their efforts to help are potent tools in securing compliance. In the following case, the network members were instrumental in ensuring that the patient would remove himself from conditioned environmental cues for substance use during the period of early abstinence.

A 23-year-old man who had insufflated heroin for a year had recently begun using it intravenously. In a psychiatric consultation that he solicited, he agreed to bring in his uncle, his cousin, and a friend for support and to take naltrexone each day under the observation of the uncle. In the ensuing session with this network, he expressed reluctance to move to his parents' house temporarily to be in a setting that would help him avoid friends who would expose him to regular drinking and marijuana use. After discussing the importance of this added security with his network members and the psychiatrist, he concurred with the consensus that he did need the move temporarily. On the basis of their input, he conceded that it was more important at the moment to avoid the drug cues of his peer group than to insist on independence from his parents.

In the network format, a cognitive framework can be provided for each session by starting with the patient's recounting events related to cue exposure or substance use since the last meeting. Network members then are expected to comment on this report to ensure that all are engaged in a mutual task with correct, shared information. Their reactions to the patient's report are addressed as well.

> An alcoholic man began one of his early network sessions by reporting a minor lapse in abstinence. This was disrupted by an outburst of anger from his older sister. She said that she had "had it up to here" with his frequent unfulfilled promises of sobriety. The psychiatrist addressed this source of conflict by explaining in a didactic manner how behavioral cues affect vulnerability to relapse. This didactic approach was adopted in order to defuse the assumption that relapse is easily controlled and to relieve consequent resentment. The psychiatrist then led members in planning concretely with the patient how he might avoid further drinking cues in the period preceding their next conjoint session.

This case illustrates the importance of maintaining an appropriate therapeutic milieu in the network sessions. In volunteering to participate, members agree to help the patient but not to subject their own motives to scrutiny. In this way the network format differs materially from the systemic family therapy approach, because the network approach avoids subjecting members to the demands of addressing their own motives. The didactic or intellectualized approach can be helpful in neutralizing excessive anger that may be felt toward the patient, without scrutinizing the reasons for a network member's anger.

In addition, the patient himself or herself is expected to help maintain amicable relations with network members to protect the supportive milieu. This expectation is made explicit in both network and individual sessions. For example, if a network member is absent for a few sessions, the patient is expected to discuss the matter with that member and to resolve any outstanding issues in an effort to promote the member's return. Any difficulty the patient may experience in carrying out this role is viewed as an issue to be addressed in individual sessions. The network therefore is conceived of as an active collaboration in which conflicts are minimized to ensure optimal function. When led effectively, members are inclined to be effective team members. They develop a positive transference toward the therapist and are willing to support the therapist's views.

Complementing Individual Therapy

Psychotherapeutic approaches have been found to yield improved outcomes when combined with certain addiction treatments, such as AA, opioid maintenance, and cocaine management techniques (Carroll 1997). In the context of network therapy, individual expressive sessions can complement the abstinence orientation of network meetings if the therapist closely attends to conditioned cues for substance use. Once abstinence is stabilized, network sessions can augment the psychotherapy with support for the patient's general social recovery.

Even after the patient's abstinence is apparently stable, it is important to examine in therapy the patient's thoughts about drinking, dreams related to substance use, and responses to environmental drinking cues. Not only do these alert the patient to the need to be aware of the long-term risk of relapse, but they provide revealing clues to ongoing conflicts, which may be apparent only in their expression in the symbolism of addiction.

Although network sessions may be terminated before long-term individual therapy comes to an end, the therapist needs to make clear that the network members should be available if the patient experiences difficulties in the future, as illustrated in the next case vignette.

> An alcoholic woman had been seen in network and individual sessions for 16 months and had been abstinent for a year. Because of her stability, a final network session was scheduled with her husband and two friends. Discussion initially focused on her successful recovery, as evidenced by her beginning employment in the previous month. Those present then agreed that any of the network members could contact the therapist if the patient relapsed in the future. The patient indicated that she would discuss any lapse in abstinence with both the network members and the therapist.

Network Therapy Contrasted With an Intervention

The Johnson Institute intervention approach, first developed by Vernon E. Johnson in the 1960s (Johnson 1986), is what people generally mean when they use the term *intervention* (see Chapter 6 for more information). Unlike network therapy, this approach initially convenes a number of people from the substance abuser's family and close friends who might otherwise constitute members of a network. In a series of preparatory meetings, the family and friends prepare letters and statements for the substance abuser describing the compromise to themselves and to the substance abuser because of the addiction. A confrontation is then planned in which the threat is explicitly made of withdrawal of support and personal contact if the patient does not agree to enter treatment, typically in a residential setting.

In some cases of network therapy, distressed family or friends may call and meet for consultation about a reluctant addicted person about whom they are concerned. The network therapist may then meet with those potential network members before an encounter with the addicted person. If the potential patient is reluctant to enter treatment, the network members can be instructed to approach the person as a group and press him or her to meet with them and with the therapist, but an aggressive confrontation is not used. The encounter is not meant to be highly confrontational like that employed in a Johnson intervention approach. This network initiation can be applied to engaging patients in both outpatient and inpatient treatment. A similar approach has been formalized in the ARISE (A Relational Intervention Sequence for Engagement) format developed by Garret et al. (1998) (see Chapter 6 for details). A strategy, however, may have to be worked out with potential network members as to how a patient who is initially reluctant will be pressed to come to treatment, as follows:

> A 40-year-old man who had managed his family-owned company had devolved into heavy cocaine use. He was now spending much of his time in his apartment ordering the cocaine, which he was using on a daily basis, by phone. When members of his family came to seek consultation, it emerged that he was sustaining himself with credit card charges from a family-managed account. The therapist said that the family members should each press him to come in, but should inform him as well that his economic resources could be cut back if he did not agree to come with them to a therapy session. Although the therapist promoted a supportive exchange between the patient and family when they all arrived at a joint session, the patient was under pressure to comply with treatment to ensure continuing access to family funds. An exchange ensued in which the patient acknowledged his problem and agreed to come to another network meeting, and to see the therapist individually. After an individual session followed by another network and individual session, an agreement was reached. He would participate in ongoing therapy, both individually and with the network. Because of implied pressure from network members, the therapist had been able to serve as a mediator in the network sessions, and avoid an unduly defensive response to him on the part of this potential patient.

Use of Alcoholics Anonymous

For the alcoholic individual, participation in AA is strongly encouraged. Groups such as Narcotics Anonymous, Pills Anonymous, and Cocaine Anonymous are modeled after AA and play a similarly useful role among drug-abusing individuals. One approach is to tell the patient that he or she is expected to attend at least two AA meetings each week for at least 1 month to become familiar with the program. After 1 month, if the patient is quite reluctant to continue and other aspects of the treatment are going well, his or her nonparticipation may have to be accepted.

Some patients are easily convinced to attend AA meetings. Others may be less compliant. The therapist should mobilize the support network as appropriate to continue pressing the patient to give participation in AA a reasonable try.

A Longer-Term Treatment Illustration

The following case illustrates the integration of multiple approaches in the network therapy treatment format.

> **Daniel,** a 22-year-old man, left a voice mail message asking to make an appointment with Dr. N. When the therapist called back, Daniel said he wanted help to address his heroin habit. He said, "I gotta get clean." In response to a few questions, he described himself as a 30-year-old single artist who clearly had aspirations of achieving wider recognition. He had been using heroin intranasally on and off for 3 years, but for the past 6 months had been "sniffing" large doses at least twice a day.
>
> At the initial encounter, given concern about Daniel's reliability, Dr. N asked to engage collateral support for the patient. He asked if they could both speak on the phone with a friend or a close family member of Daniel's who could be a resource for him until the next session. Although Daniel was somewhat wary, he agreed to their calling a cousin with whom he had a close relationship, and who had repeatedly expressed concern over Daniel's drug use. The three agreed that the cousin would meet Daniel for dinner right before the next scheduled session and then accompany him to that appointment.
>
> Daniel appeared with his cousin 4 days later. The patient was somewhat tremulous, and reported that he and a friend, also addicted to heroin, had decided to detoxify themselves abruptly with some naltrexone that his friend had acquired. They supported each other, suffering miserably over the intervening days.
>
> This patient was a good candidate for network therapy: His continuous dependence on heroin had been less than 1 year in duration, and this was less time than appropriate for maintenance therapy using buprenorphine or methadone. Also, it would be desirable to avoid his dependency for the long term on an opioid if that could be avoided, and Daniel did not want that option anyway. His network comprised three people: his cousin, a close friend, and an uncle 20 years his senior, whom he viewed as a mentor and friend. For the first 3 weeks, individual and network sessions were alternated each week. Over the subsequent weeks, the frequency of network meetings was decreased relative to Dr. N's sense of Daniel's stability in treatment. After 6 months, the network members came to a session only once every month or two.
>
> A second component of the treatment was to provide protection from relapse by having Daniel take oral naltrexone, an opioid antagonist, which blocks the effect of an agonist, heroin or otherwise, such as hydrocodone. The patient agreed to take two 50-mg pills twice weekly (Monday, Wednesday) and three on a third occasion (Friday). Daniel would do this in front of his cousin, who lived only one block away from him. This naltrexone regimen was continued over the course of the ensuing 10 months, and after that on Daniel's own recognizance.
>
> At the outset of treatment, Dr. N had stipulated that Daniel was not to use marijuana, alcohol, or other drugs, explaining to him and the network how any of these could lead to a relapse. Daniel was also expected to

give a urine sample for toxicology at random times to ensure abstinence from drugs. The patient did indeed say at one point in the treatment that he felt supported in avoiding marijuana by virtue of the fact that he did not want to have a positive urine toxicology screen.

Dr. N had often discussed with Daniel his vulnerability to alcoholism given his family history. His father drank heavily every evening, making Daniel very uncomfortable during his occasional visits home. After 3 months in treatment, however, Daniel said that he had "never bargained for not drinking at all," and that he didn't quite see himself as abstinent from alcohol for the long term. As Dr. N and Daniel discussed this, they initially agreed that it was best that he stay abstinent for at least a year, and toward the end of that time his options could be discussed. The issue was also discussed with the network members, who were wary of the patient embarking on something other than total abstinence, but Dr. N pointed out that a test of drinking was "better during treatment than afterwards." This was discussed at some length, and Daniel implemented a diary of his drinking, limited to no more than two beers a day and no wine or hard liquor.

At one point during the subsequent treatment, tragedy befell the family, when the patient's younger brother, who also drank abusively, had an auto accident while drunk and was gravely injured. Daniel continued to keep his drinking diary until a month after his brother's accident, at which point he decided that he was better off remaining abstinent and decided to do so. He did indeed maintain abstinence over a year of subsequent ongoing psychotherapy for general adaptive issues, and reported being abstinent 3 years after that.

Principles of Network Treatment

The following is a set of guidelines for applying network therapy. It can be adapted to the needs of a given patient and to the relative availability of potential network members.

Begin a Network as Soon as Possible

1. It is important to see the patient promptly, as the window of opportunity for openness to treatment generally is brief. A week's delay can result in loss of motivation or relapse to substance abuse.
2. If the patient is married, the spouse should be engaged early on, preferably at the time of the first telephone call. The therapist should point out that addiction is a family problem. The spouse generally can be enlisted in ensuring that the patient arrives at the office with a day's abstinence.
3. In the initial interview, the therapist should frame the exchange so that a good case is built for the grave consequences of the patient's addiction, and should do this before the patient can introduce his or

her system of denial. This approach avoids putting the spouse or other network members in the awkward position of having to contradict a close relative.

4. The therapist should make clear that the patient needs to be abstinent, beginning immediately. (A tapered detoxification may be necessary with some drugs, such as the sedative-hypnotics.)

5. An alcoholic patient can be started on disulfiram treatment as soon as possible, in the office at the time of the first visit if possible. The patient should be instructed to continue taking disulfiram under the observation of a network member. The therapist should obtain baseline chemistries concomitantly.

6. The therapist should start to build a network for the patient at the first visit, involving the patient's family members and close friends.

7. From the very first meeting, an important goal is to ensure the patient's abstinence until the next meeting and to plan that with the network. Initially, the network members' immediate companionship, a plan for the patient's daily attendance at a 12-step program, and planned activities all may be necessary.

Keep the Network's Agenda Focused

1. *Maintain abstinence.* The patient and the network members should report at the outset of each session any exposure of the patient to alcohol or drugs. The patient and network members should be instructed as to the nature of relapse and should work with the clinician to develop a plan to sustain abstinence. Cues to conditioned drug-seeking behavior should be examined.

2. *Support the network's integrity.* Everyone has a role: The patient is expected to ensure that network members keep their meeting appointments and stay involved with the treatment. The therapist sets meeting times and summons the network for any emergency, such as relapse. (The therapist does whatever is necessary to secure stability of the membership if the patient is having trouble doing so.) Members of the network are responsible for attending network sessions and engaging in other supportive activities with the patient.

3. *Secure future behavior.* The therapist should combine any and all modalities necessary to ensure the patient's stability. For the patient, this may involve establishing a stable, drug-free residence; avoiding substance-abusing friends; attending 12-step meetings; and using medications such as disulfiram or blocking agents. For the therapist, it may involve observing urinalysis and obtaining ancillary psychiatric care. Written agreements may be useful. This may involve a mutually ac-

ceptable contingency contract, with penalties for violation of under-standings.

End Network Therapy Appropriately

1. Network sessions can be terminated after the patient has been stably abstinent for at least 6 months to 1 year. Before network therapy is stopped, the therapist should discuss with the patient and network the patient's readiness to handle sobriety.
2. An understanding is established with the network members that they will contact the therapist at any point in the future if the patient becomes vulnerable to relapse. The network members can also be summoned by the therapist. These points should be made clear to the patient before termination, in the presence of the network, but they also apply throughout treatment.

Research on Network Therapy

Network therapy was included under the American Psychiatric Association's 1995 practice guidelines for treating substance use disorders as an approach to facilitating adherence to a treatment plan. The Substance Abuse and Mental Health Services Administration includes a description of network therapy in its National Registry of Evidence-based Programs and Practices (Substance Abuse and Mental Health Services Administration 2007), and lists network therapy as one of its Treatment Improvement Protocol–recommended substance abuse treatment and family therapy approaches (Center for Substance Abuse Treatment 2004). To date, five studies have demonstrated the effectiveness of network therapy in treatment and training. Each addressed the technique's validation from a different perspective: a trial in office-based management; studies of its effectiveness in the training of psychiatric residents and of counselors who work with cocaine-addicted persons; an evaluation of acceptance of the network approach in an Internet technology transfer course; and a trial evaluating the impact of network therapy relative to medication management in heroin-addicted persons inducted onto buprenorphine. In addition, network therapy components that have been adapted and combined with other psychosocial treatments to treat patients with opioid or alcohol dependence are described below.

An Office-Based Clinical Trial

A chart review was conducted on a series of 60 substance-dependent patients, with follow-up appointments scheduled through the period of treatment and up to 1 year thereafter (Galanter 1993c). The primary drug of dependence was alcohol for 27 patients, cocaine for 23, opiates for 6, marijuana for 3, and nicotine for 1. For all but eight of the patients, networks were fully established. Of the 60 patients, 46 experienced full improvement (i.e., abstinence for at least 6 months) or major improvement (i.e., a marked decline in drug use to nonproblematic levels). The study demonstrated the viability of establishing networks and applying them in the practitioner's treatment setting. It also served as a basis for the ensuing developmental research supported by the National Institute on Drug Abuse.

Treatment by Psychiatry Residents

We developed and implemented a network therapy training sequence in the New York University psychiatric residency program and then evaluated the clinical outcome of a group of cocaine-dependent patients treated by the residents. The psychiatric residency was chosen because of the growing importance of clinical training in the management of addiction in outpatient care in residency programs, in line with the standards set for specialty certification.

A training manual (unpublished) was prepared on the network technique, defining the specifics of the treatment in a manner allowing for uniformity in practice. It was developed for use as a training tool and then as a guide for the residents during the treatment phase. Network therapy tape segments drawn from a library of 130 videotaped sessions were used to illustrate typical therapy situations. A network therapy rating scale was developed to assess the technique's application, with items emphasizing key aspects of treatment (Keller et al. 1997). The scale was evaluated for its reliability in distinguishing between two contrasting addiction therapies, network therapy and systemic family therapy, both presented to faculty and residents on videotape. The internal consistency of responses for each of the techniques was high for both the faculty and the resident samples, and both groups consistently distinguished the two modalities. The scale was then used by clinical supervisors as a didactic aid for training and to monitor therapist adherence to the study treatment manual.

We trained third-year psychiatry residents to apply the network therapy approach, with an emphasis placed on distinctions in technique between the treatment of addiction and the treatment of other major mental illness or personality disorder. The residents then worked with a sample of 47 cocaine-addicted patients. Once treatment was initiated, 77% of the subjects did establish a network—that is, bring in at least one member for a network session. In fact, 1.47 network members on average attended any given network session, across all subjects and sessions. This is notable, because compliance after initial screening was not necessarily assured. Almost all of those who completed a 24-week regimen (15 of 17 patients) produced cocaine-negative urine in their last three toxicology screens, whereas only a minority of those who attended the first week but did not complete the sequence (4 of 18 patients) met this outcome criterion (Galanter et al. 2002). The residents, inexperienced in drug treatment, achieved results similar to those reported for experienced professionals (Carroll et al. 1994; Higgins et al. 1993). These comparisons supported the feasibility of successful training of psychiatry residents naïve to addiction treatment and the efficacy of the treatment in their hands.

To better understand the role of the therapeutic alliance in network therapy, Glazer et al. (2003) reviewed videotaped network sessions for 21 of the 47 cocaine-addicted patients and rated them on level of patient-therapist alliance using the PENN Helping Alliance Rating Scale and the Working Alliance Inventory. The tapes selected to be rated were those that represented the participants' first videotaped network therapy session. Results showed a significant positive correlation between therapeutic alliance and outcomes as measured by the percentage of cocaine-free urine toxicology screens and by eight consecutive cocaine-free urine screens.

Treatment by Addiction Counselors

Keller et al. (1999) reported on a study in a community-based addictions treatment clinic using a network therapy training sequence that was essentially the same as the one applied to the psychiatry residents. In the study, a cohort of 10 cocaine-dependent patients received treatment at the community program in a format that included network therapy along with the clinic's usual package of modalities, and an additional 20 cocaine-dependent patients received treatment as usual and served as control subjects. The network therapy was found to enhance the outcome of the experimental patients. Of 107 urinalyses conducted on the network therapy patients, 88% were negative, but only 66% of the 82 urine samples from the control subjects were negative, a significantly lower proportion. The mean retention in treatment was 13.9 weeks for the network patients, reflecting a trend toward greater retention than the 10.7 weeks for control subjects.

The results of this study supported the feasibility of transferring the network technology into community-based settings, with the potential for enhancing outcomes. Addiction counselors working in a typical outpatient rehabilitation setting were able to learn and then incorporate network therapy into their largely 12-step-oriented treatment regimens without undue difficulty and with improved outcome.

Use of the Internet

We studied ways in which psychiatrists and other professionals could be offered training by a distance-learning method using the Internet, a medium that offers the advantage of not being fixed in either time or location. An advertisement was placed in *Psychiatric News*, the newspaper of the American Psychiatric Association, offering an Internet course combining network therapy with the use of naltrexone for the treatment of alcoholism.

The sequence of material presented on the Internet was divided into three didactic "sessions," followed by a set of questions, with a hypertext link to download relevant references and a certificate of completion. The course took about 2 hours for the student to complete. Our assessment was based on 679 sequential counts, representing 240 unique respondents who went beyond the introductory Web page (Galanter et al. 1997). Of these respondents, 154 were psychiatrists, who responded positively to the course. A majority responded "a good deal" or "very much" (a score of 3 or 4 on a 4-point scale) to the following statements: "It helped me understand the management of alcoholism treatment" (56%); "It helped me learn to use family or friends in network treatment for alcoholism" (75%); and "It improved my ability to use naltrexone in treating alcoholism" (64%).

Network Therapy in Buprenorphine Maintenance

Galanter et al. (2004) evaluated the impact of network therapy relative to a control condition (medical management) among 66 patients who were inducted onto buprenorphine for 16 weeks and then tapered to zero dose. Network therapy resulted in a greater percentage of opioid-free urine screens than did medical management (65% vs. 45%). By the end of treatment, 50% of network therapy patients and 23% of medical management patients experienced a positive outcome relative to secondary heroin use. Therefore, the use of network therapy in office practice may enhance the effectiveness of eliminating secondary heroin use during buprenorphine maintenance.

Adaptations of Network Therapy Treatment

In a treatment referred to as behavioral naltrexone therapy, Rothenberg et al. (2002) adapted network therapy and combined it with relapse prevention and a voucher reinforcement system in the treatment of opioid-dependent patients who were enrolled in a 6-month course of treatment with naltrexone. The network therapy component involved one significant other who could monitor the patient's adherence to naltrexone. In addition to the patient receiving vouchers for each day of abstinence and each pill taken, the network member was reinforced with a voucher for each pill recorded as monitored. The primary treatment outcome was retention in treatment. Patients who used methadone at baseline did more poorly than those using only heroin, as demonstrated in the retention rates: 39% versus 65%, and 0% versus 31%, respectively, at 1 month and 6 months.

In a treatment they referred to as social behavior and network therapy (SBNT), Copello et al. (2002) combined elements of network therapy with social aspects of the community reinforcement approach and relapse prevention to treat persons with alcohol problems. A number of social skills training strategies are incorporated into the treatment, especially those involving social competence in relation to the development of positive social support for change in alcohol use. Every individual involved in treatment is considered a client in his or her own right, and the person with alcohol problems is referred to as the focal client. The core element of the approach is mobilizing the support of the network, even though this may involve network sessions that are conducted in the absence of the focal client. In their initial feasibility study with 33 clients, there were two cases in which sessions were held with network members in the absence of the focal client, and in both cases reengagement of the focal client in treatment was achieved. Out of the 33 clients enrolled in the study, 23 formed a network, with the mean number of network members being 1.82 and the mean number of network sessions being 5.24. In a multisite, randomized controlled trial of 742 clients with alcohol problems, the United Kingdom Alcohol Treatment Trial or UKATT, the UKATT Research Team (2005) compared SBNT to motivational enhancement therapy. Both treatment groups exhibited similar reductions in alcohol consumption and alcohol-related problems and improvement in mental functioning over a 12-month period.

Additional studies involving the UKATT sample were conducted assessing 1) cost-effectiveness (UKATT Research Team 2005), 2) client-treatment matching effects (UKATT Research Team 2008), and 3) clients' perceptions of change in alcohol drinking behaviors (Orford et al. 2009). The UKATT team evaluated the cost-effectiveness of SBNT relative to motivational enhancement therapy. SBNT resulted in a fivefold cost savings in health, social, and criminal justice service expenditures and was similar to motivational enhancement therapy in terms of cost-effectiveness estimates. The UKATT Research Team (2008) tested a priori hypotheses concerning client-treatment matching effects similar to those tested in Project MATCH. The findings were consistent with Project

MATCH in that no hypothesized matching effects were significant. Orford et al. (2009) interviewed a subset of clients ($n=397$) who participated in this trial, to assess their views concerning whether any positive changes in drinking behavior had occurred and to what they attributed those changes. At 3 months after randomization to treatment, SBNT clients made more social attributions (e.g., involvement of others in supporting behavior change), and motivational enhancement therapy clients made more motivational attributions (e.g., awareness of the consequences of drinking).

Copello et al. (2006) adapted SBNT for persons presenting with drug problems. Of 31 clients enrolled in the study, 23 received SBNT and had outcome data available at 3-month follow-up. Reductions in the amount of heroin used per day and increases in family cohesion and family satisfaction were documented. Open-ended interviews with clients, network members, and therapists were conducted in a qualitative investigation of respondents' perceptions of SBNT (Williamson et al. 2007). Major themes that emerged from analysis of the interview responses included the value of SBNT in 1) increasing network support for reducing drug use, 2) promoting open and honest communication between clients and network members about drug use, and 3) increasing network members' understanding of drugs and the focal person's behavior. Williamson et al. (2007) suggested that these features of SBNT may be more prominent when the problem is one of illicit drug use than when the problem involves alcohol use.

Conclusion

The four studies described in the preceding section support the use of network therapy as a treatment for addictive disorders. The studies are especially encouraging given the relative ease with which different types of clinicians were engaged and trained in the network approach. Because the approach combines a number of well-established clinical techniques that can be adapted to delivery in typical clinical settings, it is apparently suitable for use by general clinicians and addiction specialists.

Key Clinical Concepts

- One network member should be solicited in collaboration with the patient at the outset of treatment.
- Network members, preferably three to five individuals, should have a close ongoing relationship with the patient and should not be substance abusers.

- The addictive process and the basis for diagnosis should be explained to the patient and network members.
- The sessions should be framed to sustain abstinence, with a full explanation for the rationale.
- Discussion should be nonjudgmental, with a tone of team support for the patient.
- Ingestion of medications such as disulfiram or naltrexone should be monitored by a network member.
- If urine toxicology screens are employed, results should be shared with the network members.

Suggested Reading

Galanter M: Network Therapy for Alcohol and Drug Abuse, Expanded Edition. New York, Guilford, 1999

References

American Psychiatric Association: Practice guidelines for the treatment of patients with substance use disorders: alcohol, cocaine, opioids. Am J Psychiatry 152 (suppl 11):1–59, 1995

American Psychiatric Association: Diagnostic and Statistical Manual of Mental Disorders, 4th Edition, Text Revision. Washington, DC, American Psychiatric Association, 2000

Azrin NH, Sisson RW, Meyers R, et al: Alcoholism treatment by disulfiram and community reinforcement therapy. J Behav Ther Exp Psychiatry 13:105–112, 1982

Beckman LJ, Amaro H: Personal and social difficulties faced by women and men entering alcoholism treatment. J Stud Alcohol 47:135–145, 1986

Begleiter H, Porjesz B: Persistence of a "subacute withdrawal syndrome" following chronic ethanol intake. Drug Alcohol Depend 4:353–357, 1979

Carroll K: Manual-guided psychosocial treatment. Arch Gen Psychiatry 54:923–928, 1997

Carroll KM: A Cognitive-behavioral approach: treating cocaine addiction (NIDA Publ No 98-4308). Rockville, MD, National Institute on Drug Abuse, 1998

Carroll KM, Rounsaville BJ, Gordon LT, et al: Psychotherapy and pharmacotherapy for ambulatory cocaine abusers. Arch Gen Psychiatry 51:177–187, 1994

Center for Substance Abuse Treatment: Substance Abuse Treatment and Family Therapy. Treatment Improvement Protocol (TIP) Series, No 39 (DHHS Publ No SMA-04-3957). Rockville, MD, Substance Abuse and Mental Health Services Administration, 2004.

Copello A, Orford J, Hodgson R, et al: Social behaviour and network therapy: basic principles and early experiences. Addict Behav 27:345–366, 2002

Copello A, Williamson E, Orford J, et al: Implementing and evaluating social behaviour and network therapy in drug treatment practice in the UK: a feasibility study. Addict Behav 31:802–810, 2006

Fals-Stewart W, O'Farrell TJ, Feehan M, et al: Behavioral couples therapy versus individual-based treatment for male substance-abusing patients: an evaluation of significant individual change and comparison of improvement rates. J Subst Abuse Treat 18:249–254, 2000

Fuller RK, Branchey L, Brightwell DR, et al: Disulfiram treatment of alcoholism: a Veterans Administration cooperative study. JAMA 256:1449–1455, 1986

Galanter M: Management of the alcoholic in psychiatric practice. Psychiatr Ann 19:266–270, 1989

Galanter M: Network therapy for addiction: a model for office practice. Am J Psychiatry 150:28–36, 1993a

Galanter M: Network Therapy for Drug Abuse: A New Approach in Practice. New York, Basic Books, 1993b

Galanter M: Network therapy for substance abuse: a clinical trial. Psychotherapy 30:251–258, 1993c

Galanter M: Network Therapy for Alcohol and Drug Abuse, Expanded Edition. New York, Guilford, 1999

Galanter M, Keller DS, Dermatis H: Using the Internet for clinical training: a course on network therapy. Psychiatr Serv 48:999–1000, 1997

Galanter M, Dermatis H, Keller D, et al: Network therapy for cocaine abuse: use of family and peer supports. Am J Addict 11:161–166, 2002

Galanter M, Dermatis H, Glickman L, et al: Network therapy: decreased secondary opioid use during buprenorphine maintenance. J Subst Abuse Treat 26:313–318, 2004

Garret J, Landau J, Shea R, et al: The ARISE intervention using family and network links to engage addicted persons in treatment. J Subst Abuse Treatment 15:333–343, 1998

Glazer SS, Galanter M, Megwinoff O, et al: The role of therapeutic alliance in network therapy: a family and peer support-based treatment for cocaine abuse. Subst Abuse 24:93–100, 2003

Haley J: Problem-Solving Therapy. San Francisco, CA, Jossey-Bass, 1977

Higgins ST, Budney AJ, Bickel WK, et al: Achieving cocaine abstinence with a behavioral approach. Am J Psychiatry 150:763–769, 1993

Johnson VE: How to Help Someone Who Doesn't Want Help. Minneapolis, MN, Johnson Institute Books, 1986

Keller D, Galanter M, Weinberg S: Validation of a scale for network therapy: a technique for systematic use of peer and family support in addiction treatment. Am J Drug Alcohol Abuse 23:115–127, 1997

Keller D, Galanter M, Dermatis H: Technology transfer of network therapy to community-based addiction counselors. J Subst Abuse Treat 16:183–189, 1999

Kirby KC, Marlowe DB, Festinger DS, et al: Community reinforcement training for family and significant others of drug abusers: a unilateral intervention to increase treatment entry of drug users. Drug Alcohol Depend 56:85–96, 1999

Landau J, Stanton DM, Brinkman-Sull D, et al: Outcomes with the ARISE approach to engaging reluctant drug- and alcohol-dependent individuals in treatment. Am J Drug Alcohol Abuse 30:711–748, 2004

Liepman MR, Nierenberg TD, Begin AM: Evaluation of a program designed to help family and significant others to motivate resistant alcoholics to recover. Am J Drug Alcohol Abuse 15:209–222, 1989

McCrady BS, Stout R, Noel N, et al: Effectiveness of three types of spouse-involved behavioral alcoholism treatment. Br J Addict 86:1415–1424, 1991

Meyers RJ, Miller WR, Smith JE, et al: A randomized trial of two methods for engaging treatment-refusing drug users through concerned significant others. J Consult Clin Psychol 70:1182–1185, 2002

Meyers RJ, Smith JE, Lash DN: The community reinforcement approach. Recent Dev Alcohol 16:183–195, 2003

Miller WR, Meyers RJ, Tonigan JS: Engaging the unmotivated in treatment for alcohol problems: a comparison of three strategies for intervention through family members. J Consult Clin Psychol 67:688–697, 1999

Morgenstern J, Longabaugh R: Cognitive-behavioral treatment for alcohol dependence: a review of the evidence for its hypothesized mechanisms of action. Addiction 95:1475–1490, 2000

O'Farrell TJ: Marital therapy in the treatment of alcoholism, in Clinical Handbook of Marital Therapy. Edited by Jacobson NS, Gurman AS. New York, Guilford, 1986, pp 513–535

O'Farrell TJ, Cutter HS, Floyd FJ: Evaluating behavioral marital therapy for male alcoholics: effects on marital adjustment and communication before and after treatment. Behav Ther 16:147–167, 1985

Orford J, Hodgson R, Copello A, et al: To what factors do clients attribute change? Content analysis of follow-up interviews with clients of the UK Alcohol Treatment Trial. J Subst Abuse Treat 36:49–58, 2009

Rothenberg JL, Sullivan MA, Church SH, et al: Behavioral naltrexone therapy: an integrated treatment for opiate dependence. J Subst Abuse Treat 23:351–360, 2002

Smith JE, Meyers RJ: Motivating Substance Abusers to Enter Treatment: Working With Family Members. New York, Guilford, 2004

Speck R, Attneave C: Family Networks. New York, Vintage Books, 1974

Stark MJ, Campbell BK, Brinkerhoff CV: Hello, may we help you? A study of attrition prevention at the time of the first phone contact with substance-abusing clients. Am J Drug Alcohol Abuse 15:209–222, 1990

Stephens RS, Babor TF, Kadden R, et al: The Marijuana Treatment Project: rationale, design, and participant characteristics. Addiction 94:109–124, 2002

Substance Abuse and Mental Health Services Administration: SAMHSA's National Registry of Evidence-based Programs and Practices: Network Therapy. 2007. Available at: http://www.nrepp.samhsa.gov/programfulldetails.asp?PROGRAM_ID=61. Accessed June 16, 2010.

UKATT Research Team: Cost effectiveness of treatment for alcohol problems: findings of the randomised UK alcohol treatment trial (UKATT). BMJ 331:544–549, 2005

UKATT Research Team: UK Alcohol Treatment Trial: client-treatment matching effects. Addiction 103:228–238, 2008

Wikler A: Dynamics of drug dependence: implications of a conditioning theory for research and treatment. Arch Gen Psychiatry 28:611–616, 1973

Williamson E, Smith M, Orford J, et al: Social behavior and network therapy for drug problems: evidence of benefits and challenges. Addict Disord Their Treat 6:167–179, 2007

Wurmser L: Mrs. Pecksniff's horse? Psychodynamics of compulsive drug use, in Psychodynamics of Drug Dependence (NIDA Research Monograph 12). Edited by Blaine JD, Julius DS. Rockville, MD, National Institute on Drug Abuse, 1977

Zywiak WH, Wirtz PW: Decomposing the relationships between pretreatment social network characteristics and alcohol treatment outcome. J Stud Alcohol 63:114–121, 2002

11 | Group Therapy

David W. Brook, M.D.

Group therapy, the most commonly used psychosocial treatment for substance abuse and dependence, is the treatment of choice for many patients; it is clinically effective and cost-effective. Group therapy can deal with the psychosocial issues that are precursors to substance abuse, and with interpersonal and intrapersonal difficulties and symptoms that arise from the substance use disorders (SUDs). Because of the multifactorial etiology and sequelae of SUDs, the treatment of SUDs is often multidisciplinary. A broad biopsychosocial multidisciplinary treatment approach using a group therapy model can also include cognitive-behavioral therapy (CBT), relapse prevention, and psychopharmacological treatment.

Many groups and types of group interactions are important in the developmental pathway leading to SUDs (J.S. Brook et al. 2006). Psychosocial behavioral and cultural risk factors, as well as protective factors, may be changed through group interventions, in such developmental areas as personality, the parent-child attachment relationship, spouse and significant other attachment relationships, peer interactions, and ethnic, cultural, and environmental factors (D.W. Brook et al. 2003); group therapy can play an important role in the prevention and treatment of such risk factors.

To effectively influence treatment, the group therapist uses the *therapeutic alliance* between the group therapist and each group member, and *group cohesion*, the attachment between group members (including the group leader). Because patients with SUDs have an impaired ability to form and maintain attachments to others (Flores 2004), the attachments that form during the group process are of great importance in treatment, helping to address dysfunctions seen in these patients, including inadequate self-care, decreased self-esteem, and emotional dysregulation (Khantzian 2001). Groups help to correct the consequences of these dysfunctions, which include a loss of contact with others, self-destructive behavior, and emotional lability, as well as to address the primitive defenses often used by substance abusers, which include denial, projection, and rationalization.

During the course of the group process, group members develop mutual understanding and support, which can have a beneficial effect on relationships outside of the group, future emotional development, and health maintenance. The group's support and sharing of similar problems by group members have therapeutic effects. The group leader helps establish appropriate limits and rules for the group, which aid group members in relating to each other and which can help group members overcome feelings of isolation and shame. Over time, the group process and group interactions can help group members use more mature defenses, control substance use (Flores 2004), and alleviate symptoms. In general, better treatment results stem from a longer duration in group treatment.

Specific Issues Relevant to Group Therapy for Substance Abuse

The group therapist must pay particular attention to certain aspects of treatment. These include 1) the appropriate selection of patients for each group; 2) preparation before group meetings; 3) the establishment and maintenance of group structure and safety; 4) the utilization of supportive confrontation in the course of group process; and 5) the specific interventions of the group therapist (see D.W. Brook 2008 for a more complete discussion).

Shared group norms, goals of harm reduction and eventual abstinence, and understanding the goals of treatment all contribute to establishing the structure and safety of the group. Group members can share extremely painful feelings; supportive confrontation can provide an empathic "holding" environment (Ganzarain 1992), in which group members recognize each other's self-destructive behaviors and painful feelings with mutual understanding and support, without attribution of blame or shame.

The group therapist usually plays an active role in the treatment of substance abusers, helping group members to focus on the group structure and to comply with the group contract, which enhances the stability and cohesion of the group and advances the work of the group process. Experienced group leaders find specific methods to advance the group process despite inevitable frustrations and conflicts in the group (Vannicelli 2001). Group members learn to spot early signs of relapse by paying attention to "people, places, and things" that might be triggers or cues for the resumption of substance abuse. Here-and-now interactions in the group enable group members to gain support and guidance in coping with the often painful consequences of SUDs, which can include 1) psychosocial and interpersonal difficulties; 2) traumatic and medical consequences, including human immunodeficiency virus (HIV) and other infections; and 3) psychiatric disorders (D.W. Brook et al. 2002).

Group therapists must be aware of managed-care issues that may arise during the group treatment of substance abusers. For discussion of this topic, see Spitz 2002.

Types of Group Treatments

As described in this chapter, many kinds of groups are used to treat patients with SUDs, including self-help groups, interpersonal group psychotherapy (IGP), CBT groups, psychodynamically oriented groups using modified dynamic group therapy (MDGT), phase models of group treatment, relapse prevention groups, groups in therapeutic communities, and groups for adolescent substance abusers. Groups may also be used for the treatment of specific patient populations and patients abusing specific drugs, and group therapy is used in a wide variety of treatment settings. For further discussion, see Brook and Spitz 2002, and Flores 2007.

Self-Help Groups

The group treatments involving perhaps the greatest number of patients are self-help groups, which usually consist of large group treatments in addition to smaller groups. The most well-known example is Alcoholics Anonymous (AA). Members of self-help groups usually share a common condition and a common goal. These groups are conducted by group members, without professional group leaders, and make up a variety of types of groups. Meetings are free of charge, and relationships formed in the group are usually continued outside of the group setting. Although the primary goal is the achievement and maintenance of abstinence, 12-step programs such as AA also aid in the development of mutual support, and may lead to long-lasting personality changes. Members attend over the course of many years, some for life, either continuously or on an as-needed basis. AA has a spiritual basis, but many other self-help groups do not. Regular attendance at AA meetings has been found to reduce drinking and increase the capacity to function (Emrick et al. 1993). AA groups serve millions of members around the world. AA is discussed in Chapter 14 of this volume, "The History of Alcoholics Anonymous and the Experiences of Patients."

Interpersonal Group Psychotherapy

IGP views substance abuse and addiction as attachment disorders caused by genetic and early developmental failures, leading to defective and self-destructive efforts at self-repair. Theorists influential in the development of IGP include Flores (2007), Leszcz (1992), Vannicelli (1995), and Yalom and Leszcz (2005). According to this perspective, some people use drugs or alcohol in place of satisfactory interpersonal relationships; defects in their abilities to form object relations prevent mutually regulating relationships with other people. There are adverse effects on homeostatic neurophysiological mechanisms used by people to care for themselves, related to difficulties in relationships with other people. Physical dependence results in further impairment of function, affect regulation, self-care, interpersonal relationships, and the ability to verbalize feelings and form empathic bonds with others. However, the enhanced ability to form attachments in group psychotherapy can result in altered gene expression, which can lead to positive changes.

IGP is focused on the present, and group members' interactions with each other are encouraged. A focus on such interactions results in 1) an increase in group cohesion, 2) maintenance of therapeutic norms, and 3) further increased interactions among the group members. The group leader's ability to empathize with patients fosters the therapeutic alliance and enhances group cohesion, with a focus on individual group members rather than on the group as a whole. The support provided in IGP enables group members to achieve and maintain abstinence. IGP group members are encouraged to join 12-step programs.

IGP distinguishes different stages in the treatment of substance abusers. The early stages of treatment address developing the therapeutic alliance and helping group members learn to express their feelings. Early treatment uses more structure than later-stage treatment, and helps group members focus on relapse prevention, as well as the establishment of a safe and cohesive group environment with careful maintenance of boundaries.

Later-stage treatment focuses more on helping group members address issues of self-care. The group leader uses group cohesion and actively helps group members deal appropriately with interpersonal and intrapersonal conflicts without using substances of abuse. Group members gradually use more adaptive coping methods to handle painful affects and shame. In this corrective emotional experience, group members feel more accepted by each other, and also feel more self-acceptance and self-understanding. IGP enables members to change self-destructive interactions and to establish more empathic, fulfilling, and satisfactory relationships with other people. Eventually, this process may result in characterological change, and group members become more able to tolerate frustration in treatment as internal structural changes result in enduring external behavioral changes.

The following case demonstrates how a focus on interactions in the group can correct distortions rooted in the past. It also exemplifies the group leader's ability to use the ongoing group cohesion in a constructive manner.

Kevin, a 37-year-old lawyer, had been addicted to alcohol for the past 5 years. He had spoken in the group about his difficult childhood, complaining angrily that he felt that his parents didn't care about him, and when they did say anything to him, it always consisted of criticism. He expected other people to criticize him and not care about him in the way that he felt his parents didn't care. He had been in group psychotherapy treatment for the past 3 years; during that time he had stayed once in a 28-day rehabilitation program following a relapse. He had also resumed regular attendance at AA meetings. Upon returning to the group after discharge from the rehabilitation program, he gradually became part of the cohesive network that had been formed in the group. Although he was preoccupied with his own problems and issues, he did have the beginning of closer relationships with two other group members.

In one group session, Kevin discussed his feelings of isolation and noted the difficulty he felt in getting close to other group members. The group leader asked if he felt close to any group members and if he believed other group members cared about him. He replied that he did feel close to two particular group members but doubted that they really cared much about him.

Both group members told Kevin that they had grown to like him and that they had been particularly concerned about his relapse and his rehabilitation process. One group member commented that this was one of Kevin's blind spots, that he had difficulty in perceiving other people's feelings. Kevin became angry at this comment and said that he felt this "criticism" was one of the reasons he remained apart from other people. The group leader asked the group members about their reactions to Kevin's comment. Arthur said that he felt that Kevin was so afraid of criticism that he stayed away from other people. Arthur said that although he felt concerned about Kevin, he felt that Kevin was not concerned about him.

In subsequent group sessions, Kevin was able to reveal more of himself and his feelings in the group, and he expressed concern about Arthur when Arthur was going through a difficult period in his life. The group leader encouraged Kevin and the other group members to share their feelings with each other. Although Kevin resisted doing this, he gradually became better able to enter the cohesive interchange in the group. Kevin felt safe enough to gradually explore his feelings about other group members, and to understand that he did not have to repeat in the present the emotional isolation he had felt while he was growing up, or to use alcohol to cope with painful feelings.

Cognitive-Behavioral Group Therapy

As cognitive-behavioral approaches have become more widely known and more widespread, CBT groups have also become more commonly accepted and used (Marlatt 1985). CBT is discussed in depth elsewhere in this volume (Chapter 7, "Cognitive-Behavioral Therapies"). Group treatments that use cognitive-behavioral formulations and techniques focus on group members' cognitive processes related to SUDs, and on diverse thoughts, ideas, assumptions, and opinions. *Cognitive therapy* refers to a particular psychotherapeutic approach, developed by Dr. Aaron Beck, that attempts to modify faulty or erroneous thinking and maladaptive beliefs. It may be used as part as an overall cognitive-behavioral treatment approach. According to Carroll (1998), CBT stresses a functional analysis of substance abuse and the identification of cognitions associated with substance abuse, especially regarding beliefs about the self. CBT utilizes coping skills, with a stress on the behavioral aspects of coping. CBT has more of a didactic approach than cognitive therapy; in CBT, the goal of treatment is to change what the patient does *and* thinks, while in cognitive therapy the emphasis is on changing the way the patient *thinks.*

Cognitive processes intersect with developmental, environmental, affective, and physiological processes that result in SUDs (Beck et al. 2005). Group leaders must be aware of models of cognitive processes to better use these techniques in group treatment. Cognitive therapy group sessions may be structured to review the model of cognitive processes at each session so that group members may have a better understanding of how cognitive processes are related to their difficulties in living and substance abuse behaviors. The group leader takes an active role in helping group members to 1) set appropriate goals, 2) focus on issues relevant to cognitive restructuring, 3) use the group leader's behavior as a model, and 4) reduce substance use.

Over the course of cognitive therapy group treatment, group members review a number of different kinds of cognitions (Liese et al. 2002). Such cognitions include a number of mental activities, which together with painful affects may serve as activating stimuli and act as internal cues for people to engage in substance abuse to cope with painful affects. People, places, and things associated with substance abuse may act as external cues, and environmental triggers may also lead to substance abuse. Other types of cognitions that may be felt as physical sensations include urges and cravings. An urge may be a sudden impulse to act, whereas a craving is felt as the wish to experience the effects of an act. One goal of a cognitive therapy group is to help group members deal with urges and cravings without self-destructive behaviors such as substance abuse. The recognition of specific goals may be helpful to group members in assessing which achievements are possible, and in using internal and external resources to enhance effective coping without substances of abuse. A variety of other types of cognitions also play a role in substance abuse, such as anticipatory beliefs about the positive effects of substance abuse, relief-oriented beliefs that focus on reducing negative feelings after abusing substances, and facilitating beliefs and instrumental beliefs to begin or continue substance abuse behavior.

The group leader uses an active approach to assist group members in comprehending and restructuring cognitive processes and changing behaviors with regard to substance abuse and dependence. In addition to the group process, cognitive therapy groups also use psychoeducational techniques, and group members learn specific coping skills, including the regulation of affect, crisis management, and methods of avoiding conflicts in relationships with other people. Specific coping skills are enhanced by the use of homework assignments, which also serve to help group members reach specific goals (Center for Substance Abuse Treatment 2005, pp. 16–17).

Modified Dynamic Group Therapy

Psychodynamic psychotherapy is discussed in depth in Chapter 9; this section focuses on a particular type of psychodynamic group psychotherapy, modified dynamic group therapy. The self-medication hypothesis developed by Khantzian (Albanese and Khantzian 2002) relies on clinical findings that identify deficits in the personality structure of substance abusers that lead to impaired self-regulation, such as 1) impaired self-care, 2) poor regulation of self-esteem, 3) difficulty in regulating affect, and 4) a decreased ability to maintain ongoing interpersonal relationships. Difficulties in the regulation of affect are seen in a loss of emotional control, an inability to tolerate changes in affect, and impairment in the ability to neutralize affect, especially feelings of anger, isolation, and shame. Substance-abusing patients often experience extremes of affect (too intense or decreased affect). Some patients feel overwhelmed by anger, and loss of emotional control predominates; they may resort to substances of abuse to help themselves control painful affective states, feel more comfortable, and have better feelings about themselves. Sometimes patients are unsure of what they are feeling, because one feeling is indistinguishable from the next (alexithymia). Substance abusers often experience deficits in the parent-child relationship early in life, which may lead to later problems in forming satisfying interpersonal relationships. They may manipulate other people or become remote from others and show a lack of care for other people.

Specific substances of abuse may be used to cope with specific painful affects, or to help people feel better or feel good. For example, patients may abuse opiate drugs to cope with overwhelming angry feelings; similarly, patients with symptoms of depression may use stimulant drugs, such as cocaine. Patients who feel overwhelmed by anxiety and who fear closeness to other people may use alcohol or sedative-hypnotic drugs to overcome feelings of inhibition and shyness, and to establish a connection with other people based on a shared use of alcohol. People with attention-deficit/hyperactivity disorder may use stimulants to try to treat their symptoms themselves. Substance abusers try to achieve temporary relief from painful affects and interpersonal difficulties, but the ongoing use of such substances results in increased problems with self-regulation.

MDGT (Albanese and Khantzian 2002) focuses on interpersonal interactions in treatment. The group can help members deal with symptoms resulting from deficits in self-regulation and can provide a corrective emotional experience for group members (Khantzian 2001). The group leader attempts to provide a safe environment within the group, and group members learn to look at shared difficulties with self-regulation, shame, and isolation. The group leader acts as a model to help group members attain self-control.

Group members share examination of interactions in the group, with a focus on painful affects, loss of emotional control, and self-destructive behaviors. Group members share feelings and learn about shared symptoms and difficulties, and in doing so understand more about their own difficulties with self-care, relationships with others, low self-esteem, and regulation of affect. MDGT makes use of the interactions in the group to assist group members in the identification of internal deficits and self-destructive behaviors, with the goal of helping members to achieve better methods of coping with affects and relationships with each other. Group members help each other understand their use of specific substances of abuse, and learn effective methods of self-regulation without the use of self-destructive substances of abuse.

> **Michael** was a charming 45-year-old polydrug-abusing lawyer who had become an integral part of an ongoing cohesive group. He had mostly given up drugs, but he occasionally lapsed and used marijuana and/or cocaine. He came into one group session appearing to be high, and took his usual seat. The group members on either side of him did not seem to be aware of any difference in his mental state or behavior at the start of the session.
>
> Shortly after the group commenced, Michael spoke about the great stress he was under at work, and particularly about conflict with his immediate supervisor. The supervisor and others had noted some errors in a contract Michael had drawn up, and he was criticized for letting these

errors slip through his review of the contract. He described this situation at work with demonstrable anxiety, but also with rapid speech, which on occasion slurred. The other group members listened to him attentively, but no one commented on his presentation of his difficulties. The group leader asked if any of the other group members noted any changes in Michael. Paul, a 52-year-old alcoholic hematologist in recovery, said that he thought Michael appeared to be "stressed out," but that he understood this because Michael was being criticized at work. Janet, a 41-year-old model with a history of intermittent cocaine use, said that she knew how Michael felt, because what he said reminded her of being criticized at work, especially when she came to work high. Paul said, directed toward Janet, "You don't think that Michael is high now, do you?" Walter, a 58-year-old executive of a large corporation, in recovery from alcoholism and attending AA, said to the group, "I wonder if Michael is high now. When I was drinking, I sometimes came to work drunk, and you would be surprised how hard it was for other people to notice that." Paul said, "I wonder...Michael, are you high now?" Michael replied that he had smoked marijuana an hour before the group meeting, but that he didn't think people would notice it, and he felt too embarrassed to bring it up. The group leader asked the group members what this was all about. Another group member said that she felt that Michael was smoking marijuana because he felt stress at work, adding, "He's using it as a kind of medicine because he's stressed out."

At this point, the leader looked at Michael and asked, "Have other people felt like this?" Michael looked around at the other group members. Another group member said that he was worried that Michael would feel criticized in the group if the group focused on his being high. The group leader then asked if the members felt that it was possible to talk about issues around substance abuse without being critical. Walter commented that he had learned in therapy and in AA to accept things as they were, and not to be judgmental of himself or others. He said the important thing was to recognize a problem behavior and to change it, and he thought the group would help Michael do this in a supportive way.

This case example, a brief excerpt from a group, illustrates a number of issues that can emerge during an MDGT therapy session with substance abuse patients. Such issues include talking about "slips" and the use of substances of abuse in dealing with anxiety. Another issue concerns coming to a group meeting while intoxicated. Group support was evident in the course of the group process, as well as in the group members' use of confrontation in a supportive way. Group members understood the connection between substance abuse and difficulty at work, and members were able to relate one person's difficulty to their own lives. Group cohesion was evident in this group in which patients cared about one another, as was members' recognition of Michael's use of denial and rationalization. The use of substances of abuse to deal with impaired self-regulation is clearly seen in Michael's difficulty dealing with affect and his difficulty with low self-esteem, related to a fear of criticism. The leader used a supportive approach to help the group provide a corrective emotional experience for the group members. The group's focus on one member's self-destructive behavior was useful in helping other group members learn about their own difficulties.

Phase Models of Treatment

Several treatment models have been devised that make use of the progression of group members from one phase of treatment to the next. Each phase of treatment requires the completion of phase-specific tasks, and patients progress from one phase to the next after completing the tasks of each phase. Banys (2002) described a phase model of treatment that has four specific phases: 1) crisis, 2) abstinence, 3) sobriety, and 4) recovery. The work of treatment is aimed at repairing troubled interpersonal relationships as well as achieving and maintaining abstinence. Self-destructive behavior may lead to disturbed or disrupted relationships, and in those cases, the work of treatment may be focused on issues of loss, guilt, sorrow, and shame. Specific therapeutic techniques are used in each phase of treatment to assist group members in mastering the tasks of each specific phase. The earlier phases of treatment are centered on compliance with the requirements of the treatment program and on the management of self-destructive behavior, whereas later phases of treatment focus on helping group members identify affects and put feelings into words.

Relapse in phase models of treatment may result from a failure of treatment structure, and group members who relapse may return to earlier-phase groups, with more emphasis in the crisis phase on maintaining abstinence and controlling behavior through the use of problem-solving methods. Understanding the particular difficulties of each group member during this phase, the group leader helps group members focus on specific methods to help deal with the specific life crisis of each group member. Group members in the abstinence phase use techniques of relapse prevention, including CBT methods. The sobriety phase is viewed as an advanced phase of treatment; in this phase, the focus of the group is on difficulties with affect, particularly sorrow, grief, and depression. The recovery phase is still more advanced, and group members in this phase center their attention on the here-and-now interactions in the group and the establishment and maintenance of relationships in the group.

The group leader must view the behavior of each group member with care. What patients say is less important than how they behave, especially in the early phases of treatment, because group members may continue to abuse drugs even while giving intellectualized reasons for their behavior. The use of an insight-focused approach may not be useful and may actually serve as a risk factor for relapse. Greif (1996) has discussed several common errors in group treatment. The achievement and maintenance of behavioral change can be enhanced as group members help support one another in a cohesive group.

Relapse Prevention Groups

Relapse prevention groups address the specific stages that group members go through on the way toward recovery and the maintenance of abstinence. Rawson and Obert (2002) presented a method for the use of relapse prevention groups based on the work of Marlatt (1985), which views the treatment of substance abuse and addiction as necessitating a change in habits. This approach is different from the AA view of addiction as a disease. Relapse is viewed as having clearly identified precursors, and as being the result of a sequence of cognitive and behavioral steps. Specific risks for relapse can be identified using this approach, and treatment focuses on diverse methods of coping to avoid risks and achieve constructive behaviors. Cognitive and behavioral methods are often used in a psychoeducational approach, to provide information, help group members cope with risks for relapse, and make constructive changes in behavior and relationships with other people.

Motivational methods may be used in relapse prevention groups (Walters et al. 2002) so that members may explore and understand the rationale for changing self-destructive substance abuse behaviors. Group motivational interviewing for dually diagnosed inpatients has been studied by Santa Ana et al. (2007). Relapse prevention groups may also explore factors related to abstinence to help group members in the action stage of change alter behavior and stop substance use (Prochaska and DiClemente 1986).

Relapse prevention groups may be time limited, and may address the maintenance of abstinence by using such CBT techniques as psychoeducation, peer support, and an active therapeutic approach. Sometimes, a harm-reduction approach may be useful (Marlatt and Carlini-Marlatt 2005). A group leader using an active approach to treatment may help group members to choose topics for discussion and to learn more effective methods of dealing with difficulties. The group leader's interventions may focus on any behavioral issues that arise in the group or that may be raised by group members. Group members make a commitment to maintain abstinence during the group treatment and are also encouraged to participate in self-help groups. Group members unable to make such a commitment to abstinence may use preparatory groups. Each type of preparatory group uses specific techniques and goals focused on the specific needs of the group members.

To appreciate the processes seen in relapse prevention groups, the group leader benefits from familiarity with the transtheoretical stages-of-change model (Prochaska and DiClemente 1986). This model can specify stages of change experienced by patients during the course of altering substance abuse behaviors, and is described elsewhere in this volume (see especially Chapter 5, "Motivational Enhancement"). Prochaska and DiClemente (1986) identified the following stages of change: 1) the *precontemplation* stage, in which the person is not aware that substance abuse behavior is causing difficulties; 2) the *contemplation* stage, when the person is aware that substance abuse behavior is problematic but also has difficulty in coping with this behavior; 3) the *preparation* stage, when the person determines to change behavior and prepares to take action needed to achieve change; 4) the *action* stage, when the person determines to follow a particular path to achieve change and undertakes action to change behavior; and 5) the *maintenance* stage, during which the person focuses on avoiding relapse and maintaining abstinence. In this formulation using stages of change, relapse may be viewed as a regression back from one stage of change to a previous stage of change. This model enables the group therapist to specify individualized interventions most appropriate for patients in each stage of change. More nuanced stages of change as described by Velasquez et al. (2001) may also be used for this purpose.

Preparatory group treatment interventions may be necessary for those people in the stages of precontemplation, contemplation, or preparation. Learning methods of abstinence is appropriate for people in the action stage, whereas formal relapse prevention techniques may be most helpful for people in the maintenance stage. Washton (2002) espoused preliminary or beginning time-limited group treatments for certain specific people, including a self-evaluation group and an initial abstinence group. Supervised urine testing is done to assess abstinence (Washton 2004), in order to evaluate each group member's progress and to deter further substance use.

After deciding on the goal of abstinence and achieving initial abstinence, people may become members of formal relapse prevention groups. The goal of such structured groups is to help group members maintain abstinence and avoid risky behavior and slips. The therapeutic aspects of such groups include psychoeducation, group support, the continued development of coping skills, and involvement in ongoing recovery-based treatment. Some longer-term relapse prevention groups help group members to assess self-destructive patterns of thinking and behavior, and may lead to more appropriate and satisfying relationships with others.

In a relapse prevention group, the leader utilizes the cohesive group process to help group members talk about how difficult it is to pursue recovery, and how important it is for people to avoid risks related to people, places, and things from their previous drinking or drug-using lives. The leader helps the group members share experiences in a useful way, without confrontation or direct advice. Group sessions may be organized around specific topics, presented in written form or read by the group members. Topics focus on sharing information about addiction and recovery, and about helping people change behavior. Group sessions should be firmly structured as to time and content, so that the group members understand that the leader is in charge of the group session. Successful group leaders need certain attributes (Grotjohn 1983). These include reliability, responsiveness, trustworthiness, a firm sense of identity, humor, and the ability to be human and relate with compassion and empathy.

Group Therapy in Therapeutic Communities

A variety of groups are used in therapeutic communities. The group process in the therapeutic community of peers serves to bring about change. The types commonly used in therapeutic communities include educational groups (e.g., seminars, tutorials) and community groups (e.g., encounter groups, marathon groups). These groups and others use special techniques to encourage patient participation and self-awareness. Therapeutic communities are used in many settings with diverse patient populations. Such groups are described at length elsewhere (e.g., De Leon 2002; Jainchill 1994).

Group Therapy for Adolescent Substance Abusers

The group therapy of adolescent substance abusers requires an understanding of both adolescents and the development of substance abuse during adolescence. Adolescent developmental milestones include psychosexual development and pubertal growth, accompanied by gender-specific psychological and physiological changes; the growth of significant and close relationships with peers of both genders; the gradual separation from parents and the family of origin; the beginning of independence; and important steps on the pathway toward reaching vocational and educational goals. School plays a central role during this time, and peer and school groups assume a more central role during adolescence.

Substance abuse during adolescence has particularly adverse effects on the course of adolescent development, because the psychosocial and cultural impact of substance abuse and the psychopharmacological effects of substances of abuse interfere with developmental tasks of adolescence, or may contribute to the onset of concurrent or later psychiatric disorders. Substance dependence, with some exceptions (e.g., tobacco), is less frequent than substance abuse during this time. Adolescent substance abuse occurs in a dysfunctional family setting, and some therapists advise the use of family therapy, either alone or with group therapy; however, the use of group therapy alone for the treatment of adolescent substance abuse is "safe and effective" (Burleson et al. 2006). Family therapy is discussed in depth in Chapter 13 of this volume.

The extensive psychosocial risk and protective factors for adolescent substance abuse have been described in the literature (D.W. Brook et al. 2003; J.S. Brook et al. 2006). Polysubstance abuse, problem behaviors, and co-occurring psychiatric disorders are common (J.S. Brook et al. 1998). Common comorbid psychiatric disorders during adolescence include anxiety disorders, affective disorders, and conduct disorders (Kaminer and Bukstein 2005). Substance abuse is related to gender, as well as to adolescent suicide, physical and sexual abuse, and risky sexual behavior (D.W. Brook et al. 2003).

Group therapy has become the most frequently used method of treatment for adolescent SUDs (Kaminer and Bukstein 2005). A variety of kinds of groups may be used to treat adolescents. Network therapy, described in Chapter 10, is an innovative treatment combining aspects of group and family therapy that have been tested empirically and proven effective (Galanter 2008). The goals of group therapy for the treatment of adolescent substance abuse are the following: 1) appropriate and satisfactory relationships with other people, 2) affective control (with a focus on anger), 3) responsible and non-self-destructive behavior (e.g., avoiding risky sexual behavior), and 4) abstinence from substances of abuse (Spitz and Spitz 1996). Some therapists use homogeneous groups, whereas others treat one or two patients who are substance abusers as part of a mixed-diagnosis group.

With regard to technique, interventions focused on behavior in the here and now of the group may prove more helpful than interpretations (Galanter 2008); behavioral change may occur in spite of emotional outbursts, denial, and interpersonal conflicts. Sometimes, self-disclosure may be useful, whereas the confrontation of denial and limit setting may prove to be more effective through the interventions of other group members rather than the group therapist. Although the primary goal is to help adolescent group members cease substance abuse, it is also important for the therapist to help the group with interpersonal conflicts and the expressions of emotions. The group therapist helps adolescent group members look at the group and group issues, as well as the issues of individual group members. Peer support and supportive peer confrontation are important. Structured guidelines and limit setting help provide safety and support, especially with regard to impulsivity and acting out. These behaviors may be seen in all adolescents, but especially in adolescent substance abusers, and must be a focus of attention, to limit possible iatrogenic effects of the group (Kaminer 2005).

> **The group** consisted of eight adolescents: four boys and four girls. The group took place in a structured day program for the treatment of adolescents with substance abuse and comorbid psychiatric diagnoses. The adolescents were William, a 16-year-old chronic marijuana user who also was severely depressed; Elizabeth, a 17-year-old who was a polydrug abuser and who had had inpatient treatment for severe depression prior to joining the group; Susan, a 15-year-old who had tried heroin and had been in an inpatient rehabilitation program and who was angry and depressed; George, a 16-year-old polydrug abuser and heavy cigarette smoker who was severely depressed; Lamont, a 17-year-old alcoholic who was depressed and had had a couple of episodes of disorientation; Jennifer, a 14-year-old polydrug abuser who had been diagnosed with borderline personality traits and was from an upper-class family; Jason, an 18-year-old high school dropout whose drug of choice was marijuana and who had episodes of anxiety and depression; and Juanita, a 16-year-old who abused alcohol and cocaine, and who also had a conduct disorder. The group was led by Dr. B, an experienced adolescent and addiction psychiatrist (male), and Dr. S, a developmental psychologist and a recent Ph.D. recipient (female).
>
> Prior sessions of the group had been devoted primarily to testing the therapists' limit-setting abilities, and struggling with difficulties in controlling emotional outbursts during the sessions. Before the group began, George approached Lamont and asked for a cigarette (smoking during the group was prohibited). Lamont gave him a cigarette but responded, "You know you can't do that here." Jennifer started to giggle, and Elizabeth said, "I need a joint." At that point Dr. B entered the room and said, "I'm sorry I'm a couple of minutes late; we'll start the group now." Elizabeth said, "This is not the first time you are late" to Dr. B. Juanita said, "Come on, he's already apologized for being late."
>
> The group members talked about whether the therapists had been late before, and expressed some anger toward the therapists, primarily focused on Dr. B. Susan said that her mother was often late and kept her waiting, and William said that when he had to wait for things, he smoked pot. A silence ensued, and Dr. S commented, "Waiting for someone can be difficult." Susan talked about how angry she was with her mother, and the group members talked about feeling angry and neglected by teachers and friends. Jason stood up and walked around the room. Juanita asked him to sit down, saying, "You make me nervous when you walk around like that." Elizabeth said that in her previous inpatient group, group members were not allowed to walk around. Susan asked her what happened if someone walked around during a group, and Elizabeth said, "Sometimes they were asked to leave the group for the rest of the session." Dr. B asked if

group members found it difficult to stay seated. A couple of group members said that they knew they had to learn to control themselves, and that people had to follow rules even if they didn't agree with them. Jennifer and Juanita started to talk about not liking rules, and Jennifer talked about sexual activity in school, which was not allowed. The group members talked about sexual activity, and Elizabeth asked Dr. S what she felt about it. Dr. S asked the group members if they wanted to talk about sex during the group. The group members responded by saying that some people felt uncomfortable talking about sex and other things in group. Dr. B asked if it was difficult to talk about emotions as well as sex. Juanita talked about how angry she was at her mother when her mother wouldn't let her stay overnight at a friend's house. Lamont said that he didn't let his parents tell him what to do. Dr. B said that it could be hard to listen to parents, especially if people felt they were being criticized. George said that sometimes he felt that the therapists had a critical attitude, and that he resented that. Dr. S said that sometimes caring about people could be interpreted as criticism. The group ended on that note.

Homogeneous Groups for Therapy

Homogeneous groups are sometimes useful, such as for female substance abusers (Greenfield et al. 2007; Najavits et al. 1996), elderly substance abusers, and gay men and lesbians. Groups are also helpful for medically ill substance abusers and psychiatric patients who abuse substances. Homogeneous groups for patients abusing specific substances are useful, as are ethnically homogeneous groups (D.W. Brook 2002).

Research on Group Therapy for Substance Abuse

Some authors have reviewed research on group therapy for substance abuse (Stinchfield et al. 1994) and have found few well-designed and well-conducted studies. Many research studies lack clarity about treatment methods, parameters, and outcomes, and have methodological limitations; some have been centered on the use of a cognitive-behavioral approach but have omitted a more thorough evaluation of the group process (Greene 2002).

Weiss et al. (2004) provided a thoughtful review of research in "Group Therapy for Substance Use Disorders: What Do We Know?" This overview assessed 24 prospective treatment outcome studies of the effectiveness of group therapy for SUDs that compared types of group therapy or compared group therapy with other types of treatment. Three patterns emerged: 1) the addition of specialized group therapy enhanced the effectiveness of "treatment as usual"; 2) no differences were seen between group therapy and individual therapy; and 3) few differences were noted between different types of group therapies, and no particular type of group therapy was more effective than any other type. Group therapy did not offer a "unique benefit" for substance abusers. The authors pointed out that failure to detect differences does not signify equivalence; perhaps insufficient statistical power contributed to the lack of differences.

Although many clinicians are enthusiastic about group therapy in the treatment of patients with SUDs, much remains to be learned (Leshner 1997). The field lacks well-designed, carefully conducted, carefully analyzed studies, and the effectiveness of specific treatment approaches remains unclear (Weiss et al. 2004). However, Weiss et al. (2007) showed the utility of integrated group treatment of comorbid substance abuse and psychiatric disorders; Bradley at al. (2007) studied group intervention for comorbid disorders; and James et al. (2004) studied group intervention for dually diagnosed patients in a randomized controlled trial. Recent research has shown the value of manual-based group treatments; for example, Greenfield et al. (2007) studied manualized group therapy for women substance abusers, and found value in a single-gender group treatment for women with SUDs.

Research on group therapy for substance abuse is difficult to conduct. Difficulties include 1) finding adequate and appropriate numbers of groups and group members, 2) maintenance of group membership during a study, 3) maintenance of a treatment plan appropriate for all group members, and 4) management of the effects of group membership changes over time.

Many clinicians believe they understand the processes of change leading to effective treatment, but little clinical research underlies these beliefs. Future research efforts may overcome the many difficulties in research in processes of change and in outcome and effectiveness in this area; the use of innovative conceptual and statistical approaches may increase understanding of both group process and group outcome. Both kinds of studies can contribute to more effective group treatment methods. As stated by Greene (2002), further research can increase knowledge of "how, when, why, and for whom group treatment works" (p. 406). It is encouraging that the National Institute on Drug Abuse (2003) has an ongoing interest in research in this area.

Conclusion

Clinicians have found that the group treatment of substance abusers is both therapeutically effective and cost-effective. An individualized treatment plan for each patient can determine the techniques and goals of treatment and the type of group utilized. The therapist's ability to understand and use the therapeutic alliance and group cohesion as well as the group members' interactions can lead to beneficial therapeutic changes. Sociocultural factors, ethnicity, and linguistic and cultural understanding and competence must be considered in substance abuse group treatment (D.W. Brook 2002). Because of increasing immigration to the United States and the changing demographic composition of the population, multicultural treatment programs are of great importance. Group treatment can provide corrective emotional experiences for substance abusers (Khantzian 2001) with regard to many aspects of their lives, especially difficulties in relationships with other people, the regulation of emotions, self-esteem, and self-care.

Key Clinical Concepts

- Substance use disorders (SUDs) are chronic, relapsing disorders of the brain, with biopsychosocial, behavioral, and cultural antecedents and consequences.

- Psychosocial and cultural risk factors (and corresponding protective factors) that play a role in the development and course of SUDs include the parent-child mutual attachment relationship, peer and significant other interactions (occurring in families and groups), and personality and behavioral issues.

- Group therapy is a special kind of psychosocial intervention for the treatment of these issues and these disorders. Group therapy may be used as part of a comprehensive treatment program, which may also include individual therapy, psychopharmacological approaches, and attendance at 12-step programs.

- SUDs may require repeated group treatment interventions. Most clinicians agree that the goal of treatment should be abstinence, although a harm-reduction approach may be of use on the way to the achievement of abstinence. Generally speaking, the effectiveness of treatment is related to the duration of treatment, and a long-term treatment approach over the course of the patient's lifetime may be necessary.

- Regardless of the kind of group therapy approach used, the therapist should be active, with a focus on effective communication in the group. Poor communication may result in poor treatment outcome and early dissolution of the therapy group. Early-stage and later-stage treatment techniques and goals differ. Many different types of group therapy use similar techniques with many points in common.

- In the course of successful group treatment, relationships in the group and the group interactions come to take the place of "relationships" with substances of abuse and interactions with people, places, and things that act as risk factors for relapse. The group process may serve as a corrective emotional experience for group members.

Suggested Reading

Brook DW (guest ed): Special issue on group therapy and substance abuse. Int J Group Psychother 51(1):322, 2001

Brook DW, Spitz HI (eds): The Group Therapy of Substance Abuse. New York, Haworth Medical Press, 2002

Center for Substance Abuse Treatment: Substance Abuse Treatment: Group Therapy. Treatment Improvement Protocol (TIP) Series, No 35 (DHHS Publ No SMA-05-3991). Rockville, MD, Substance Abuse and Mental Health Services Administration, 2005

Daley DC, Douaihy A, Weiss RD, et al: Group therapies, in Principles of Addiction Medicine, 4th Edition. Edited by Ries RK, Fiellin DA, Miller SC, et al. Philadelphia, PA, Lippincott Williams & Wilkins, 2009, pp 757–768

Flores PJ: Addiction as an Attachment Disorder. Lanham, MD, Jason Aronson, 2004

Flores PJ: Group Psychotherapy With Addicted Populations: An Integration of Twelve-Step and Psychodynamic Theory, 3rd Edition. New York, Haworth, 2007

Washton AN: Group treatment with outpatients, in Substance Abuse: A Comprehensive Textbook, 4th Edition. Edited by Lowinson JH, Ruiz P, Millman RB, et al. Philadelphia, PA, Lippincott Williams & Wilkins, 2004, pp 671–680

Weiss RD, Jaffee WB, de Minil VP, et al: Group therapy for substance use disorders: what do we know? Harv Rev Psychiatry 12:339–350, 2004

Weiss RD, Griffin ML, Kolodziej ME, et al: A randomized trial of integrated group therapy versus group drug counseling for patients with bipolar disorder and substance dependence. Am J Psychiatry 164:100–107, 2007

References

Albanese MJ, Khantzian EJ: Self-medication theory and modified dynamic group therapy, in The Group Therapy of Substance Abuse. Edited by Brook DW, Spitz HI. New York, Haworth Medical Press, 2002, pp 79–96

Banys P: Group therapy for alcohol dependence within a phase model of recovery, in The Group Therapy of Substance Abuse. Edited by Brook DW, Spitz HI. New York, Haworth Medical Press, 2002, pp 59–77

Beck JS, Liese BS, Najavits LM: Cognitive therapy, in Clinical Textbook of Addictive Disorders, 3rd Edition. Edited by Frances RJ, Miller SI, Mack AH. New York, Guilford, 2005, pp 547–573

Bradley AC, Baker A, Lewin TJ: Group intervention for coexisting psychosis and substance use disorders in rural Australia: outcomes over 3 years. Aust N Z J Psychiatry 41:501–508, 2007

Brook DW: Ethnicity and culture, in The Group Therapy of Substance Abuse. Edited by Brook DW, Spitz HI. New York, Haworth Medical press, 2002, pp 225–242

Brook DW: Group therapy, in The American Psychiatric Publishing Textbook of Substance Abuse Treatment, 4th Edition. Edited by Galanter M, Kleber HD. Washington, DC, American Psychiatric Publishing, 2008, pp 413–427

Brook DW, Brook JS, Zhang C, et al: Drug use and the risk of major depressive disorder, alcohol dependence, and substance use disorders. Arch Gen Psychiatry 59:1039–1044, 2002

Brook DW, Brook JS, Richter L, et al: Risk and protective factors of adolescent drug use: implications for prevention programs, in Handbook of Drug Abuse Prevention: Theory, Science, and Practice. Edited by Sloboda Z, Bukoski WJ. New York, Plenum, 2003, pp 265–287

Brook JS, Cohen P, Brook DW: Longitudinal study of co-occurring psychiatric disorders and substance use. J Am Acad Child Adolesc Psychiatry 37:322–330, 1998

Brook JS, Brook DW, Pahl K: The developmental context for adolescent substance abuse intervention, in Adolescent Substance Abuse: Research and Clinical Advantages. Edited by Liddle HA, Rowe CA. New York, Cambridge University Press, 2006, pp 25–51

Burleson JA, Kaminer Y, Dennis ML: Absence of iatrogenic or contagion effects in adolescent group therapy: findings from the Cannabis Youth Treatment (CYT) study. Am J Addict 15 (suppl 1):4–15, 2006

Carroll KM: Therapy manuals for drug addiction. Manual 1: A cognitive-behavioral approach: treating cocaine addiction (NIH Publ No 98-4308). Bethesda, MD, U.S. Department of Health and Human Services, National Institutes of Health, National Institute on Drug Abuse, 1998, p 9

Center for Substance Abuse Treatment: Substance Abuse Treatment: Group Therapy. Treatment Improvement Protocol (TIP) Series, No 35 (DHHS Publ No SMA-05-3991). Rockville, MD, Substance Abuse and Mental Health Services Administration, 2005

De Leon G: Groups in therapeutic communities, in The Group Therapy of Substance Abuse. Edited by Brook DW, Spitz HI. New York, Haworth Medical Press, 2002, pp 155–172

Emrick CD, Tonigan JS, Montgomery H, et al: Alcoholics Anonymous: what is currently known? in Research on Alcoholics Anonymous: Opportunities and Alternatives. Edited by McCrady BS, Miller WR. Piscataway, NJ, Rutgers Center of Alcohol Studies, 1993, pp 41–76

Flores PJ: Addiction as an Attachment Disorder. Lanham, MD, Jason Aronson, 2004

Galanter M: Network therapy, in The American Psychiatric Publishing Textbook of Substance Abuse Treatment, 4th Edition. Edited by Galanter M, Kleber HD. Washington, DC, American Psychiatric Publishing, 2008, pp 401–412

Ganzarain R: Introduction to object relations group psychotherapy. Int J Group Psychother 42:205–224, 1992

Greene LR: Research in group psychotherapy for substance abuse: fiction, fact and future, in The Group Therapy of Substance Abuse. Edited by Brook DW, Spitz HI. New York, Haworth Medical Press, 2002, pp 391–410

Greenfield SF, Trucco EM, McHugh RK, et al: The Women's Recovery Group Study: a Stage I trial of women-focused group therapy for substance use disorders versus mixed-gender group drug counseling. Drug Alcohol Depend 90:39–47, 2007

Greif GL: Ten common errors beginning substance abuse workers make in group treatment. J Psychoactive Drugs 28:297–299, 1996

Grotjohn M: The qualities of the group psychotherapist, in Comprehensive Group Psychotherapy. Edited by Kaplan HI, Sadock BJ. Baltimore, MD, Williams & Wilkins, 1983, pp 294–301

Jainchill N: Co-morbidity and therapeutic community treatment, in Therapeutic Community: Advances in Research and Application (NIDA Res Monogr 144, NIH Publ No 94-3633). Edited by Tims FM, De Leon G, Jainchill N. Rockville, MD, National Institute on Drug Abuse, 1994, pp 209–231

James W, Preston NJ, Koh G, et al: A group intervention which assists patients with dual diagnosis reduce their drug use: a randomized controlled trial. Psychol Med 34:983–990, 2004

Kaminer Y: Challenges and opportunities of group therapy for adolescent substance abuse: a critical review. Addict Behav 30:1765–1774, 2005

Kaminer Y, Bukstein OG: Treating adolescent substance abuse, in Clinical Textbook of Addictive Disorders, 3rd Edition. Edited by Frances RJ, Miller SI, Mack AH. New York, Guilford, 2005, pp 559–587

Khantzian EJ: Reflections on group treatments as corrective experiences for addictive vulnerability. Int J Group Psychother 51:11–20, 2001

Leshner AI: Drug abuse and addiction treatment research: the next generation. Arch Gen Psychiatry 54:691–694, 1997

Leszcz M: The interpersonal approach to psychotherapy. Int J Group Psychother 42:37–62, 1992

Liese BS, Beck AT, Seaton K: The cognitive therapy addictions group, in The Group Therapy of Substance Abuse. Edited by Brook DW, Spitz HI. New York, Haworth Medical Press, 2002, pp 37–57

Litt MD, Kadden RM, Cooney NL, et al: Coping skills and treatment outcomes in cognitive-behavioral and interactional group therapy for alcoholism. J Consult Clin Psychol 71:118–128, 2003

Marlatt GA: Relapse prevention: theoretical rationale and overview of the model, in Relapse Prevention: Maintenance Strategies in the Treatment of Addictive Behaviors. Edited by Marlatt GA, Gordon TR. New York, Guilford, 1985, pp 3–67

Marlatt GA, Carlini-Marlatt B: Harm reduction: a pragmatic approach for alcohol-related problems, in Alcohol Use and Prevention: A Resource for College Students. Edited by Fearnow-Kenney M, Wyrick DL. Greensboro, NC, Tanglewood Research, 2005, pp 61–70

Najavits LM, Weiss RD, Liese BS: Group cognitive behavioral therapy for women with PTSD and substance abuse disorder. J Subst Abuse Treat 13:13–22, 1996

National Institute on Drug Abuse, National Institute on Alcohol Abuse and Alcoholism: Request for applications for group therapy for individuals in drug abuse or alcoholism treatment (DHHS Publ No RFA-DA-04-008). Washington, DC, Department of Health and Human Services, 2003

Prochaska JO, DiClemente CD: Toward a comprehensive model of change, in Treating Additive Behaviors: Processes of Change. Edited by Miller WR, Miller N. New York, Plenum, 1986, pp 3–27

Rawson RA, Obert JL: Relapse prevention groups in outpatient substance abuse treatment, in The Group Therapy of Substance Abuse. Edited by Brook DW, Spitz HI. New York, Haworth Medical Press, 2002, pp 121–138

Santa Ana EJ, Wulfert E, Nietert PJ: Efficacy of group motivational interviewing (GMI) for psychiatric inpatients with chemical dependence. J Consult Clin Psychol 75:816–822, 2007

Spitz HI: The impact of managed care on the group therapy of substance abuse, in The Group Therapy of Substance Abuse. Edited by Brook DW, Spitz HI. New York, Haworth Medical Press, 2002, pp 3–18

Spitz HI, Spitz SI: A five-phase model for adolescents who abuse substances, in Group Therapy With Children and Adolescents. Edited by Halperin DA, Kymissis P. Washington, DC, American Psychiatric Press, 1996, pp 265–279

Stinchfield R, Owen PL, Winters KC: Group therapy for substance abuse: a review of the empirical research, in Handbook of Group Psychotherapy: An Empirical and Clinical Synthesis. Edited by Fuhriman A, Burlingame G. New York, Wiley, 1994, pp 458–488

Vannicelli M: Group psychotherapy with substance abusers and family members, in Psychotherapy and Substance Abuse: A Practitioner's Handbook. Edited by Washton AM. New York, Guilford, 1995, pp 337–356

Vannicelli M: Leader dilemmas and countertransference considerations in group psychotherapy with substance abusers. Int J Group Psychother 51:43–62, 2001

Velasquez MM, Mauer GG, Crouch C, et al: Group Treatment for Substance Abuse: A Stages-of-Change Therapy Manual. New York, Guilford, 2001

Walters ST, Ogle R, Martin JE: Perils and possibilities of group-based motivational interviewing, in Motivational Interviewing: Preparing People for Change, 2nd Edition. Edited by Miller WR, Rollnick S. New York, Guilford, 2002, pp 377–390

Washton AM: Outpatient groups at different stages of substance abuse treatment: preparation, initial abstinence, and relapse prevention, in The Group Therapy of Substance Abuse. Edited by Brook DW, Spitz HI. New York, Haworth Medical Press, 2002, pp 99–119

Washton AM: Group treatment with outpatients, in Substance Abuse: A Comprehensive Textbook, 4th Edition. Edited by Lowinson JH, Ruiz P, Millman RB, et al. Philadelphia, PA, Lippincott Williams & Wilkins, 2004, pp 671–680

Weiss RD, Jaffee WB, de Minil VP, et al: Group therapy for substance use disorders: what do we know? Harv Rev Psychiatry 12:339–350, 2004

Weiss RD, Griffin ML, Kolodziej ME, et al: A randomized trial of integrated group therapy versus group drug counseling for patients with bipolar disorder and substance dependence. Am J Psychiatry 164:100–107, 2007

Yalom ID, Leszcz M: The Theory and Practice of Group Psychotherapy, 5th Edition. New York, Basic Books, 2005

12 | Twelve-Step Facilitation for Co-occurring Addiction and Mental Health Disorders

Richard K. Ries, M.D.
Marc Galanter, M.D.
J. Scott Tonigan, Ph.D.
Penelope P. Ziegler, M.D.

The goal of this chapter is to help clinicians better engage and support patients who have co-occurring or primary alcohol or drug problems through use of 12-step programs to enhance treatment outcomes and recovery. Twelve-step facilitation (TSF) is an evidence-based practice with a large research base, a therapy manual (Nowinski et al. 1995), and a World Wide Web–based training site (Sholomskas and Carroll 2006). TSF is a valuable technique easily available to practicing psychiatrists and other mental health professionals. The research base of TSF has been reviewed by Moos and Timko (2008). This chapter provides a condensed presentation of some of the key techniques and concepts of TSF, with special adaptations useful for psychiatric practice. An important concept to recognize at the outset is that TSF is a therapist's technique to help patients engage in and maximize their response to 12-step meetings, such as Alcoholics Anonymous (AA). (TSF is not AA, and as far as we know, it is not officially endorsed by AA or other 12-step programs.) TSF can also be applied to treat individuals who are dependent on substances other than

This chapter was developed in conjunction with the American Academy of Addiction Psychiatry at their December 2006 annual meeting. Support for the workshop was provided by the National Institute on Alcohol Abuse and Alcoholism and the National Institute on Drug Abuse.

alcohol, such as opioids, sedatives, or stimulants. Such individuals can be encouraged to go to Narcotics Anonymous (NA) meetings or meetings of other mutual-help fellowships, where the 12 steps are applied as well.

It should be noted that there are many approaches to self-help that clinicians can promote through TSF that have parallels to group mutual help. Norcross (2006), for example, has described a variety of self-help techniques and available resources, including meditation, readings, and film.

Defining the Problem

Why should clinicians be interested in TSF? Fifteen percent of the general population may be diagnosed with a substance use disorder (13% with alcohol abuse, with or without other drug abuse) at some time in their lives (Kessler et al. 2005), and somewhere between 20% and 50% of typical psychiatric inpatients or outpatients will have a current, episodic, or past history of a substance use disorder (Center for Substance Abuse Treatment 2005). For example, approximately 50% of patients with bipolar disorder will experience alcohol or other drug problems, and research has shown that those with active substance use are more likely to be medication nonadherent and experience a wide variety of other problems, including suicide attempts and more frequent decompensations (Comtois et al. 2004). Other research shows that these other problems improve with sobriety (Weiss et al. 2005). When treating a patient with bipolar disorder who has relapsed to or developed substance dependence, the clinician is faced with several options: trying to manage the patient on his or her own, referring the patient for outside substance use treatment while continuing to treat him or her, or referring the patient to another service or an addiction specialist for management of both the bipolar disorder and substance use problems. In our experience, many clinicians would rather continue to work with most of their patients; however, many assess their weekly, biweekly, or monthly visits as just not potent enough to deal with active addiction as well as the bipolar issues.

For patients who have developed major addiction, have lost control, and are at serious risk for adverse consequences, referral to a specialized inpatient or outpatient program may be the best choice. However, many patients may not be so out of control, or they may not want addiction treatment to show up on their insurance or health records. Furthermore, participating in concurrent, outside professional treatment may present other problems, including problems with cost, location, transportation, time, and potentially conflicting treatment messages (Walitzer et al. 2009; Ziedonis 2004). Even if an outside referral is made but the patient returns to the referring clinician when stable, there is a good chance that

12-step programs will be part of his or her ongoing treatment plan. Almost all accredited residential and intensive outpatient treatment programs in the United States have a strong 12-step orientation and are invested in orienting their patients to continuation with 12-step attendance after discharge. Thus, for the practicing psychiatrist, knowing about TSF is likely to be helpful.

Adding TSF to Ongoing Treatment

A typical treatment plan would be to integrate the patient's usual therapy and medications with the principles, content, and support offered in 12-step meetings. TSF is a method for helping the patient both get to and productively use 12-step meetings, as well as a method for the clinician to learn and use key concepts about 12-step recovery as part of an overall therapeutic intervention. This integrated treatment plan, although not indicated or possible for all patients, has some significant advantages in terms of its addictions impact: no or low cost, ready availability in most communities, anonymity to insurance systems and others, long-term support that will not go away with a change or end of insurance benefits, and, importantly, the patient's ongoing relationship with the treating clinician while experiencing the benefits of the 12-step program. Additionally, patients with alcohol and/or other substance dependence and psychiatric disorders may have become socially isolated and will benefit from 12-step meetings' social support, particularly support that does not endorse substance use. For example, research has shown that nondrinking support from other 12-step meeting participants is associated with abstinence over three times greater than support from the patient's own family (Kaskutas et al. 2002). Addiction treatment programs that are 12-step based have been shown to yield reduced cost in continuing care (Humphreys and Moos 2007). Further evidence of the benefit of 12-step-oriented approaches in treatment programs was provided by Morgenstern (2002), who found that promotion of a 12-step orientation was associated with a greater decrease in substance use at 6 months posttreatment than was the orientation of cognitive-behavioral therapy. Brown et al. (2006) demonstrated the effectiveness of TSF in a population of substance-dependent, depressed adults.

Furthermore, 12-step programs endorse personal responsibility for recovery behavior, loss of denial of illness (denial of illness also occurs for many psychiatric disorders), and helping others to recover (thus developing both empathy and self-esteem). These elements of 12-step recovery are applicable to the treatment of and recovery from any psychiatric disorder in addition to addiction recovery (Minkoff 1989). Nevertheless, patients and physicians may resist this approach due to some common misperceptions, such as the idea that 12-step programs are antimedication and require certain religious beliefs. We address these issues in later sections.

AA is most appropriate for alcohol-dependent individuals, not alcohol abusers. That is to say, many people who meet DSM-IV-TR (American Psychiatric Association 2000) criteria for alcohol abuse (not dependence) can learn to drink in a controlled manner. For such individuals, alcohol may be associated with certain social situations or even mood states and can be limited; such people may be managed in a psychotherapy situation, where they learn to moderate their drinking. Most alcoholics, however, can stop drinking for a period of time before they fall into problematic use again; what they cannot do is moderate their consumption in a consistent manner over the long term. Clinicians must therefore clarify the distinction between the two patterns of consumption in deciding whether AA membership is indicated.

The Background of TSF

As with most manualized, evidence-based practices for psychotherapies, the elements of TSF come from good clinicians working with astute academicians to put together a manual that is based on their experiences with 12-step treatment. In this case, Kathleen Carroll, Ph.D., from Yale worked with two talented addiction counselors, Joseph Nowinski, Ph.D., and Stuart Baker, M.A., to develop a manual for use as a treatment condition in Project MATCH (Matching Alcoholism Treatment to Client Heterogeneity; Mattson et al. 1998), the largest addiction treatment trial of the early 1990s, which compared outcomes of motivational interviewing, cognitive-behavioral therapy, and TSF. What follows is based on this manual but has substantial input from several other sources, including clinician focus groups organized by the American Academy of Addiction Psychiatry and other referenced sources. It also includes our experience teaching psychiatry residents to do a psychiatric version of TSF with patients, using the TSF manual as a basis.

Starting Out

The first step in helping patients go to 12-step meetings is for the therapist to work on a simple program to enhance his or her own familiarity with meetings as well as 12-step content. There are three easy ways to do this:

1. *Read AA material.* First, the therapist should go to the AA Web site (www.aa.org) and read through the introductory material, or read

printed material. The therapist will be in a much stronger position in referring patients to AA, and to this site, if he or she can talk to them about his or her actual experience with this material and with this site. Basic orientation requires 15–30 minutes. Additional material is on the Web site, including *Alcoholics Anonymous*, the "Big Book" of AA. Printed materials can be obtained by calling a local AA phone number. This same approach applies to NA materials (www .na.org) and material from other 12-step programs, such as Cocaine Anonymous (www.ca.org), Pills Anonymous (www.pillsanonymous.org), and Marijuana Anonymous (www.marijuana-anonymous.org). An additional resource is available in a brief course on AA on the New York University Langone Medical Center Web site (www.med .nyu.edu).

2. *Read the TSF manual.* This 120-page manual can be obtained in print from the National Institute on Alcohol Abuse and Alcoholism, Publications Distribution Center, P.O. Box 10686, Rockville, MD 20849-0686, or online at www.niaaa.nih.gov/publications.

3. *Go to a meeting as a professional guest.* There is no better way for a therapist to learn about AA than by going to an actual AA (or other 12-step) meeting as a professional guest. This can be easily accomplished by calling the AA phone number in virtually any directory throughout the United States (and many other countries) and identifying oneself as a doctor or other health care provider who would like a guide to take him or her to a local AA meeting as a professional guest. Most AA communities have standing committees of members whose job it is to do this, and some of them are recovering health care professionals themselves. It works best to meet with one or two of these guides for half an hour before the meeting to hear their views and get oriented to what happens in meetings. The therapist can attend an open meeting (i.e., one where guests [i.e., nonalcoholic individuals] are allowed), then meet with the guides afterward to talk about the meeting and ask questions about what went on. Meetings typically run for 60–90 minutes. At most meetings, free pamphlets are available about various aspects of AA recovery. If the therapist finds this meeting interesting and helpful, he or she might want to ask the guides about attending a meeting of a different socioeconomic, cultural, racial, or other specific group—AA meetings reflect the general communities from which they spring. Matching patients to the right AA meeting, where they feel more comfortable with others, is often key to their becoming regular members. It is hard to appreciate these differences without experiencing them. It also substantially strengthens the therapist's suggestion to patients to attend if the therapist can discuss his or her experience with attending AA meetings as

a professional guest and comment on the fact that one meeting can feel quite different from another.

Core Elements of the TSF Manual

In the remainder of this chapter, we present material from the Project MATCH *Twelve Step Facilitation Therapy Manual* (Nowinski et al. 1995). This chapter does not review the manual in full. What is offered might be considered a primer for the manual, with editorial comments and additions for psychiatrists regarding treating patients with co-occurring psychiatric issues. In Project MATCH, TSF was designed to be accomplished in 12 sequential sessions over about 3 months. However, for the practicing clinician, it is more likely that real-world TSF will occur off and on over the course of treatment, which for some may be weeks or months, and for others could be many years.

The following material set in block text is quoted or paraphrased from the TSF manual (Nowinski et al. 1995, pp. ix–18) and is primarily from the introductory material and therapist guidelines. *The italic text indicates our edits to the original material.* Our discussion of the TSF materials (and of *our edits*) is presented in regular paragraphs. Our comments may help the psychiatrist starting out with TSF by adding material and approaches that harmonize with psychiatric practice and psychiatric patients. For the sake of brevity, we have used the psychiatric example of bipolar disorder in most cases, rather than invoking many different diagnostic examples.

TSF Treatment Goals

The primary TSF treatment goals are acceptance and surrender. These are discussed below. The next section describes more specific objectives in TSF.

Acceptance

> Acceptance by patients that they suffer from the chronic and progressive illness of alcoholism.

It is very important that clinicians who refer patients to AA or other 12-step programs make sure that the message given to patients about their addictions harmonizes with what patients hear at 12-step meetings, because receiving conflicting information is not a good way to make a productive integration. A pharmacological analogy would be that one should not prescribe medications that negatively interact. Some clinicians will have a hard time swallowing the acceptance phrase above as it is written; however, most clinicians can endorse the statement if the following phrase is added at the end: *if they continue to drink harmfully and dangerously, and do not participate in recovery activities.* The corollary for psychiatric patients can be useful: for example, in the case of bipolar disorder, it would read, *acceptance by patients that they suffer from bipolar disorder and that their disease will likely become chronic and progressive if they do not take their medications or participate in recovery (therapeutic) activities.* Dual Recovery Anonymous [DRA] (2004) and "Double Trouble" are 12-step programs created by persons with both psychiatric and addiction disorders. The first of DRA's 12 steps is "We admitted we were powerless over our dual illness of chemical dependency and emotional or psychiatric illness—that our lives had become unmanageable." Importantly, this means that individuals are

- Powerless over being born with the illnesses or managing them without help, and
- Powerless to predict behavior once drinking, in a manic episode, or both; but
- Not powerless to get to meetings or therapy appointments,
- Not powerless to take medications regularly and avoid bars, and
- Not powerless to participate in recovery from both disorders.

> Acceptance by patients that they have lost the ability to control their drinking.

Research has shown that persons with more severe dependence do better in AA than those with episodic abuse (Tonigan et al. 2006) because of the concept of loss of control stated above, as well as other issues. This means that if a patient has only mild abuse and can control his or her drinking most of the time with a therapist's support, then he or she is probably not the most likely AA candidate. In terms of bipolar behavior, the correlate would be *acceptance by patients that they have lost the ability to control their behavior when manic or severely depressed.* In talking to patients about this concept or phrase excerpted above, one can add the word *reliably* just before "control their drinking." For example, with the alcohol-dependent bipolar patient, the clinician would ask, "Can you reliably control your drinking well enough that you are willing to take the risk of decompensating with both your alcohol and manic behavior and ending up back in the hospital, jail, or both? Can you reliably control your manic behavior (if you stop your medications) such that you are willing to take the risk of decompensating, or going back to drinking, or both?"

Acceptance by patients that since there is no effective cure for alcoholism, the only viable alternative is complete abstinence from the use of alcohol.

If patients with major mental illness can reliably control their drinking to one small glass of wine a day, then by definition, they do not have dependence, and TSF is not for them. However, if they do have dependence with episodic or regular dyscontrol if they drink, it is much easier for them to not drink at all than to prime the pump with attempts at controlled drinking. The analogy here is *acceptance by patients that since there is no effective cure for bipolar or schizophrenic disorder, the only viable alternative is to take daily medications and participate in healthy recovery behaviors (such as seeing their psychiatrist and attending 12-step meetings if they have substance dependence).*

> **Geoffrey,** a 34-year-old businessman with a long history of heavy drinking and three hospitalizations for manic episodes, sees Dr. T for psychiatric follow-up after his most recent hospital stay. When Dr. T inquires about his drinking, the patient becomes defensive and states, "Don't start up about this 'powerless' stuff! I can control my drinking when I want to." However, in describing his recent hospital admission, he states that he had started drinking with friends at a ball game and got too intoxicated to walk home. Someone called a cab for him, but when he got home, his wife wouldn't let him in and he had to sleep in the garage. He then decided to "show her" by continuing to drink, and he is unsure whether he took any of his lithium and aripiprazole over the next few days. Within 3 days, he was arrested for disrobing in public and was involuntarily committed to the hospital in a full-blown manic state.
>
> Dr. T asks, "Was that part of your plan when you decided to have a beer at the ball game?" Geoffrey responds, "No, of course not! Things just got away from me. And my wife pissed me off." Dr. T comments, "OK, that sounds terrible, but for whatever reason, you kept drinking, probably stopped or forgot your medications, became manic, then off to the races." Geoffrey says, "But that doesn't happen every time I drink beer." Dr. T says, "Right. Maybe sometimes—maybe even usually—you can have a few and stop, but can you *reliably* predict which time you might lose control?" The patient admits, "No, I guess not. I see what you mean about not being able to *reliably* control it. I guess it's sort of like Russian roulette. Why do I keep taking these crazy chances?"

Surrender

Acknowledgment on the part of the patient that there is hope for recovery, but only through accepting the reality of loss of control (*from alcohol dependence/major mental illness*) and by having faith that some higher power (*AA meetings, the psychiatrist, medications, support groups for the mentally ill, a spiritual higher power*) can help the individual whose own willpower has been defeated by alcohol/ *major mental illness*.

Most psychiatrists are unfortunately familiar with the mentally ill patient who understands his or her disorder one month, accepts it, and does everything possible to stay in remission, but who over time begins to believe that he or she no longer has a disorder and then decreases or stops taking medications and receiving therapy and decompensates to depression or mania. The same process can hold for addictions. Clinical experience shows that relapsing back into denial of illness happens for both psychiatric and addiction disorders and is not something that is dealt with once and for all. Quite often, denial can creep back intermittently and lead to serious problems. By continually concentrating on acceptance of illness, 12-step members reinoculate themselves against denial. For example, each time members of AA, DRA, or another 12-step program speak in meetings, they introduce themselves by saying, for example, "Hi, my name is Rick, and I am a recovering alcoholic." In dual-disorder AA or DRA meetings, the speaker might say, "Hi, my name is Rick, and I am a recovering bipolar alcoholic." The power in this phrase is the direct challenge to denial; 12-step meetings strongly promote that denial can reemerge if it is not actively and regularly challenged.

> Acknowledgment by the patient that the fellowship of AA has helped millions of alcoholics to sustain their sobriety and that the patient's best chances for success are to follow the AA path. *Furthermore, the 12-step approach can be a valuable approach to dealing with any other potentially chronic and relapsing condition, such as most psychiatric disorders.*

Two key issues are represented in this statement. First, by merely examining a schedule book of meetings in any community and going to a meeting or two, one recognizes that many, many people go to AA meetings. For example, in Seattle there are about 1,200 meetings per week, and an average meeting has 15–100 attendees. Observing this mass of people all going in the same healthy direction has a potency that cannot be captured by the academic discussion of a research finding. Second, *sustain* is a key word in the excerpt above. Although research shows that most psychiatric and addiction disorders are chronic and relapsing in nature, most treatment structures are short term or episodic (e.g., with limits on study lengths, limits on payment for an episode of treatment, managed care limits on number of sessions). Twelve-step meetings are available without cost, without end, and almost without boundary, because they are now easily available almost anywhere in the United States and are becoming more available throughout much of the world. As Mark Twain reportedly said, "Stopping smoking is easy. I've done it hundreds of times." Without the power of continual reinforcement, denial returns and relapse is likely.

In this regard, it is useful to explain to the patient how the speakers' presentations ("qualifications") are useful in putting the illness into context. The narratives and personal stories that one hears at meetings have an important psychological role in promoting both the speakers' and listeners' recovery (Mankowski et al. 2001). Their relevance, however, often needs to be clarified for the new attendee, who might say something like, "I don't like those meetings. All they ever talk about is alcohol and drinking. What's the point of that?"

> **Rachel,** a 27-year-old divorced nurse, has been hospitalized after a suicide attempt involving taking an overdose of clonazepam and superficially cutting her wrist. During the initial evaluation, Dr. W determines that although Rachel has a valid diagnosis of recurrent major depressive disorder (established before she abused any substances), she is currently in withdrawal from both benzodiazepines and opioids. Rachel gives a long history of intermittent abuse of these and other prescription medications, some of which she obtained from her physicians and some of which were diverted from hospital supplies. She says she has tried therapy, medications (antidepressants and anxiolytics), and AA, but "nothing works for me!" With further gentle probing, Rachel acknowledges that she only attended a few sessions with two different therapists and did not tell them about her drug use. She also didn't take any medications as prescribed, discarding the antidepressants because she didn't like the side effects and maneuvering her doctors into giving benzodiazepines because she liked the effect. At AA, what she *heard* was that she really didn't belong because she preferred pills, not alcohol. Although she had attended a good number of AA meetings, she never got a sponsor, hung out with the people who came late to meetings and sat in the back, and became involved in an affair with a man she met at AA, who was later abusive to her soon after both relapsed to drug use.
>
> After completing detoxification, Rachel admitted she had never given treatment a chance. She agreed to attend a minimum of three meetings per week of Dual Recovery Anonymous and Pills Anonymous, and to get a female sponsor with at least 5 years of recovery; to take mood-stabilizing medication as prescribed; and to see a therapist weekly. After 3 months, Rachel also agreed to start attending a dialectical behavior therapy group. After a short relapse on pills, she was able to establish abstinence and recently picked up a 1-year chip, and she started the nurses' professional recovery program in her area. Dr. W focused on supporting Rachel's 12-step recovery by also facilitating dialectical behavior therapy involvement and providing some translation of concepts between these two mutually supportive therapies. In addition, no dependence-inducing medications were given to Rachel during the search for the right type and dose of antidepressant.

Objectives

The two major treatment goals of acceptance and surrender are reflected in a series of specific objectives that are congruent with the AA view of individuals with alcoholism. These specific objectives are cognitive, emotional, behavioral, social, and spiritual in nature.

Cognitive Objectives

Patients need to understand some of the ways in which their thinking has been affected by alcohol, *other drugs, or mental disorders.*

Clinicians who conclude that TSF might be helpful to their patients are likely driven by observing behaviors and negative consequences that have resulted from alcohol or other drug use. At times, the patients themselves may conclude they have an addiction problem, but it is more likely that the clinician will be led to such a conclusion based on the patient's substance-related problems and consequences. In such cases, although the patient may have sought treatment for only a psychiatric problem, the clinician may decide that the patient also has a co-occurring problem with addiction, which needs to be a focus in the overall treatment plan.

Patients need to understand how their thinking may reflect denial and thereby contribute to continued drinking (*or psychiatric relapse*) and resistance to acceptance (Step 1 [see Table 12–1 later in this chapter]), *which can lead to decompensation of addiction, psychiatric disorder, or both conditions.*
   The therapist remains vigilant for signs of denial *of either disorder,* patient accounts of slips, and *medication nonadherence or missing appointments, and explains these slips in terms of denial.*
   The therapist suggests recovery tasks that will enhance the patient's understanding of *addiction and his or her psychiatric disorder, as well as how both of these can benefit from active participation in AA or other 12-step programs.*

Denial of illness by a previously substance-dependent person usually leads to experimentation, which may then lead to increased use (in an effort to match previous effects as tolerance to the substance builds). This may lead fairly rapidly to problematic and dependent use. In the case of relapse, this process may start with a drop-off in attendance at 12-step meetings, even before the actual substance use begins. The clinician should therefore be attentive to a patient's attendance at 12-step meetings and view a decline in attendance as an indication both to encourage renewed attendance on the part of the patient and to look for circumstances potentially associated with relapse.

For individuals with a psychiatric disorder, denial of illness may lead to a refusal to initiate treatment. Similarly, individuals in denial of their relapse to substance use may begin canceling treatment appointments or decreasing or stopping medications—either of which may occur before recurrence of major psychiatric symptoms.

Certain psychiatric conditions display denial in different manners. For example, grandiosity in mania leads the patient to believe that he or she knows better and can handle anything; nihilism in depression leads the patient to believe that he or she is not worth treatment and nothing matters anyway; posttraumatic stress disorder leads the patient to believe that his or her symptoms are becoming worse because he or she is seeing a specialist and concentrating on the memories; delusions in schizophrenia may lead the patient to believe that it is the medications that are causing, for example, electric rays from the sky that torture him or her.

> Patients need to see the connection between their alcohol abuse and the negative consequences that result...which may be physical, social, legal, psychological, financial, or spiritual; *and, further, patients need to analyze in detail how their co-occurring psychiatric problems have been affected by their addictions, and vice versa. Common problems include aggravated symptoms, decompensations, medication adherence problems, suicide attempts, and monetary problems.*

Emotional Objectives

> Patients need to understand the AA view of emotions and how certain emotional states (e.g., anger and loneliness) *or a relapsing psychiatric disorder* can lead to drinking.

A version of the AA view of emotions and how to deal with them is described in Topic 8 of the *Twelve Step Facilitation Therapy Manual* (Nowinski et al. 1995, p. 79) but is too lengthy to fully review here. The reader may be surprised to find that many elements of Marlatt's relapse prevention (Marlatt and Gordon 1985) and Linehan's dialectical behavioral therapy (Linehan 1993) overlap a good deal with AA content and principles, in terms of analyzing how certain emotions lead to certain behaviors and how to handle them.

HALT (Hungry, Angry, Lonely, Tired) is an AA mnemonic and slogan that not only captures common emotional relapse states but also suggests action, as in "HALT before you do something you do not really want to do." Interestingly, this model is quite compatible with the cognitive-behavioral approach that many therapists apply in treating addictive disorders. Feelings such as anxiety and depression may regularly lead to the self-administration of a drug of abuse; these feelings may then become conditioned stimuli that produce a response experienced as craving, thereby precipitating drug taking without a conscious decision on the part of the addicted person. The same is true for a particular setting in which alcohol or drugs were repeatedly taken; it may become a conditioned stimulus for drug-seeking behavior on subsequent occasions of exposure. For this reason, the recovering alcoholic individual is warned in 12-step groups to watch out for negative feelings and avoid bars and drug-related social situations; these have become conditioned stimuli for alcohol-seeking behavior, leaving the alcoholic person more vulnerable to "needing" a drink.

When reviewing a patient's psychiatric symptoms or substance use or craving since the last visit, the psychiatrist might integrate TSF by asking, "Have there been any episodes of feeling hungry, angry, lonely, or tired since your last visit, and if so, how did you handle them?" By using the AA verbiage, the psychiatrist is telling the patient that he or she supports AA and that the psychiatrist's therapy is meant to be integrated with what the patient is getting through AA.

> Patients need to be informed regarding some of the practical ways AA suggests for dealing with emotions so as to minimize the risks of drinking.

The most common and obvious way for a patient to become informed of these methods is to attend AA meetings (Cloud and Kingree 2008). In fact, the methods by which a patient learns how to deal with emotions are so numerous that they are included in almost every story, vignette, step description, and other literature that AA publishes. (Topic 8 from the *Twelve Step Facilitation Therapy Manual* [Nowinski et al. 1995, pp. 79–86] has very practical materials in a workbook format.) For individuals who are seeing a therapist, AA methods present a way to deal with problematic emotions other than taking medication or using drugs.

Behavioral Objectives

> Patients need to understand how the powerful and cunning illness of alcoholism has affected their whole lives and how many of their existing or old habits have supported their continued drinking. *They also need to understand how their addiction and psychiatric conditions have interacted and adversely affected each other.*

The behavioral approach associated with conditioned stimuli is a useful cognitive-behavioral technique for addiction treatment to frame changes in the activities associated with drug use (Brown et al. 2006; Carroll 2004). The issue of self-medication may emerge and has the potential to confuse both the psychiatrist and the patient.

Virtually all research conducted on the matter shows that addictive use of substances makes major psychiatric disorders worse, resulting in increased symptoms, decompensations, emergency room visits, homelessness, and suicide, among other problems (Substance Abuse and Mental

Health Services Administration 2005). Furthermore, patients who invoke the term *self-medication* have an increased likelihood of suicidal ideation and suicide attempts (Bolton et al. 2006). To equate substance abuse with what psychiatric medications are supposed to do is like equating electricity used for home heating to electricity in a lightning bolt that destroys someone's house. Research has shown that when an individual with bipolar disorder who is in a manic state claims to be self-medicating, he or she is most likely aiming to get even more euphoric, and that patients with bipolar disorder who use the term *self-medication* have worse prognoses for recovery (Weiss 2004). Using the term *self-medication* when *addiction* or *abuse of substances* is more accurate can be confusing to both the patient and the psychiatrist. Such use allows concrete-thinking patients to think, "Well, the psychiatrist said I self-medicated, so I guess I will take his medications [lithium, antipsychotics, etc.] on Monday through Friday and my medications [crack and alcohol] on the weekend. After all, it's all medication."

We will deal with this topic more in the later section "Facilitation," when we give concrete examples of how to talk to patients about meetings.

Social Objectives

> Patients need to turn to the fellowship of AA and make use of its resources and practical wisdom in order to change their alcohol behavior.
> Patients need to "get active" in AA as a means of sustaining their sobriety.
> Patients need to attend and participate regularly in meetings of various kinds, including AA-sponsored social activities.
> Patients need to obtain and develop a relationship with an AA sponsor.
> Patients need to access AA whenever they experience the urge to drink or suffer a relapse.
> Patients need to reevaluate their relationships with "enablers" and fellow alcoholics/addicts.

It is easy to understand the need for an individual who is trying to stay sober to avoid spending time with friends who are still drinking or using substances. Similarly, an individual who is receiving treatment for a psychiatric disorder might have well-meaning but uninformed friends or relatives who suggest that the patient stop taking his or her medications because they are chemicals and not natural. Identifying persons who are supportive of recovery and avoiding or working to change those who are not are important elements of TSF. This is especially important in choosing certain AA meetings that may be more supportive of co-occurring issues and in choosing a sponsor. The sponsor should either have co-occurring disorders or should be supportive and understanding of these issues.

Spiritual Objectives

Patients need to experience hope that they can arrest their alcoholism *and manage and recover from their psychiatric disorder(s)*.

Patients need to develop a belief and trust in a power greater than their own willpower.

The above statements hold for both addictions and psychiatric disorders. If the willpower of the individual seeking treatment were adequate, he or she would not need to see the psychiatrist, take medications, or use the 12-step programs. These types of "power greater than oneself" are pretty concrete; however, what about the role of spirituality or God?

The issue of God in TSF. *Spirituality* has been defined as "that which gives people meaning and purpose in life" (Puchalski et al. 2004, p. 689). The element of spirituality is what distinguishes AA from orientations that approach addiction recovery on the basis of physical and behavioral consequences of disease alone as well as from formal religious practices. The book *Alcoholics Anonymous* repeatedly mentions a "program of recovery" and associates it with terms such as *spiritual experience* and *spiritual awakening* (Alcoholics Anonymous 1976). A spiritual orientation is inherent in four of the 12 steps, which include the word *God*. However, both key AA texts (Alcoholics Anonymous 1976, 1984) dedicate great effort to differentiating traditional concepts of God from the AA spiritual concept of a higher power.

Both *spirituality* and *God* can have many different meanings, and a patient who balks at interpretation of these terms might be open to working under another interpretation. Either word can attract or repel individuals, depending on their associations with the terms. During discussions with a patient about his or her previous experiences with 12-step programs (or simply what he or she might have heard about these programs), the issue of the spiritual element in these programs is raised quickly. (Special care needs to be taken in these discussions with psychotic patients who have religious delusions.) One should try to explore the person's associations to key words with open-ended questions:

- What do you know or think about the term *spirituality*? How do you think it is used in AA [or another 12-step program the individual may have attended or heard about]?
- How about the term *higher power*? Was this concept helpful to you? If not, let's see if we can figure out how it might be.
- Your dependence on alcohol [or] drugs, by definition, is clearly stronger than your own willpower. Do you recognize your dependence as a power greater than yourself? If so, then what are some examples of this?

–   Recovery from this dependence can also be seen as greater than
    yourself; what does this mean to you?
–   The wisdom and experience from those in 12-step meetings with
    successful long-term recovery are clearly greater than your own;
    are you willing to use this help?
–   How do you feel about the term *God*?
–   What does this term mean to you?

When speaking with an individual who seems resistant to discuss God,
one may find it helpful to explain that the use of this term is not a requirement for membership in AA or other 12-step programs and that
others prefer the terms *my higher power* or *the power of my AA group.* Most
larger AA communities even have agnostic and atheist groups, for those
for whom hearing the term *God* is too disruptive.

Matthew, a 47-year-old clothing store manager, consults Dr. C about managing his depression. He had been taking antidepressant medication prescribed by his internist, but continues to be both depressed and nearly
hopeless. Dr. C learns that Matthew was also taking antiretroviral medication for HIV. He has a long history of alcoholic drinking and a more recent history of binges on crystal methamphetamine several times per year,
during which he engaged in sexual activity (and was later very ashamed of
this). He says he uses protection, but hates it when he goes on these
binges and hates himself because he is unable to stop. Although he has attended AA in the past, he did not talk at meetings in any detail about his
drug use/sex pattern, being ashamed to talk about this with the group.
Also, as he tells Dr. C, "I just can't stomach the God stuff." When encouraged to say more, he relates, "I hate religion, and I don't believe in God.
All my life I've been told that what I am is an abomination, and if my family found out I was gay, they would disown me in the name of Jesus! To me,
God is just an excuse for hate crimes." Dr. C explains to Matthew that any-
body would feel depressed, hopeless, and isolated in his circumstances,
dealing with this kind of conflict and guilt. Furthermore, Dr. C says that
he has some other patients with histories not exactly the same, but also
not too different from Matthew's, and that he would like to have Matthew
try a local gay-lesbian AA meeting, but with a recovering AA guide who
goes to these meetings. [A guide can be a local AA volunteer, obtained
through a therapist's intergroup, a recovering former patient, or a member of the local gay community group.] Dr. C tells Matthew, "Give yourself
a chance by attending the meetings for a month; each week we will discuss
what you heard and how it might apply to you. If at the end of a month you
still can't find anything there, we will go in another direction, but please,
just give this a chance—I think you will be surprised."

After the first meeting, Matthew tells Dr. C how amazed he is at how
open the people were at this different kind of AA meeting, and that although he didn't hear his exact story, he did see and hear a number of

people with stories fairly like his. These people seemed both much happier and more hopeful; in fact, some of them would laugh at their previous crazy behavior. By the end of the month, Matthew is going to several meetings a week, and says he can't believe how crazy and isolated he was. His mood improves markedly; in fact, Dr. C and Matthew both decide to hold off on psychiatric medications for now. With Dr. C's encouragement, Matthew obtains a sponsor and begins to do step work. In working on Step 4 ("Made a searching and fearless moral inventory of ourselves"), he realizes that he has a deep resentment against a God that he doesn't even believe in. Admitting this brings him a huge sense of relief that he can stop destroying himself over guilt and shame and he tells Dr. C, "Maybe I need to reevaluate this spirituality stuff too."

In the context of the 12-step process, spirituality can be thought of as the willingness to change. It can also be defined as connectedness with other people and what is meaningful in someone's life.

How is the discomfort with the use of *God* addressed in AA? First, the issue of God is qualified with "as we understood him" (Alcoholics Anonymous 1976, 1984). Second, flexibility on the concept of God is made clear in one chapter of *Alcoholics Anonymous* that addresses any alcoholic person who feels that he or she is an atheist or agnostic, encouraging his or her membership. The text points out for these potential members that "we Agnostics…had to face the fact that we must find a spiritual basis for life" in order to achieve recovery, thereby alluding to AA's distinction between spirituality and theistic religion.

Universality of spirituality.   All people across cultures have had exposure to spirituality. Patients should be encouraged to reflect on past spiritual experiences and to build on them. Also, clinicians should encourage patients to find comfort in spiritual experiences.

Resistance to religion or spirituality.   When working with patients who express resistance to religion or spirituality, the therapist should talk to them after they have been to a few 12-step meetings to determine if there is anything they can connect with.

Spirituality from a different perspective.   For patients who are not inclined toward the spiritual aspects of AA, the clinician can suggest that they do some other things that have similar spiritual foundations. For example, patients can volunteer for the Salvation Army or a rescue mission to experience spirituality from another perspective.

Spirituality and morality.   The TSF manual specifies acknowledgment of wrongdoing:

Patients need to acknowledge character defects including specific immoral or unethical acts, and harm done to others as a result of *the patients' alcoholism or psychiatric disorders.*

The moral tone of this statement may cause discomfort for many psychiatrists; however, looking at the "wreckage of the past"—a typical AA phrase—is something that should be done as part of taking any good history. This task helps to challenge patients' denial. Although it is clear that the cocaine-abusing patient who sold his or her parents' television should acknowledge substance use problems and make restitution, what about the manic patient who by choice cuts down on medications to "get an edge," then spends the entire limit of the family's credit cards on unnecessary, impulsive items? Is this an illness issue, a moral issue, or both? The AA approach says that although an individual may not be responsible for having the illness, he or she is very responsible for managing its recovery. Facing up to the wreckage of the past, whether from addictions, psychiatric illness, or both, is a basic part of recovery. Although restitution of money or other concrete objects can be made, self-forgiveness for hurting others, such as in the examples above, is more difficult. Both the individual and the therapist must work together on this task (Kaskutas 2009).

Role of the Therapist

The primary role of the therapist is as a facilitator of patients' acceptance of their alcoholism and commitment to the fellowship of AA as the preferred path of recovery. However, when the facilitator is also a psychiatric practitioner (and often a prescriber), explaining the nature of co-occurring psychiatric illnesses, medications, and other therapies is also a key facilitation issue.

Education

The therapist acts as a resource and advocate of the 12-step approach to recovery.

The 12-step therapist explains the AA view of alcoholism and interprets slips and resistance to AA in terms of the power of alcoholism and the dynamics of denial.

The 12-step therapist introduces several of the 12 steps and their related concepts and helps the patient to understand key AA themes and concepts (e.g., denial, powerlessness) by identifying the patient's personal experiences that illustrate them.

For patients with comorbid disorders, the therapist adds the context of a patient's psychiatric disorder to these same conditions (e.g., the role of denial in bipolar illness, the similarity between a return to drinking and psychiatric medication nonadherence).

Introduction of steps is probably best done in actual meetings or by the patient's sponsor, unless the psychiatrist wants to get much more involved. Table 12–1 lists the Dual Recovery Anonymous steps.

The therapist introduces, explains, and advocates reliance on the fellowship of AA as the foundation for recovery, which should be thought of as an ongoing process of "arrest" (as opposed to cure). *The concepts of arrest and recovery versus cure hold for most psychiatric disorders.*

In the clinical context, recovery is based on an individual's behavior and medical status, which can be assessed by recourse to diagnostic criteria in DSM-IV-TR. Some of these criteria are also given in the items listed in the Addiction Severity Index (McLellan et al. 1992), which is used

TABLE 12–1. The 12 steps of Dual Recovery Anonymous

1. We admitted we were powerless over our dual illness of chemical dependency and emotional or psychiatric illness—that our lives had become unmanageable.
2. Came to believe that a Higher Power of our understanding could restore us to sanity.
3. Made a decision to turn our will and our lives over to the care of our Higher Power, to help us to rebuild our lives in a positive and caring way.
4. Made a searching and fearless personal inventory of ourselves.
5. Admitted to our Higher Power, to ourselves, and to another human being, the exact nature of our liabilities and our assets.
6. Were entirely ready to have our Higher Power remove all our liabilities.
7. Humbly asked our Higher Power to remove these liabilities and to help us to strengthen our assets for recovery.
8. Made a list of all persons we had harmed and became willing to make amends to them all.
9. Made direct amends to such people wherever possible, except when to do so would injure them or others.
10. Continued to take personal inventory, and when wrong promptly admitted it, while continuing to recognize our progress in dual recovery.
11. Sought through prayer and meditation to improve our conscious contact with our Higher Power, praying only for knowledge of our Higher Power's will for us and the power to carry that out.
12. Having had a spiritual awakening as a result of these Steps, we tried to carry this message to others who experience dual disorders and to practice these principles in all our affairs.

Source. Reprinted from Dual Recovery Anonymous: "The Twelve Steps of Dual Recovery Anonymous." 1993–2004. Available at: http://www.draonline.org/dra_steps.html. Accessed January 20, 2008. Used with permission.

widely in research to evaluate recovery. Behavior and medical status can be assessed relatively easily because they are premised on observable behavior or symptoms described by the patient, family member, or clinician. However, a spiritually grounded definition of recovery can be useful as well. Different sets of criteria can be used to diagnose addiction and to describe the spiritual aspects of recovery associated with the 12-step experience, such as relief of guilt and shame, expression of gratitude, and finding purpose in life (Galanter 2007). These aspects are particularly relevant in helping the patient understand what is meant by recovery from the broader perspective of the 12-step experience.

> *The therapist* explains the role of a sponsor and helps patients identify what they would most benefit from in a sponsor.
> *The therapist* answers questions about material found in the "Big Book," The Twelve and Twelve, and other readings.

Again, it is possible for a psychiatrist to help his or her patients to attend AA meetings and get something out of them without having to read the "Big Book" (Alcoholics Anonymous 1976) in its entirety. However, reading it can be both helpful and interesting and can help the psychiatrist to better understand addiction and the AA model of recovery. Most of this type of more concrete AA work is best done by the patient's sponsor.

Facilitation

> The therapist uses patients' reports of their experience between sessions to actively facilitate their involvement in AA. The 12-step therapist... encourages attendance at AA meetings, monitors patient involvement in AA, and actively promotes a progression toward greater involvement in AA, for example in going to meetings that require more personal involvement, such as "step" meetings and "discussion" meetings. *The psychiatric practitioner can productively use his or her patient's behavior and understanding of meeting discussions as therapeutic material for both disorders.*

A therapist can spend a great deal of time on the issue of active involvement in AA. It is important for patients to understand that participation is necessary for recovery (Kaskutas et al. 2009). On the other hand, for first-time attendees or patients with social anxiety, it may be understandable that they are reluctant to speak or meet with other members. When this is clearly the case for a particular patient, the situation should be addressed in a supportive way. The therapist should emphasize that if the patient keeps going back, he or she will feel more comfortable in time; however, sitting in the back of the meeting room and not speaking is an acceptable first step toward later involvement.

Some basic meeting involvement coaching might include asking such questions as the following: What meetings did you attend since last session? Did you arrive early, on time, or late for meetings? Where exactly were the meetings? Where did you sit? Did you stay for the whole meeting? Were you able to pay attention the whole time?

Discussing answers to these questions uncovers resistance and nonattendance as well as psychiatric problems that might be interfering with attendance, such as paranoia or social phobia. Dealing with the causes of nonattendance and resistance then becomes part of therapeutic work, involving medications, motivational interviewing strategies, cognitive-behavioral techniques, or other specific cognitive approaches. Initiating discussion about AA involvement using such approaches is briefly illustrated here.

- *Motivational interviewing.* "So you thought about going to a meeting last night, but didn't quite get there. What do you think you might have gained if you had gone? What would have been the downside of going?"
- *Cognitive-behavioral therapies and AA facilitation.* "So you thought about going to a meeting last night, but didn't quite get there. Let's examine what you said to yourself to convince yourself not to go, and then work out a strategy to get you there."
- *Twelve-step disease model facilitation.* "So you thought about going to a meeting last night, but didn't quite get there. What was responsible for your not getting there—was it you or was it your disease? That kind of experience is the illness at work; it's the disease that tells you that you don't have a disease. Whom could you have called?"
- *More detailed attendance questions.* "Did you offer to help with setup or cleanup at the meeting? Did you talk to anyone before or after the meeting? What were some key issues you heard discussed at the meeting? How did these issues apply to you? Did you say something in the meeting? What was it like to talk, or want to talk but be unable or afraid to talk? Let's rehearse right here what you could say."
- *An example of a specific co-occurring disorders intervention (panic disorder and social phobia).* "So you thought about going to a meeting last night, but were afraid you would panic if you were called on, so you didn't go. Let's work out a strategy."
  - Prescribe medications for social phobia (e.g., selective serotonin reuptake inhibitor, gabapentin). Note that an alcoholic patient should not receive benzodiazepines (see Alcoholics Anonymous 1984).

- Rehearse something very simple to say in meetings (in the patient's words) with visualization, such as, "Hi, I'm Rick and I'm glad to be here." Have the patient carry a written card or have this phrase written on his or her hand. Rehearse this again and again in session and have the patient do this at home. Let the patient know that there is no requirement for individuals to say anything during meetings; even if called on, he or she can just pass.
- For highly anxious, performance-challenged patients, a 10- to 20-mg dose of propranolol before meetings may help, until the patient is more comfortable.

The therapist clarifies the role of therapist versus sponsor and refuses to become a sponsor while helping the patient to find one.

Naturally, a number of other types of issues can arise with respect to initiating AA treatment. Table 12–2 presents some common problems and offers solutions that may guide a clinician in his or her facilitation of AA participation. Table 12–3 provides specific questions and topics whose discussion can further help to facilitate patients' involvement in treatment.

Some clinicians may choose to meet a patient's sponsor so that both sponsor and clinician know they are on the "same side" and are providing consistent information to the individual seeking treatment. Such a meeting should occur only with the patient's approval and during a session with the patient present. Other clinicians prefer not to meet the patient's sponsor but to still encourage a constructive relationship between patient and sponsor. A patient may not feel comfortable with the initial choice of sponsor and may discuss this in therapy. In this situation, the therapist can explore the patient's concern. This discussion may help the patient relate more comfortably to his or her sponsor. AA members can arrange to get a new sponsor if they feel that would be best for them.

Some patients are resistant to the idea of getting a sponsor, and this can be a problem. For those with more serious psychiatric disorders, it is best, though not absolutely necessary, that their sponsors also have co-occurring disorders or have experience sponsoring individuals with co-occurring psychiatric issues; then, problems around psychiatric diagnosis, symptoms, and treatments, especially medications, are avoided, and psychiatric treatments are reinforced rather than resisted by the sponsor. Patients are more likely to meet such sponsors by going to DRA, dual-diagnosis AA meetings, or other variants of 12-step meetings that focus on persons with co-occurring disorders. Many AA schedules in larger communities even list dual diagnosis as a qualifier for certain meetings.

TABLE 12–2. Engaging those with resistance to involvement in Alcoholics Anonymous (AA)

Problem	Solution
The patient has had previous bad experiences with treatment for alcohol dependence, and AA is guilty by association.	Explore these issues and interpret the resistance of guilt by association.
The patient has had a previous bad experience with AA directly (e.g., the patient might have met someone at a meeting and then drunk with that person; the patient might have gone to a meeting and felt that he or she did not fit with the other attendees).	Explore what happened and the patient's role in this. Talk about matching meetings to the patient.
The patient has had a previous bad experience due to symptoms of co-occurring psychiatric problems (e.g., social phobia, paranoia).	Explore this experience, and explain that you will develop a strategy to deal with these symptoms. Explain to the patient that an AA meeting is about the safest place there is to exhibit symptoms publicly because it is a supportive and nonconfrontational environment.
The patient has had very little previous experience with AA but stopped attending meetings, used alcohol or drugs, and concluded that meetings "don't work."	Explain that the patient's previous attendance and involvement wasn't an adequate "dose." Illustrate this point with the following analogies, selecting the analogy that the patient is most likely to hear or understand given his or her clinical history: *Antibiotic model.* Would it be safe to conclude that an antibiotic was ineffective after taking only one-third of the dose for only one-third of the time prescribed? *Diabetes model.* Would it be safe to conclude that a diabetes treatment was ineffective after taking the medicine only half the time and eating chocolate cake in between doses? *Bipolar model.* Would it be safe to conclude that a bipolar medication was ineffective after taking just one-third of the prescribed dose or skipping doses altogether for weeks at a time?

TABLE 12–3.　**Examples of working with patients**

Examine the patient's previous experiences with the following core topics. Stay focused not so much on illness as on the patient's previous attempts at quitting, treatment, and AA participation.

Sobriety

"Tell me about the times you have been abstinent from both drugs and alcohol."

"What seemed to work and what did not work for 1) addictions, 2) psychiatric problems, and 3) both problems?"

Treatment

"Tell me about times you have stopped or cut down use in the past."

"Tell me about your previous treatments. What seemed to work and what didn't?"

Twelve-step meetings

"What have been your experiences with Alcoholics Anonymous (AA)?"

"Have you ever gone to meetings? If so, when?"

"How involved and committed were you? Did you ever try '90 in 90' (90 meetings in 90 days)?"

"Did you go to the same meeting regularly (e.g., weekly for several months)? Tell me about these meetings and the people you met there."

"Did you get a sponsor? If so, how, and what was he or she like? Did he or she help, and if so, how? If not, why not—what got in the way? Did this sponsor know you have a dual disorder or that you are also on medications?"

"Did you ever work the steps? If so, which steps?"

"How fully 'plugged-in' did you ever get with AA? Did people know you? Did you know them? Did you ever do any 'service'? If so, tell me about your service."

If the patient answers mostly "yes" to the above 12-step questions, analyze what happened to the patient's 12-step relationship.

If the patient answers mostly "no" to the above 12-step questions, make your position clear on why you are a strong advocate of AA by stating, "Most people with more than a few months of sobriety are regularly using AA" and "The more involved with AA you are, the more likely it is you will have a positive outcome and the more likely your psychiatric disorder will improve."

Desired Therapist Characteristics

Twelve-step therapists, being professionals whose goal is to facilitate and encourage active participation in AA, need not be personally in recovery; however, they must be knowledgeable of and comfortable with the foundation of 12-step recovery as described in AA-approved literature. Therapist self-disclosure of recovery status is to some extent a clinical issue, but generally speaking the authors encourage honesty in the therapeutic relationship.

If they are not in recovery, it is strongly recommended for therapists to attend at least 10 open AA meetings and an equal number of Al-Anon or Families Anonymous meetings, and to be thoroughly familiar with AA reading materials.

In addition, to be maximally effective as a facilitator, the therapist is advised to develop a network of AA contacts—men and women—who are active in AA and who could be called on to assist in getting a shy or ambivalent patient to their first meetings, giving advice about particular meetings, providing directions, and so forth. Persons who have been sober and active in AA for at least a year are candidates for doing this type of 12-step work as part of their own recovery. Therapists can develop working relationships with these people by going to AA meetings on some regular basis, or by talking with recovering persons they know. First-hand knowledge of such contact people is desirable.

ACTIVE, SUPPORTIVE, AND INVOLVED: 12-step therapists are expected to be interactionally active and nonjudgmentally confrontational during therapy sessions, as opposed to merely reflective. This does not mean that the therapist lectures the patient, does more talking than the patient, or chastises the patient for slips. Rather, the therapist utilizing this approach should be prepared to identify denial and confront the patient consistently in a frank but respectful manner regarding the patient's attitudes or behaviors, to actively encourage the patient to get involved in the fellowship of AA, and to help the patient understand key AA concepts as they are reflected in the patient's actual experience.

Patients can be expected to interpret the AA concepts presented here in light of their own experience. This is consistent with the AA approach, which allows for a great deal of individuality of interpretation within broad guidelines. For example, the 12 steps specifically allow for individuality in conceptualizing a higher power ("God as we understand him"). Similarly, what represents unmanageability (Step 1) for one patient may not be meaningful to another. What is most important is not whether patients interpret these concepts in the same way; rather, what counts is the end result: active involvement in the fellowship of Alcoholics Anonymous.

CONFRONTATION: In the context of this program, confrontation is something that therapists can think of as helpful and honest mirroring. The most appropriate form of confrontation is to share frankly but respectfully what you see the patient doing. Most often this involves confronting the patient about some form of denial. Confrontation that is patronizing or harsh or implies that the patient has a character problem as opposed to a powerful and cunning illness is likely to be counterproductive.

We discussed therapist preparation earlier in this chapter, in "Starting Out." Realistically, we doubt that many practicing clinicians will go to 10 meetings, and we have observed many residents become at least moderately 12-step adept by attending a couple of meetings, reading the TSF manual, and working intensively with a few patients who go to 12-step meetings, making sure to spend a good deal of each session talking about what went on at meetings. In this review of meetings, the therapist should bring up psychiatric symptoms, relationship matters, and cognitive challenges, providing ample material to attend to during the session. This concentration on what goes on at meetings also conveys the idea that meetings are important.

Key Clinical Concepts

- Co-occurring and substance-induced disorders are common in psychiatric patients, and mental health practitioners can enhance outcomes from both disorders by applying 12-step facilitation (TSF).

- TSF is not AA and it is not endorsed by AA. It is an evidence-based therapy performed by the clinician to help a patient begin to attend and benefit from 12-step meetings, including AA.

- Co-occurring disorders TSF is a practical enhancement of TSF that includes typical psychiatric issues and treatment but has not been separately tested.

- Twelve-step approaches and meetings are ubiquitous, inexpensive, and evidence based, and they provide long-term, recovery-based help for patients with substance use disorders.

- Twelve-step approaches to acceptance and denial for the chronic and often relapsing illness of addiction are appropriate for and benefit most psychiatric disorders.

- AA has no official policy on seeing a psychiatrist or taking medication for a mental health disorder—it is an outside issue and not part of the AA program. According to AA, "Alcoholics Anonymous has no opinion on outside issues; hence the AA name ought never be drawn into public controversy." However, members of AA and other 12-step communities may have strong opinions on psychiatric medication and other issues. Therefore, patients need to be prepared for the possibility that they may hear disturbing ideas and receive advice in 12-step contexts that contradicts their psychiatrists' recommendations. AA does have a helpful pamphlet, "The AA Member—Medications and Other Drugs," on this topic.

- Developing TSF skills for co-occurring disorders is an effective way for the mental health practitioner to stay productively involved with his or her patient who has co-occurring disorders. Use of these skills provides a good model of integrated care and offers the patient a great deal of low-cost, high-frequency psychosocial support.

Suggested Reading

Bogenschutz MP: Specialized 12-step programs and 12-step facilitation for the dually diagnosed. Community Ment Health J 41:7–20, 2005

Double Trouble in Recovery: Double Trouble in Recovery. 2010. Available at: http://www.doubletroubleinrecovery.org. Accessed February 23, 2010.

Nowinski J: The Twelve Step Facilitation Outpatient Program Facilitator Guide. Center City, MN, Hazelden, 2006

Nowinski J, Baker S: The Twelve Step Facilitation Handbook: A Systematic Approach to Early Recovery From Alcoholism and Addiction. Center City, MN, Hazelden, 2003

Nowinski J, Baker S, Carroll K: Twelve Step Facilitation Therapy Manual. Rockville, MD, National Institute on Alcohol Abuse and Alcoholism, 1995

References

Alcoholics Anonymous: Alcoholics Anonymous. New York, Alcoholics Anonymous World Services, 1976

Alcoholics Anonymous: Twelve Steps and Twelve Traditions. New York, Alcoholics Anonymous World Services, 1984

American Psychiatric Association: Diagnostic and Statistical Manual of Mental Disorders, 4th Edition, Text Revision. Washington, DC, American Psychiatric Association, 2000

Bolton J, Cox B, Clara I, et al: Use of alcohol and drugs to self-medicate anxiety disorders in a nationally representative sample. J Nerv Ment Dis 194:818–825, 2006

Brown SA, Glasner-Edwards SV, Tate SR, et al: Integrated cognitive behavioral therapy versus twelve-step facilitation therapy for substance-dependent adults with depressive disorders. J Psychoactive Drugs 38:449–460, 2006

Carroll KM: Behavioral therapies for co-occurring substance use and mood disorders. Biol Psychiatry 56:778–784, 2004

Center for Substance Abuse Treatment: Treatment Improvement Protocol (TIP), Series No 42 (DHHS Publ No SMA-05-3992). Rockville, MD, Substance Abuse and Mental Health Services Administration, 2005

Cloud RN, Kingree JB: Concerns about dose and underutilization of twelve-step programs: models, scales, and theory that inform treatment planning. Recent Dev Alcohol 18:283–301, 2008

Comtois KA, Russo JE, Roy-Byrne P, et al: Clinicians' assessments of bipolar disorder and substance abuse as predictors of suicidal behavior in acutely hospitalized psychiatric inpatients. Biol Psychiatry 56:757–763, 2004

Dual Recovery Anonymous: The twelve steps of Dual Recovery Anonymous. 1993–2004. Available at: http://www.draonline.org/dra_steps.html. Accessed February 23, 2010.

Galanter M: Spirituality and recovery in 12-step programs: an empirical model. J Subst Abuse Treat 33:265–272, 2007

Humphreys K, Moos RH: Encouraging posttreatment self-help group involvement to reduce demand for continuing care services: two-year clinical and utilization outcomes. Alcohol Clin Exp Res 31:64–68, 2007

Kaskutas LA: Alcoholics Anonymous effectiveness: faith meets science. J Addict Dis 28:145–157, 2009

Kaskutas LA, Bond J, Humphreys K: Social networks as mediators of the effect of Alcoholics Anonymous. Addiction 97:891–900, 2002

Kaskutas LA, Subbaraman MS, Witbrodt J, et al: Effectiveness of making Alcoholics Anonymous easier: a group format 12-step facilitation approach. J Subst Abuse Treat 37:228–239, 2009

Kessler RC, Chiu WT, Demler O, et al: Prevalence, severity, and comorbidity of 12-month DSM-IV disorders in the National Comorbidity Survey Replication. Arch Gen Psychiatry 62:617–627, 2005

Linehan MM: Cognitive Behavioral Treatment of Borderline Personality Disorder. New York, Guilford, 1993

Mankowski ES, Humphreys K, Moos RH: Individual and contextual predictors of involvement in twelve-step self-help groups after substance abuse treatment. Am J Community Psychol 29:537–563, 2001

Marlatt GA, Gordon JR (eds): Relapse Prevention: Maintenance Strategies in the Treatment of Addictive Behaviors. New York, Guilford, 1985

Mattson ME, Del Boca FK, Carroll KM, et al: Compliance with treatment and follow-up protocols in Project MATCH: predictors and relationship to outcome. Alcohol Clin Exp Res 22:1328–1339, 1998

McLellan AT, Kushner H, Metzger D, et al: The fifth edition of the Addiction Severity Index. J Subst Abuse Treat 9:199–213, 1992

Minkoff K: An integrated treatment model for dual diagnosis of psychosis and addiction. Hosp Community Psychiatry 40:1031–1036, 1989

Moos RH, Timko C: Outcome research on 12-step and other self-help programs, in The American Psychiatric Publishing Textbook of Substance Abuse Treatment. Edited by Galanter M, Kleber HD. Washington, DC, American Psychiatric Publishing, 2008, pp 511–521

Morgenstern J, Bux D, Labouvie E, et al: Examining mechanisms of action in 12-step treatment: the role of 12-step cognitions. J Stud Alcohol 63:665–672, 2002

Norcross JC: Personal integration: an N of 1 study. Journal of Psychotherapy Integration 16:59–72, 2006

Nowinski J, Baker S, Carroll K: Twelve Step Facilitation Therapy Manual. Rockville, MD, National Institute on Alcohol Abuse and Alcoholism, 1995

Puchalski CM, Dorff RE, Hendi IY: Spirituality, religion, and healing in palliative care. Clin Geriatr Med 20:689–714, vi–vii, 2004

Sholomskas DE, Carroll KM: One small step for manuals: computer-assisted training in twelve-step facilitation. J Stud Alcohol 67:939–945, 2006

Tonigan JS, Bogenschutz MP, Miller WR: Is alcoholism typology a predictor of both Alcoholics Anonymous affiliation and disaffiliation after treatment? J Subst Abuse Treat 30:323–330, 2006

Walitzer KS, Dermen KH, Barrick C: Facilitating involvement in Alcoholics Anonymous during out-patient treatment: a randomized clinical trial. Addiction 104:391–401, 2009

Weiss RD: Treating patients with bipolar disorder and substance dependence: lessons learned. J Subst Abuse Treat 27:307–312, 2004

Weiss RD, Ostacher MJ, Otto MW, et al: Does recovery from substance use disorder matter in patients with bipolar disorder? J Clin Psychiatry 66:730–735, 2005

Ziedonis DM: Integrated treatment of co-occurring mental illness and addiction: clinical intervention, program, and system perspectives. CNS Spectr 9:892–904, 925, 2004

13 | Family Therapy

Timothy J. O'Farrell, Ph.D.

Any review of the development and applications of the family treatment model for addictions over the last half century reveals a rapid progression in the acceptance of family-involved therapy as an important component of treatment for alcoholism and drug abuse. For example, the treatment literature from the 1950s and early 1960s primarily conceptualized substance abuse as an individual problem that was best treated on an individual basis (e.g., Jellinek 1960). However, during the 1960s this view was gradually supplanted by what has become the prevailing clinical wisdom, that family members can play a central role in the treatment of alcoholic individuals and drug abusers (Stanton and Heath 1997). By the early 1970s, couples and family therapies were described by the National Institute on Alcohol Abuse and Alcoholism as "one of the most outstanding current advances in the area of psychotherapy of alcoholism" (Keller 1974, p. 161). By the late 1970s, family therapy for substance abuse was embraced by the majority of substance abuse treatment programs and community mental health settings (e.g., Coleman and Davis 1978; Kaufman and Kaufman 1992). During the last two decades, family-based assessment and intervention has become widely viewed as part of standard care for alcoholism and drug abuse. In fact, many have argued that the only reason not to include family members in the treatment of a substance-abusing patient is refusal by the patient or members of the family to have them be involved (e.g., O'Farrell 1993b).

In addition, the popular literature on families and substance abuse has grown into its own cottage industry, filling the bookstores with a wide

Preparation of this chapter was supported by the National Institute on Alcohol Abuse and Alcoholism (Grant K02 AA00234) and by the Department of Veterans Affairs.

range of books describing codependency, enabling, and adult children of alcoholics. The role of family factors in the etiology and maintenance of addictive disorders and the application of family therapy in substance abuse treatment have indeed come a long way.

Historically, family interventions used to treat alcoholism grew out of couples therapy approaches and focused primarily on the spousal system. In contrast, family treatments for drug abuse evolved from systemic family therapy, focusing on the entire family. More recently this distinction has blurred, with both alcoholism and drug abuse treatment programs often providing a wide array of family therapy services for the patients and their family members.

In this chapter, we describe different types of family therapy commonly used in the treatment of alcoholism and drug abuse. We also summarize the evidence base for each type of family therapy described. We focus on the use of family-involved treatments to assist the family, initiate change when the substance-abusing individual refuses to seek help, and aid recovery once the substance abuser has sought help.

Helping the Family When the Substance Abuser Refuses to Get Help

Spouses and other family members often experience many stressors and heightened emotional distress caused by the negative consequences of the substance abuser's drinking and drug use. Stress is highest for the family when the substance abuser refuses to get help. The therapist can use two approaches to try to help family members cope with their emotional distress and concentrate on their own motivations for change rather than trying to motivate the substance abuser to change. These approaches are 1) to help the family member use the concepts and resources of Al-Anon and 2) to teach specific coping skills to deal with alcohol- and drug-related situations involving the substance abuser.

Al-Anon Facilitation and Referral

Al-Anon is a 12-step program that is by far the most widely used source of support for family members troubled by a loved one's substance abuse. Al-Anon advocates that family members detach themselves from the substance abuser's drinking and drug use in a loving way, accept that they are powerless to control the substance abuser, and seek support from other members of the Al-Anon program (Al-Anon Family Groups 1985). There are two ways in which a psychiatrist or other addictions professional might use Al-Anon to help family members.

The first is *referral of family members to Al-Anon*. This includes providing information about times and locations of nearby Al-Anon meetings and discussing any concerns the family members may have about Al-Anon. Arranging for them to go to their first few meetings with an established Al-Anon member can be particularly effective. Like any other referral, checking back to see if the person has followed through is important.

The second is *Al-Anon facilitation therapy*, which is a therapist-delivered counseling method designed to encourage involvement in Al-Anon. Nowinski (1999) developed and tested a therapist's manual for this approach. It consists of 10–12 sessions designed to engage the family member in the program and concepts of Al-Anon. Each session explores one of Al-Anon's 12 steps (e.g., admitting one is powerless over another person's addiction) or a closely related Al-Anon concept (e.g., detaching with love). There are also has recovery tasks the person is asked to pursue between sessions, including attending Al-Anon meetings and reading Al-Anon literature.

Coping Skills Therapy

Coping skills therapy (CST) teaches family members of substance abusers how to deal with alcohol- and drug-related situations involving the substance abuser. Rychtarik and McGillicuddy (2005) developed and tested a therapist's manual for an eight-session CST group for spouses and family members of substance abusers. Based on a family stress and coping perspective, CST helps group members apply a problem-solving approach to substance-related problem situations commonly experienced by families of substance abusers (e.g., dealing with intoxicated behavior, partner violence, failure to maintain household responsibilities). In each CST session, the group leader presents a stressful situation drawn from a master list of such situations, leads the group in problem solving, and provides situation-specific skill hints. For example, the situation could involve the substance abuser's asking for money when in the past he has used these occasions to go out and drink. Responses discussed might range from passive acquiescence to assertively declining the request. The therapist then models the recommended response, group members role-play the situation, and the therapist and group provide feedback. Participants keep a diary of personal problematic situations encountered, and these are discussed and role-played in the group as well.

Evidence for Family Therapy to Help the Family When a Substance Abuser Refuses Help

Al-Anon referral, Al-Anon facilitation therapy, and coping skills therapy all produce improvements in family members' emotional distress and coping that are greater than those in a wait-list control group. Evidence that Al-Anon facilitation and referral help family members, as intended and believed by its many adherents, comes from controlled studies (e.g., Barber and Gilbertson 1996; Miller et al. 1999) that support this widely used approach.

Although they produce similar improvements in emotional distress, CST leads to less drinking and less violence by the alcoholic than does Al-Anon facilitation therapy. Specifically, compared with female spouses of alcoholics who participated in Al-Anon facilitation therapy, female spouses who participated in CST received less violence from their male alcoholic partners, and their male partners drank less in the year after treatment (Rychtarik and McGillicuddy 2005). These advantages of CST over Al-Anon facilitation therapy are important because one-half to two-thirds of male substance abusers have been violent toward a female partner in the past year (O'Farrell et al. 2003, 2004). In addition, reduced drinking by the alcoholic who was not in treatment is an important indirect effect of CST. Although CST is not widely used, these findings suggest that it should receive more attention from clinicians and program administrators.

Table 13–1 summarizes key points about family-based methods to help the family when the substance abuser refuses to get help.

Initiating Change When the Substance Abuser Refuses to Get Help

Many if not most substance abusers seek treatment in response to external pressure. With the possible exception of legal system coercion, pressure by a family member is the most powerful inducement for substance abusers to enter treatment (Stanton 1997). Several family-based methods have been developed to motivate resistant substance abusers to enter treatment. These include the Johnson Institute intervention, A Relational Intervention Sequence for Engagement (ARISE), Pressures to Change (PTC), and Community Reinforcement and Family Training (CRAFT).

Johnson Institute Intervention

The best known of these family-involved motivational techniques is the Johnson Institute intervention (Johnson 1986; Liepman 1993). "The intervention," as it is most commonly called, involves three to four educational and rehearsal sessions to prepare family members and others (e.g., neighbors, friends) for a confrontation meeting. After these preparation sessions, the confrontation meeting is scheduled and the substance user is brought to this meeting, typically not knowing the agenda of the group. Once the substance user is in their midst, family members share their

TABLE 13–1.   **Family-based methods to help the family when the substance abuser refuses to get help**

Major approaches to help the family

- Al-Anon facilitation and referral—Family member is engaged in program and concepts of Al-Anon.
- Coping skills therapy—Family member is taught how to deal with common alcohol- and drug-related situations involving the substance abuser.

Evidence for these approaches

- Both Al-Anon and coping skills therapy reduce emotional distress and improve coping of family member.
- Coping skills therapy leads to less drinking and less violence by substance abuser than does Al-Anon.

concerns and feelings; these are to be presented in a sincere, nonjudgmental fashion. The intervention team members also express their hope that the substance user will enter treatment, outline the consequences if the substance user refuses, and openly discuss the desired outcome of both the intervention itself and the recommended treatment. A referral to treatment is then made. Often, the members of the intervention team meet with the therapist at a later date to go through a debriefing and discuss a plan for change to be followed by the family members and others in the substance user's social network.

A Relational Intervention Sequence for Engagement

ARISE (Landau and Garrett 2006) was developed as a less coercive alternative to the traditional Johnson intervention. ARISE is a three-level approach, with each successive level including greater family involvement, therapist involvement, and coercion. The ARISE model advocates use of less coercive steps early in the process and gradually proceeds to the use of greater counselor and family involvement if the lower-intensity steps are not successful in motivating the substance abuser to engage in treatment.

Level I involves one or more telephone sessions with the family member who contacts the treatment agency, followed by an in-person meeting of the family and other network members with the therapist to mobilize them in support of treatment for the substance abuser. Level II involves an informal "invitational intervention" with a therapist present. This meeting is not a surprise to the substance abuser and does not involve consequences for refusing treatment. Family and relevant others and the substance abuser are invited to attend this meeting, although the meeting can still be conducted without the substance abuser present. In the meeting, the members collectively consider possible approaches that might be used to motivate the substance abuser to enter treatment. If, after repeated attempts, the substance user remains unwilling to seek help, the process moves to Level III, which involves a formal intervention similar to the Johnson intervention.

Pressures to Change

James G. Barber (e.g., Barber and Crisp 1995) developed the PTC approach for partners living with heavy drinkers who deny their alcohol problem and refuse treatment. PTC makes use of learning theory to train partners in coping responses that are designed to empower the non-substance-abusing partner and to provide incentive for the alcoholic partner to change.

PTC involves five to six structured counseling sessions to instruct the non-substance-abusing partner in how to use five gradually increasing levels of pressure on the drinker to seek help or moderate his or her drinking. Over the course of these five levels, the non-substance-abusing partner 1) receives feedback from the therapist about the seriousness of the drinker's problem and education on PTC; 2) plans incompatible activities during times when the drinker usually drinks (e.g., taking children to an amusement park, going to dinner with friends or relatives who do not drink); 3) responds to drinking by withdrawing reinforcers and to drinking-related crises by suggesting treatment; 4) establishes a contract in which the partner agrees to exchange some reinforcer for sobriety; and 5) when prior steps have been unsuccessful, confronts the drinker with the negative effects of the drinking and a simple, direct request to seek change or seek help.

Community Reinforcement and Family Training (CRAFT)

The CRAFT approach (Smith and Meyers 2004) involves six to eight sessions that draw heavily on learning theory. CRAFT teaches a family member how to use positive reinforcement and negative consequences to discourage drug use or drinking by the substance abuser. For example, positive reinforcement might include the family member engaging in pleasant activities (e.g., discussing enjoyable topics, giving gifts) when the substance abuser is not drinking or using drugs. In addition, the family member would expressly state that reinforcement is being given because the substance user is not drinking or using drugs. Negative consequences for intoxication might include withholding reinforcements and explaining why, and ignoring the substance abuser during periods of intoxication. Emphasis is also placed on the family member to decrease stress in general and to increase positive aspects of his or her own life by, for example, establishing new friendships, engaging in positively rewarding activities outside of the relationship with the substance abuser, or joining a therapy group.

A unique aspect of CRAFT is its emphasis on identifying dangerous situations as behavioral changes are introduced at home. The family member is taught how to identify potentially violent situations so that he or she can take immediate action before getting hurt. The therapist helps the family member identify the sequence of events that lead to violence and teaches him or her to identify significant "cues" before physical violence begins. The family member develops a specific plan for leaving these situations until it is safe to return.

Finally, CRAFT teaches the family member effective ways to suggest treatment to the substance abuser. The family member is taught to pick a time and situation when the substance abuser may be highly motivated to enter treatment because the substance use has caused unacceptable behavior. These may include times after the substance abuser has engaged in embarrassing behavior when drinking, has disappointed his or her children, or has been arrested for drunk driving.

Evidence for Family Therapy to Initiate Change When a Substance Abuser Refuses Help

Of these family-based methods to promote change and treatment entry by the resistant substance abuser, CRAFT has the strongest evidence base. Across four randomized trials, two for alcoholics and two for drug abusers (Kirby et al. 1999; Meyers et al. 2002; Miller et al. 1999; Sisson and Azrin 1986), the average treatment engagement rate for CRAFT was 68% (range 59%–85%), which was significantly and substantially higher than engagement rates for Al-Anon facilitation therapy or Al-Anon referral (20%) or the Johnson intervention (30%). Thus, CRAFT is a more effective alternative to engage substance abusers in treatment than popular confrontational or detachment approaches.

The Johnson Institute intervention showed a disappointing treatment engagement rate of 30% in the first randomized, controlled study of this popular method (Miller et al. 1999). This was similar to the 25% rate in an uncontrolled study (Liepman et al. 1989), not much higher than that for Al-Anon, which does not try to change the substance abuser's behavior. The reason for these disappointing findings is that 70% of families in these two studies who started the intervention process did not go through with the family confrontation meeting. When family members completed the confrontation in these two studies, most succeeded in getting their substance abuser into treatment. Adherents of the Johnson intervention have cited a 90% success rate, which we now know does not apply for an intent-to-treat basis (which has a 25%–30% success rate) but only for the minority of families willing and able to use the method.

ARISE has a less coercive multistep process that is conceptually appealing and may lead to better engagement rates than the Johnson intervention. However, although ARISE has shown promise in uncontrolled studies (e.g., Landau et al. 2004), controlled studies have not been reported.

In three controlled studies, PTC was better than wait-list control for initiating change, defined as treatment entry or reduced drinking for the rather brief period of 2 weeks (Barber and Crisp 1995; Barber and Gilbertson 1996, 1998). Treatment entry rate (31%) was less than half that found for CRAFT. PTC has been used with spouses of heavy drinkers, but not with spouses of drug abusers or with other family members. Nonetheless, PTC may be a promising approach. It is brief, and it is well specified in a manual for therapists and a self-help manual for spouses. If PTC can be shown to produce durable reductions in the drinker's alcohol use, it may be of particular use in countries without extensive alcohol treatment systems.

Table 13–2 summarizes key points about family-based methods to initiate change when the substance abuser refuses treatment.

Family Therapy to Aid Recovery When a Substance Abuser Has Sought Help

In the preceding sections, we have examined interventions to help the family and support the substance abuser's entry into treatment. Regardless of the impetus for seeking help, once the substance abuser has entered treatment, family therapy interventions are often used as part of the treatment to aid the substance abuser's recovery and to help the family. Network therapy, family systems therapy, and behavioral couples therapy (BCT) are three influential approaches. In this section, we examine these hallmark therapy techniques and the evidence base for these approaches.

Network Therapy

Network therapy (Galanter 1999) involves key members of the patient's social network at the outset and at regular intervals during treatment to support the patient's recovery. Network therapy is not considered further here because Chapter 10 in this volume is devoted to a detailed consideration of this approach.

TABLE 13–2.   **Family-based methods to initiate change when the substance abuser refuses to get help**

Major approaches to initiate change

- Johnson Institute intervention—Therapist helps family plan and conduct surprise family confrontation meeting called an *intervention.*
- A Relational Intervention Sequence for Engagement (ARISE)—This three-step model starts with low-pressure methods and ends with Johnson intervention if earlier steps are unsuccessful.
- Pressures to Change (PTC)—Therapist teaches coping responses to empower family member and provide incentives for alcohol abuser to change.
- Community Reinforcement and Family Training (CRAFT)—Family member learns to use positive reinforcement and negative consequences to discourage substance use and encourage treatment.

Evidence for these approaches

- CRAFT is most effective, averaging a 68% treatment engagement rate across four randomized trials.
- Although popular, Johnson intervention has only a 25%–30% engagement rate because many families do not follow through with the confrontation.
- PTC reduces drinking for brief period, but durability of changes is unknown.
- ARISE is promising but lacks controlled studies.

Family Systems Therapy

Family systems therapy has incorporated many core concepts of family systems theory as applied to substance abuse (Stanton et al. 1982; Steinglass et al. 1987). Therapy focuses on the interactional rather than the individual level, using a variety of techniques to affect interactions within the family. The greatest emphasis is on identifying and altering family interaction patterns that are associated with problematic substance use.

The family systems approach views substance abuse as a major organizing principle for patterns of interactional behavior within the family system. A reciprocal relationship exists between family functioning and substance abuse, with an individual's drug and alcohol use being best understood in the context of the entire family's functioning. According to family systems theory, substance abuse often evolves during periods in which the individual family member is having difficulty addressing an important developmental issue (e.g., leaving the home) or when the family is facing a significant crisis (e.g., marital discord). During these periods, substance abuse can serve to 1) distract family members from their central problem or 2) slow down or stop a transition to a different developmental stage that is being resisted by the family as a whole or by one of its members.

From a family systems perspective, substance abuse represents a maladaptive attempt to deal with difficulties that develop a homeostatic life of their own and regulate family transactions. The substance abuse itself serves an important role in the family, and once the therapist understands the function of the substance abuse for the family, the therapist can then explain how the behavior has come about and the function it serves. In turn, treatment is aimed at restructuring the interaction patterns associated with the substance abuse, thereby making the drinking or drug use unnecessary in the maintenance of the family system functioning. To accomplish this aim, a variety of therapy techniques are used by family systems therapists. These techniques fall into two broad categories, joining and restructuring.

Joining With the Family in Family Systems Therapy

Joining consists of techniques designed to promote the therapeutic alliance and increase the therapist's leverage within the family. The therapist alternates between joining that supports the family system and its members and joining that challenges the system. Joining involves making a connection with each family member engaged in treatment and instilling a sense of confidence that the therapist has a firm commitment to working together with the family members on identified problems. In the joining process, the therapist typically solicits from each family member his or her perception of the problems in the family and his or her feelings about the issues raised. By attending to each person's views, the therapist conveys that each family member's viewpoint is important and that differences in perception about the identity, nature, and severity of problems are acceptable. The therapist attempts to communicate that he or she 1) understands each family member's perceptions of the problems and 2) has a clear idea about how to address the issues raised by the family member.

The process of joining may involve the therapist in promoting areas of strength in the family, supporting a threatened member of the family, and using the family member's methods of communicating (e.g., humor, touching) to introduce new ideas and concepts (Minuchin 1974). Of course, joining is an ongoing process, which is ultimately supported and reinforced as the therapist demonstrates his or her understanding and helpfulness throughout the course of treatment.

Restructuring Family Alliances and Interactions in Family Systems Therapy

Unlike joining, the second category of intervention techniques, restructuring, involves challenging the family's homeostasis and takes place through modifications in the family's bonding and power alignments among individuals and subsystems in the family (e.g., Haley 1976; Minuchin 1974). Several different techniques are used in the process of restructuring, including contracting, enactment, reframing, restructuring, and marking boundaries. *Contracting* is an agreement to work on agreed-upon issues, with an emphasis on helping the substance abuser with his or her problems prior to expanding to and probing other issues. The contract is developed at the end of the first interview and is maintained throughout treatment. As part of the contract, the family must choose to develop a family system that is conducive to abstinence by the substance abuser and agree to pursue the contract after it has been agreed upon as part of the initial evaluation.

Enactment involves the therapist eliciting, observing, and interrupting recurring problematic behavioral sequences in family interaction patterns. To do this, the therapist requires family members to talk to each other about problems during sessions rather than directing their communications to the therapist. The therapist carefully observes these enactments. Once the therapist has observed problematic interactions, he or she can interrupt and destabilize these customary behavioral exchanges among family members.

Reframing requires the therapist to help family members understand the interrelatedness of their behaviors and to see and understand how the substance abuse serves an important function in the family. *Restructuring* involves shifting family interaction patterns and establishing new, healthier behaviors. For example, this might include changing seating arrangements to strengthen the role of parents in the family, restating problems in solvable form, and teaching methods of communication and problem solving that preclude triangulation or conflict avoidance.

Marking boundaries is accomplished by clearly delineating individual and subsystem boundaries. For example, the parental subsystem should be protected from intrusion by children and other adults who may be inside or outside the family. To strengthen the parental subsystem, sessions may be held that include parents and exclude other family members.

Family systems therapy is more than a set of techniques. It involves a conceptual framework that explains common puzzling clinical phenomena (e.g., a family member seeming to sabotage a patient's newfound sobriety) and guides interventions. From this perspective, substance abuse by a family member serves an important function for the family, helping to maintain the homeostasis of the family system. Thus, if a family has functioned as a stable unit with a substance-abusing member, subsequent sobriety would likely threaten homeostasis and may be resisted on some level.

Behavioral Couples Therapy

Behavioral couples therapy (O'Farrell and Fals-Stewart 2006) works directly to increase relationship factors conducive to abstinence. A behavioral approach assumes that family members can reward abstinence, and that alcoholic and drug-abusing individuals from happier, more cohesive relationships with better communication have a lower risk of relapse.

BCT is designed for married or cohabiting individuals seeking help for alcoholism or drug abuse. The purposes of BCT are to build support for abstinence and to improve relationship functioning. BCT promotes abstinence with a "recovery contract" that includes a daily ritual to reward abstinence. BCT improves the relationship with techniques for increasing positive activities and improving communication. Finally, BCT helps the couple plan for continuing recovery to prevent or minimize relapse.

In BCT, the therapist sees the substance-abusing patient together with the spouse or live-in partner, typically for 12–20 weekly outpatient sessions over a 3- to 6-month period, followed by periodic maintenance contacts. BCT usually is an adjunct to individual or group counseling for the substance abuser. Generally, couples have been married or cohabiting for at least 1 year; the individuals do not have current psychosis; and one member of the couple has a current problem with alcoholism and/or drug abuse. The couple starts BCT soon after the substance abuser seeks help.

The BCT Recovery Contract

Before the substance abuser seeks help, the problems from substance abuse lead the couple into an intense, hostile struggle in which the spouse tries desperately to control the substance abuse, whereas the substance abuser, although at times promising to reform or staying abstinent for short periods, continues to drink or use drugs. The repeated unkept promises to change, and problems caused by the substance abuser's continued use, lead to a high level of distrust and conflict in the relationship.

The BCT recovery contract specifies behaviors that each member of the couple can do to reduce distrust and conflict about substance abuse and to reward abstinence and actions leading toward abstinence. The recovery contract starts with the "trust discussion," in which the patient states his or her intent not to drink or use drugs that day, in the tradition of 1 day at a time from Alcoholics Anonymous (AA). Then the spouse expresses support for the patient's efforts to stay abstinent, and the patient thanks the spouse for encouragement and support. For a patient taking a recovery-related medication (e.g., disulfiram, naltrexone), the spouse witnesses and verbally reinforces the daily medication ingestion during the trust discussion. The couple performs the trust discussion in each

BCT session to highlight its importance and to let the therapist observe the couple's performance of this important ritual.

Self-help meetings and drug urine screens are part of the contract for most patients. The patient and spouse mark performance of the trust discussion and other recovery activities (self-help meetings, drug screens, medication) on a calendar that is provided. At the start of each BCT session, the therapist reviews the recovery contract calendar to see how well each spouse has done his or her part. The calendar provides an ongoing record of progress that is rewarded verbally at each session. The couple also agrees not to discuss substance-related conflicts that can trigger relapse, reserving these discussions for the counseling sessions.

The following case examples illustrate the use of the BCT recovery contract. The first case illustrates BCT with a highly motivated, compliant couple. The second case illustrates that when both members of a couple have a current substance use problem and both want abstinence, then BCT often is workable. The third case illustrates BCT with an uncooperative substance abuser.

> **Mary and Jack.** Mary was an addicted daily drinker and marijuana smoker who came to treatment after being suspended from her job for drinking. Her husband, Jack, was a light drinker with no drug involvement. Their recovery contract had 1) a daily trust discussion, 2) at least two AA meetings per week, and 3) drug urine screens at each BCT session. They were very compliant, as shown by their calendar.
>
> However, Jack was upset about the positive urine screens for marijuana in the first few weeks. The counselor explained that marijuana could stay in the system for some time and suggested that Jack go to Al-Anon to help with his distress over Mary's suspected drug use. Soon, however, Mary's drug screens were negative for marijuana and stayed that way. Jack found Al-Anon helpful, so they added to the contract 1 night per week going together to a local church where Mary attended AA and Jack went to Al-Anon.
>
> **Sue and Gene.** Sue came to BCT after detoxification for heavy daily drinking plus cocaine and marijuana use three or four times per week. Gene had similar problems but did not need detoxification. Both wanted to "quit for good" to get their three school-age children back. Sue's parents were given temporary custody when Gene was arrested for drunk driving; Sue, who was also intoxicated, and the kids were in the car. Sue and Gene had 6 months of weekly BCT. Their dual recovery contract had 1) a daily trust discussion, 2) taking disulfiram daily together, 3) three AA meetings per week, and 4) weekly urine screens.
>
> About 5 weeks after starting BCT, Sue used cocaine on a Friday night when she went to the local bar with a girlfriend. At the next BCT session, her urine was positive for cocaine. The following Friday, both Gene and Sue went to the bar. They planned to just socialize, but when cocaine was

offered, they didn't refuse and did one line each. The next night they went to the bar again, and each used multiple lines of cocaine. This relapse was a turning point. They became more committed to their recovery. They planned things to do on Friday and Saturday nights, starting with an AA meeting together on Friday night. Each got a sponsor and some sober friends.

After weekly BCT, they had quarterly checkups for 2 more years. They regained custody of their children and stayed abstinent except for a few isolated days for Gene and a 5-day relapse for Sue, which led to a few crisis sessions with the BCT counselor to help them get back on track.

James and Cindy. James, a 27-year-old unemployed white male, was referred for treatment by his probation officer after being arrested during a police raid on a local crack house. James started an intensive outpatient program with urine screens at all appointments, and was referred to BCT. His wife, Cindy, was seriously considering taking their 2-year-old daughter and moving in with her parents. Problems in this case included high levels of distrust in the couple, and a substance-abusing patient who was court-mandated to treatment, lied about substance use, and falsified his urine samples.

The initial recovery contract for James and Cindy had 1) a daily trust discussion, 2) at least two AA meetings a week, 3) urine drug screens at each BCT session, and 4) job training classes. For the first month, all urine screens were negative, but Cindy wasn't convinced. Many BCT sessions focused on Cindy's suspicions that James was still using drugs and on James's anger over being accused of lying.

James's lying was discovered about 1 month after the couple started BCT, when the probation officer caught James submitting someone else's urine for analysis. When the probation officer supervised the urine sample more carefully, it was positive for cocaine. The probation officer told James that another positive urine sample would lead the officer to recommend jail time. Also, the probation officer started doing more frequent regular and random urine screening in addition to the ones done for BCT.

James admitted he had been using cocaine since starting BCT. Cindy said she would "give this another month," but only if they moved in with her parents so "if he screws up again, it's him who gets kicked out, not me." Their revised recovery contract gave more structured support for abstinence: 1) increase to daily AA meetings at least for the next 2 months, 2) get an AA sponsor and contact him at least twice weekly, 3) attend job training classes faithfully (James had been missing some) until he graduated, and 4) continue the daily trust discussion. Also, the BCT counselor began calling each member of the couple between the weekly BCT sessions to check on compliance with the recovery contract and other assignments.

Although Cindy remained understandably suspicious, after another month of BCT, she noted that James was not seeing his old friends and was very involved with AA, his sponsor, and trade school. BCT sessions moved toward increasing positive activities and better communication. James completed job training and got a full-time job. He stayed abstinent from cocaine and alcohol. He completed weekly BCT, outpatient treatment, and probation. During quarterly checkup visits for the year after BCT, the couple reported that they were still doing the daily trust discussion and James was attending at least two AA meetings a week. As this example shows, the combination of a patient, persistent BCT counselor, a willing couple, and external pressure to encourage abstinence can often overcome even major difficulties.

Other Support for Abstinence in BCT

BCT also supports abstinence by 1) reviewing substance use or urges to use since the last session; 2) decreasing exposure to alcohol and drugs (e.g., deciding whether to have alcohol in the house); 3) addressing stressful life problems to reduce relapse risk and make abstinence more rewarding; and 4) decreasing partner behaviors that trigger or reward substance use. These aspects are part of many types of substance abuse counseling. In BCT, they are carried out with the participation of the spouse.

Improving Relationship Functioning in BCT

Using a series of behavioral assignments, BCT increases positive feelings and activities and teaches constructive communication because these relationship factors are conducive to abstinence. Three methods focus on increasing positive feelings and activities. First, in "Catch Your Partner Doing Something Nice," each person is asked to notice and acknowledge one nice thing each day that his or her partner did. Second, "Caring Day" involves each person planning ahead to surprise his or her partner with a day when they do some special things to show their caring. Third, "Shared Rewarding Activities" encourage couples to have fun together, either by themselves or with their children or other couples, to help bring the couple closer together. Such shared activities are associated with positive recovery outcomes (Moos et al. 1990).

Teaching communication skills can help the substance abuser and spouse deal with stressors in their relationship and their lives, and this may reduce the risk of relapse. BCT includes basic communication skills of effective listening and speaking, and use of planned communication sessions. Couples also learn more advanced skills of conflict resolution, negotiating agreements for desired changes, and problem-solving skills.

Continuing Recovery in BCT

Most couples who attend BCT sessions faithfully show substantial improvement. However, when the structure of the weekly BCT sessions ends, there is a natural tendency for backsliding. Therefore, it is critical to help couples maintain the gains they made in BCT and prevent or minimize relapse. Near the end of weekly sessions, the BCT counselor helps the couple make a continuing recovery plan that specifies what aspects of BCT (e.g., trust discussion) they wish to continue and an action plan of steps to prevent or minimize relapse. Having couple checkup visits every few months for an extended period can encourage continued progress. Finally, those with more severe problems may benefit from periodic couple relapse prevention sessions in the year after weekly BCT ends (O'Farrell 1993a).

Evidence for Family Therapy to Aid Recovery When a Substance Abuser Has Sought Help

Research reviewed in detail elsewhere (Epstein and McCrady 1998; O'Farrell and Fals-Stewart 2001, 2003, 2006; Powers et al. 2008) shows that of these family-based methods to aid recovery when the substance abuser has sought help, BCT has the strongest evidence base. Over 15 randomized trials have compared substance abuse and relationship outcomes for alcoholic and drug-abusing patients treated with BCT or individual counseling. Many of the studies compare equally intensive treatments of BCT plus individual counseling with individual counseling alone. The studies show a fairly consistent pattern of results. Compared with patients who received only individual-based treatment, substance-abusing patients who received BCT had more abstinence and fewer substance-related problems, happier relationships, and lower risk of couple separation and divorce (e.g., Fals-Stewart et al. 1996, 2006; O'Farrell et al. 1992; Winters et al. 2002). Although earlier studies of BCT were done with white male alcoholic and drug-abusing patients and their female partners, more recent studies have shown the same pattern of superior results for black and Hispanic patients, heterosexual female patients, and both male and female same-sex couples with a substance-abusing member. Finally, compared with individual-based treatment, BCT produces greater improvements in compliance with recovery-related medication (disulfiram for alcoholic patients, naltrexone for opioid-using patients), intimate partner violence, and emotional problems of the couple's children (e.g., Fals-Stewart and O'Farrell 2003; Fals-Stewart et al. 2002; Kelley and Fals-Stewart 2002).

Evidence also supports the clinical utility of family systems therapy. Evidence for the effectiveness of family systems therapy is strongest for adolescent substance abusers (e.g., Szapocznik et al. 1988) and heroin-dependent young adults (Stanton et al. 1982). Although family systems concepts have influenced clinicians' work with adult alcoholic patients and their families (e.g., Steinglass et al. 1987), the evidence base supporting this practice is not very extensive. Only a small number of studies have been reported, and these generally had small sample sizes and no consistent pattern of favorable results. Interestingly, however, one study (Shoham et al. 1998) found family systems therapy was superior to BCT at retaining in treatment those couples with more seriously disturbed communication patterns. If replicated, these findings might implicate a patient-treatment matching effect.

Table 13–3 summarizes key points about family-based methods to aid recovery when the substance abuser has sought help.

Conclusion

In this chapter, we have described a variety of family interventions to help the family and to initiate change when the substance abuser resists treatment and to aid recovery once treatment has begun. We also showed that popular approaches may or may not have a strong evidence base, and vice versa. In helping the family, Al-Anon facilitation and referral help family members as intended and believed by its many adherents. However, coping skills training, which not only helps the family but also reduces violence and drinking better than Al-Anon does, is virtually unknown. For initiating change, the Johnson Institute intervention is very popular, and proponents often state that the approach is very effective, but research has

TABLE 13–3. **Family-based methods to aid recovery when the substance abuser has sought help**

Major approaches to aid recovery

- Network therapy—This therapy involves the patient's social network in treatment to support the patient's recovery (see Chapter 10).

- Family systems therapy (FST)—This therapy involves joining with the family and restructuring family alliances and interactions.

- Behavioral couples therapy (BCT)—Recovery contract and daily trust discussion support abstinence; positive activities and communication skills improve relationship.

Evidence for these approaches

- BCT has the strongest evidence base in over 15 randomized trials.

- Compared with individual-based treatment, BCT produces more abstinence, happier relationships, better compliance with recovery-related medication, and greater reductions in partner violence and emotional problems of the couple's children.

- Evidence supports FST for adolescent substance abusers and young adult heroin-using patients.

- Evidence supporting FST with adult alcoholism is not very extensive.

demonstrated that methods such as CRAFT are far more effective. For aiding recovery, BCT appears to be a very effective treatment for married or cohabiting substance-abusing patients, but it is rarely used by substance abuse treatment providers in non-research-based settings (Fals-Stewart and Birchler 2001).

Dissemination of effective family-based treatment methods is a shared responsibility between researchers and treatment providers. Investigators need to examine family treatment techniques that providers can adopt, given the economic and system constraints faced by community programs. For example, the involvement of managed care in substance abuse treatment has resulted in the more routine use of brief interventions. Thus, family-based treatment methods that require multiple therapy sessions over the course of several months may not be adopted, regardless of effectiveness. Conversely, it is the responsibility of providers and treatment programs to consider using family-based treatment methods that may be less familiar (e.g., behavioral interventions) but nonetheless more effective than traditional approaches. This would require challenging preconceived notions about what long-standing clinical wisdom may dictate as effective. Although these changes may be difficult to implement, the beneficiaries are likely to be substance-abusing patients and their families.

Key Clinical Concepts

- Family therapy interventions have been designed for three main purposes: 1) to help the family when the substance abuser refuses help, 2) to initiate change when the substance abuser resists treatment, and 3) to aid recovery once treatment has begun.

- Major approaches to help the family when the substance abuser refuses help are 1) Al-Anon facilitation and referral and 2) coping skills therapy (CST). Studies show that both Al-Anon and CST reduce emotional distress and improve coping of family members. However, CST leads to less drinking and less violence by the substance abuser than does Al-Anon.

- Major approaches to initiate change when the substance abuser resists treatment are 1) the Johnson Institute intervention, 2) A Relational Intervention Sequence for Engagement (ARISE), 3) Pressures to Change (PTC), and 4) Community Reinforcement and Family Training (CRAFT).

- Studies have shown that CRAFT is the most effective approach for initiating change for substance abusers who resist treatment. Although popular, the Johnson intervention has a lower engagement rate because many families do not follow through with the confrontation meeting that is the hallmark of this approach.

- Major approaches to aid recovery once treatment has begun are 1) network therapy, 2) family systems therapy, and 3) behavioral couples therapy (BCT).
- Studies show that BCT is effective with alcoholism and drug abuse. Compared with individual-based treatment, BCT produces more abstinence, happier relationships, better compliance with recovery-related medication, and greater reductions in partner violence and in emotional problems of the couple's children.
- Studies support family systems therapy (FST) for adolescent and young adult drug abusers, but evidence supporting FST with adult alcoholism is not very extensive.

Suggested Reading

Landau J, Garrett J: Invitational Intervention: A Step by Step Guide for Clinicians Helping Families Engage Resistant Substance Abusers in Treatment. New York, Haworth Press, 2006

Nowinski JK: Family Recovery and Substance Abuse: A Twelve-Step Guide for Treatment. Thousand Oaks, CA, Sage, 1999

O'Farrell TJ, Fals-Stewart W: Behavioral Couples Therapy for Alcoholism and Drug Abuse. New York, Guilford Press, 2006

Rychtarik RG, McGillicuddy NB, Duquette JA: Coping skill training program for women with alcoholic partners: therapist manual. Unpublished manuscript, University at Buffalo, State University of New York, 1995. (Available from Robert Rychtarik, Ph.D., Research Institute on Addictions, 1021 Main St, Buffalo, NY 14203.)

Smith JE, Meyers RJ: Motivating Substance Abusers to Enter Treatment: Working With Family Members. New York, Guilford Press, 2004

Steinglass P, Bennett L, Wolin S, et al: The Alcoholic Family. New York, Basic Books, 1987

References

Al-Anon Family Groups: Al-Anon Faces Alcoholism. New York, Al-Anon Family Groups, 1985

Barber JG, Crisp BR: The "Pressure to Change" approach to working with the partners of heavy drinkers. Addiction 90:269–276, 1995

Barber JG, Gilbertson R: An experimental study of brief unilateral intervention for the partners of heavy drinkers. Res Soc Work Pract 6:325–336, 1996

Barber JG, Gilbertson R: Evaluation of a self-help manual for the female partners of heavy drinkers. Res Soc Work Pract 8:141–151, 1998

Coleman SB, Davis DT: Family therapy and drug abuse: a national survey. Fam Process 17:21–29, 1978

Epstein EE, McCrady BS: Behavioral couples treatment of alcohol and drug use disorders: current status and innovations. Clin Psychol Rev 18:689–711, 1998

Fals-Stewart W, Birchler GR: A national survey of the use of couples therapy in substance abuse treatment. J Subst Abuse Treat 20:277–283, 2001

Fals-Stewart W, O'Farrell TJ: Behavioral family counseling and naltrexone for male opioid dependent patients. J Consult Clin Psychol 71:432–442, 2003

Fals-Stewart W, Birchler GR, O'Farrell TJ: Behavioral couples therapy for male substance-abusing patients: effects on relationship adjustment and drug-using behavior. J Consult Clin Psychol 64:959–972, 1996

Fals-Stewart W, Kashdan TB, O'Farrell TJ, et al: Behavioral couples therapy for male drug-abusing patients and their partners: the effect on interpartner violence. J Subst Abuse Treat 22:1–10, 2002

Fals-Stewart W, Birchler GR, Kelley ML: Learning sobriety together: a randomized clinical trial examining behavioral couples therapy with female alcoholic patients. J Consult Clin Psychol 74:579–591, 2006

Galanter M: Network Therapy for Alcohol and Drug Abuse, Expanded Edition. New York, Guilford, 1999

Haley J: Problem-Solving Therapy. San Francisco, CA, Jossey-Bass, 1976

Jellinek EM: The Disease Concept of Alcoholism. New Haven, CT, Hillhouse Press, Yale Center of Alcohol Studies, 1960

Johnson VE: Intervention: How to Help Someone Who Doesn't Want Help. Minneapolis, MN, Johnson Institute Books, 1986

Kaufman E, Kaufman P: Family Therapy of Drug and Alcohol Abuse, 2nd Edition. Needham Heights, MA, Allyn & Bacon, 1992

Keller M: Trends in treatment of alcoholism, in Second Special Report to the U.S. Congress on Alcohol and Health. Washington, DC, Department of Health, Education, and Welfare, 1974, pp 145–167

Kelley ML, Fals-Stewart W: Couples versus individual-based therapy for alcoholism and drug abuse: effects on children's psychosocial functioning. J Consult Clin Psychol 70:417–427, 2002

Kirby KC, Marlowe DB, Festinger DS, et al: Community reinforcement training for family and significant others of drug abusers: a unilateral intervention to increase treatment entry of drug users. Drug Alcohol Depend 56:85–96, 1999

Landau J, Garrett J: Invitational Intervention: A Step by Step Guide for Clinicians Helping Families Engage Resistant Substance Abusers in Treatment. New York, Haworth Press, 2006

Landau J, Stanton MD, Ikle D, et al: Outcomes with the ARISE approach to engaging reluctant drug- and alcohol-dependent individuals in treatment. Am J Drug Alcohol Abuse 30:711–748, 2004

Liepman MR: Using family influence to motivate alcoholics to enter treatment: the Johnson Institute intervention approach, in Treating Alcohol Problems: Marital and Family Interventions. Edited by O'Farrell TJ. New York, Guilford, 1993, pp 54–77

Liepman MR, Nirenberg TD, Begin AM: Evaluation of a program designed to help family and significant others to motivate resistant alcoholics into recovery. Am J Drug Alcohol Abuse 15:209–221, 1989

Meyers RJ, Miller WR, Smith JE, et al: A randomized trial of two methods for engaging treatment-refusing drug users through concerned significant others. J Consult Clin Psychol 70:1182–1185, 2002

Miller WR, Meyers RJ, Tonigan JS: Engaging the unmotivated in treatment for alcohol problems: a comparison of three strategies for intervention through family members. J Consult Clin Psychol 67:688–697, 1999

Minuchin S: Families and Family Therapy. Cambridge, MA, Harvard University Press, 1974

Moos RH, Finney JW, Cronkite RC: Alcoholism Treatment: Context, Process, and Outcome. New York, Oxford University Press, 1990

Nowinski JK: Family Recovery and Substance Abuse: A Twelve-Step Guide for Treatment. Thousand Oaks, CA, Sage, 1999

O'Farrell TJ: Couples relapse prevention sessions after a behavioral marital therapy couples group program, in Treating Alcohol Problems: Marital and Family Interventions. Edited by O'Farrell TJ. New York, Guilford, 1993a, pp 305–326

O'Farrell TJ (ed): Treating Alcohol Problems: Marital and Family Interventions. New York, Guilford, 1993b

O'Farrell TJ, Fals-Stewart W: Family involved alcoholism treatment: an update, in Recent Developments in Alcoholism, Vol 15: Services Research in the Era of Managed Care. Edited by Galanter M. New York, Plenum, 2001, pp 329–356

O'Farrell TJ, Fals-Stewart W: Alcohol abuse. J Marital Fam Ther 29:121–146, 2003

O'Farrell TJ, Fals-Stewart W: Behavioral Couples Therapy for Alcoholism and Drug Abuse. New York, Guilford, 2006

O'Farrell TJ, Cutter HS, Choquette K, et al: Behavioral marital therapy for male alcoholics: marital and drinking adjustment during two years after treatment. Behav Ther 23:529–549, 1992

O'Farrell TJ, Fals-Stewart W, Murphy M, et al: Partner violence before and after individually based alcoholism treatment for male alcoholic patients. J Consult Clin Psychol 71:92–102, 2003

O'Farrell TJ, Murphy CM, Stephen S, et al: Partner violence before and after couples-based alcoholism treatment for male alcoholic patients: the role of treatment involvement and abstinence. J Consult Clin Psychol 72:202–217, 2004

Powers MB, Vedel E, Emmelkamp PM: Behavioral couples therapy (BCT) for alcohol and drug use disorders: a meta-analysis. Clin Psychol Rev 28:952–962, 2008

Rychtarik RG, McGillicuddy NB: Coping skills training and 12-step facilitation for women whose partner has alcoholism: effects on depression, the partner's drinking, and partner physical violence. J Consult Clin Psychol 73:249–261, 2005

Shoham V, Rohrbaugh MJ, Stickle TR, et al: Demand-withdraw couple interaction moderates retention in cognitive-behavioral versus family systems treatments for alcoholism. J Fam Psychol 12:557–577, 1998

Sisson RW, Azrin HH: Family-member involvement to initiate and promote treatment of problem drinkers. J Behav Ther Exp Psychiatry 17:15–21, 1986

Smith JE, Meyers RJ: Motivating Substance Abusers to Enter Treatment: Working With Family Members. New York, Guilford, 2004

Stanton MD: The role of family and significant others in the engagement and retention of drug-dependent individuals, in Beyond the Therapeutic Alliance: Keeping the Drug-Dependent Individual in Treatment (NIDA Res Monogr 165, NIH Publ No 97-4142). Edited by Onken LS, Blaine JD, Boren FJ. Rockville, MD, National Institute on Drug Abuse, 1997, pp 157–180

Stanton MD, Heath AW: Family and marital treatment, in Substance Abuse: A Comprehensive Textbook, 3rd Edition. Edited by Lowinson JH, Ruiz P, Millman RB, et al. Baltimore, MD, Williams & Wilkins, 1997, pp 448–454

Stanton MD, Todd TC, and associates: The Family Therapy of Drug Abuse and Addiction. New York, Guilford, 1982

Steinglass P, Bennett L, Wolin S, et al: The Alcoholic Family. New York, Basic Books, 1987

Szapocznik J, Perez-Vidal A, Brickman AL, et al: Engaging adolescent drug abusers and their families in treatment: a strategic structural systems approach. J Consult Clin Psychol 56:552–557, 1988

Winters J, Fals-Stewart W, O'Farrell TJ, et al: Behavioral couples therapy for female substance-abusing patients: effects on substance use and relationship adjustment. J Consult Clin Psychol 70:344–355, 2002

14 The History of Alcoholics Anonymous and the Experiences of Patients

Edgar P. Nace, M.D.

Today, the general public knows that Alcoholics Anonymous (AA) is where people go when they cannot handle alcohol and need to quit drinking. Almost everyone knows somebody who goes or has gone to AA. Relatively little stigma is attached to participating in AA programs today, although those approaching it for the first time may not agree. As familiar as AA is in North America and Europe, few people likely know about its origins and fewer still appreciate its impact on so many lives.

On June 10, 1935, an Akron, Ohio, surgeon named Bob Smith took his last drink, a beer, to steady his nerves prior to performing surgery. This date is considered the founding date of AA (White 1998).

Bob Smith and Bill Wilson, the cofounders of AA, had met in May 1935 in Akron. Bill, a New York stockbroker who was newly sober, was about to drink while on business in Akron. He desperately sought a meeting of the Oxford Group (a predecessor of AA), realizing that he might stay sober if he had another alcoholic person to talk to. In the course of his search, he was introduced to "Dr. Bob," a struggling alcoholic surgeon.

Followers of AA and most students of alcoholism are familiar with the names Bill Wilson and Dr. Bob Smith. Their fateful meeting in Ohio spawned the formation of the most successful grassroots self-help movement known.

Why has this program been so successful? What happens to people who go to AA? Easy answers do not follow from these questions. Regarding its success, many AA members would say what they say to newcomers: "Keep coming back. It works!" What makes it work is no doubt multifaceted and variable from person to person.

AA meetings include testimonials from recovering alcoholics who tell what their life was like while drinking, what they had to do to get sober, and what their life is like now. Both those in AA and those who observe the work of AA often reflect on how such a change occurs.

Modern concepts of behavior change typically embrace the transtheoretical model of change explicated by Prochaska and DiClemente (1984). This very apt model of behavior change emphasizes gradual shifts in motivation that occur in stages: precontemplation (not really considering change); contemplation (considering the need to change); decision (deciding that change is necessary); action (putting into effect strategies and behaviors that will accomplish the desired change); and maintenance (maintaining behaviors necessary to sustain the desired change).

For example, an alcohol-dependent person may be in denial about the impact of his drinking on himself or others and see no need for change (precontemplation). An episode of pancreatitis may alert him to the need to consider change (contemplation). When his employer confronts him with increasing absenteeism because of alcohol-related medical complications, he decides he has to do something about his drinking now (decision). A coworker takes him to an AA meeting (action), and he finds support and friendship that assist him in giving up a chronic pattern of alcohol dependence (maintenance).

The transtheoretical model recognizes that the motivation to change behavior waxes and wanes and that first or second efforts are not necessarily successful. Individuals will "recycle" back to decision and action stages when they fail at maintenance. Most persons who overcome an addiction or attempt other significant behavior change (e.g., weight loss) will experience and reexperience the stages of change referred to above.

This model, however, does not capture the totality of experience in recovery from alcoholism. A qualitatively different experience characterizes change for some. This "transformational" type of change occurs suddenly, is experienced as profound, and yields enduring shifts in values and behaviors (Forcehimes et al. 2008). Miller and C'de Baca (2001) describe such changes as "vivid, surprising, benevolent and enduring personal transformation" (Miller and C'de Baca 2001, p. 4). Such an experience may lead directly to sobriety or may first impact values and character before leading to sobriety.

Spiritual awakenings (a type of transformational change) are the emphasized means of change in the AA literature. Bill Wilson, one of the previously mentioned cofounders of AA, had a dramatic spiritual experience while hospitalized (described in "Forerunners of AA" below). Change may also occur abruptly, without the trappings of a spiritual experience (e.g., white light, rushing wind). More commonly, however, change is experienced gradually.

The Experiences of Patients

Laura was adopted into an upper-middle-class professional home. She is her parents' only child and has no knowledge of her biological parents. Her adopting mother was chronically ill and verbally abusive to Laura, especially during Laura's adolescence. Laura would become enraged at her mother and struck her on several occasions. Marijuana, lysergic acid diethylamide (LSD), and alcohol were Laura's escape mechanisms. She was sent to a psychiatric hospital briefly after an altercation with her mother. She said that her junior year in high school was "ruined" by this hospitalization. Then she was enrolled in an intensive outpatient program to deal with her substance abuse. This failed. Laura ridiculed 12-step programs. Her intelligence enabled admittance into an excellent 4-year liberal arts college; however, cycles of depression, drinking, and drug use led to her expulsion after 3½ years, without a degree. Her father relied on her for companionship as her mother became increasingly medically ill. The enmeshed family life, Laura's sense of failure, and her turn to intensive drinking led to a 30-day rehabilitation program. While she was off alcohol, Laura's mood stabilized and she agreed to a long-term outpatient program. Over her initial 12-month period of sobriety, she gradually warmed up to the step work and the teachings of AA. By her 4-year sobriety date, she had acquired a good employment record and completed her college degree.

Laura, now focused on a career path and graduate school, slowly overcame dependence on alcohol and drugs, a turbulent depressing family environment, and several failed attempts at treatment. Her acceptance of AA was fitful and gradual, but now she is a stalwart AA member and a sponsor. There was neither a profound moment of insight nor an experience of sudden transformation. Steady exposure to AA, constructive psychotherapy, and increasing autonomy shifted the balance in favor of a productive future for Laura.

Greg never knew his biological father and was raised by a schizophrenic mother. He was physically abused and predictably abused drugs and alcohol by his early teens. Two suicide attempts during adolescence led to psychiatric hospitalizations. He used cocaine, alcohol, and cannabis continuously, and by his late teens he was diagnosed with bipolar disorder. He first married at age 20 and soon divorced. When his mother committed suicide, Greg attempted suicide again. This attempt led to a second divorce and another psychiatric hospitalization. Eventually he was sentenced to a treatment program after a felony arrest for driving while intoxicated. In this program, he attempted suicide again and was rehospitalized. Divorced, jobless, and a felon, Greg explained that he *suddenly* figured that all his problems were of his own making. *It dawned on him.* He is not sure why. He knew alcohol and drugs depressed him or made him manic. He quit and decided to work the 12 steps. He also quit his medications. Three years later, he remains sober, is self-employed, and follows AA and the 12-step program of Celebrate Recovery. He endures custody court battles with equanimity as his ex-wives fight his efforts to resume his role as a responsible father.

Forerunners of AA

Just as individual experiences of change may be either gradual or sudden, so it is with the concepts and experiences that shaped AA over decades. The Washingtonian Total Abstinence Society gradually informed the structure of AA. Also, the experience of Bill Wilson in Towns Hospital exemplifies an abrupt personal change that contributed enormously to the forming of AA.

In 1840, nearly 100 years before the meeting of Bob Smith and Bill Wilson, six members of a drinking club in Baltimore, Maryland, who were inspired to turn from drink after attending a lecture on temperance, decided to quit their club and form what they would call the Washingtonian Total Abstinence Society. The men resolved to meet nightly, just as they previously had drunk nightly. These meetings involved sharing experiences. The men valued drama, and avoided debates and formal speeches. Local alcoholic persons were encouraged to attend and to say a few words. Later, dues were assessed. The Washingtonians started with private meetings, but because of increasing public interest, they began holding public meetings as well. Their slogan—"Let every man be present, and every man bring a man"—conveys the zeal this organization had for recruiting new members; they have since been described as "secular missionaries." They formed ward committees to recruit more alcoholic individuals and required that members sign a pledge of abstinence (Tyrell 1979).

The Washingtonians—named after George Washington in honor of his character, and not the fact that he distilled liquor—grew at an impressive rate. Their numbers increased more rapidly in their first few years than did AA's membership a century later. (In fact, by mid-1841, an organization for women was established, known as the Martha Washington Society [Maxwell 1950]; however, that group's momentum was not sustained.) Individuals who were not alcoholic could also attend the meetings, and soon they began to outnumber the alcoholic members. The message of the Washingtonians was carried largely by a few charismatic speakers who pursued their own independent agendas. Debates about alcohol prohibition divided the Washingtonians, and no central organizational structure was sustained (Maxwell 1950). By 1847, most Washingtonian societies had ceased to exist (White 1998). Nevertheless, the Washingtonian Total Abstinence Society laid the groundwork for several features that would eventually characterize AA: mutual self-help, sharing of the drinking experience and the recovery experience, focus on the welfare of the alcoholic person, the power of personal shared commitment to abstinence, and the use of religious and/or spiritual foundations for recovery.

Fraternal temperance societies and reform clubs soon emerged. These organizations tended to emphasize anonymity and secrecy, which allowed alcoholic members to seek support without public acknowledgment. (The importance of anonymity would later be adopted by AA.) Some of these societies and clubs focused only on the reform of the alcoholic person, whereas others joined the political debate on prohibition. The Independent Order of Good Templars, founded in 1851, claimed to have 400,000 alcoholic members by 1876, half of whom were purported to have kept their pledge of abstinence (Fahey 1996). These societies emphasized maintenance of sobriety, and breaks of abstinence could lead to expulsion. Some were racially integrated. Similar societies were formed for women.

Reform clubs later overtook the fraternal temperance societies. These groups did not have restrictive membership, were less inclined to participate in prohibition issues, and were more informal. No particular religion was endorsed, but personal change was expected to include prayer and church attendance. The clubs' ability to recruit members was impressive; 50,000 members were reported in Philadelphia, Pennsylvania, alone by 1870 (White 1998).

By the turn of the twentieth century, a variety of mutual-aid organizations had arisen to assist alcoholic persons who were willing to try to quit drinking. White (1998) described many of these groups, most of whose legacies have fallen into the cracks of social, religious, or medical history; the Keeley Leagues, the United Order of Ex-Boozers, and the Emmanuel Clinic are little remembered today. However, one movement, now also out of existence, avoided obscurity by its seminal role in the origin of AA: the Oxford Group.

Founded by a Lutheran minister in the early 1900s, the Oxford Group hoped to reestablish the fervor and enthusiasm of first-century Christianity: the group was not founded to address alcoholism but became active in helping alcoholic persons largely through the leadership of a New York City Episcopal priest, Rev. Sam Shoemaker. The Oxford Group emphasized personal spiritual change as a solution to people's problems. It endorsed "four absolutes": absolute honesty, absolute purity, absolute unselfishness, and absolute love. It also endorsed the "five C's": confidence, confession, conviction, conversion, and continuance (White 1998).

To better appreciate the role of the Oxford Group as the immediate forerunner of AA, one must briefly divert attention to Roland H, who was from a wealthy Connecticut family and had exhausted his family fortune through drinking. He sought treatment with Dr. Carl Jung and spent an uncertain amount of time in Zurich under analysis with Jung. Confident that his obsession with alcohol was resolved, Roland H returned to the United States and promptly became drunk (Thomsen 1975). He then returned to Zurich. Jung explained that medicine and psychiatry could do no more for him. A spiritual or religious conversion, Jung explained, had brought recovery for some alcoholic persons, and this was Roland's only remaining hope, albeit somewhat unlikely to occur (Kurtz 1979).

Roland joined the Oxford Group, which was also very active in Europe at that time. He underwent a conversion experience, returned to New York City, and never drank again. He became active at the headquarters of the Oxford Group, the Calvary Episcopal Church in New York, which was headed by Rev. Sam Shoemaker. Rev. Shoemaker has been described as erudite, enthusiastic, eager, and honest. He was known to discuss his own shortcomings in preference to faulting others. People from all walks of life were drawn to him (Thomsen 1975).

Under the auspices of the Oxford Group, Roland shared his conversion experience with those in need. This "mission" of Roland's led him to intervene with an old friend, Edwin Thacher, or Ebby T, who in 1934 was about to be committed to a long-term institution. Roland, along with another alcoholic individual, reached out to Ebby and led him to the Oxford Group, whereupon Ebby established his first period of sobriety and found "friendship and fellowship of a kind he had never known" (Kurtz 1979, p. 10). Ebby sought out another hopeless alcoholic, his friend Bill Wilson. As Kurtz (1979) described it, Ebby and Bill were talking over the kitchen table at Bill's house in Brooklyn. Bill was drinking that November afternoon and offered Ebby the same. Ebby refused Bill's repeated offers, finally explaining that he had found religion. Bill is described as being "not exactly insulted, but embarrassed, and somehow strangely betrayed" (Thomsen 1975, p. 207). Ebby explained that he had joined the Oxford Group, which had originated on the Princeton campus and had later moved to Oxford and beyond. Bill had heard of the group but considered them too zealous for Christ, too social, and too rich. Ebby explained that the situation was different; he had learned to pray and to maintain an open mind about the benefit of prayer, and he felt that the desire to drink had been lifted from him. Ebby must have sensed that religious terms were averse to Bill. According to Thomsen (1975), instead of repeating the word *God* in their conversation, Ebby used terms such as "another power" and "higher power" (p. 209). Perhaps this is the origin of AA's embracing of the concept of a higher power in lieu of more precise religious terminology.

Bill continued his drinking. Ebby stopped by a few days later with another Oxford Group member who was newly sober. They reiterated the power of prayer and meditation, giving of oneself, and finding a new sense of purpose. Bill remained disparaging of the religious promptings of these men, but he could not deny that his friend Ebby had changed. Days later, Bill decided to investigate the Oxford Group and found his way to a meeting while intoxicated. The dregs of the city were there. The odor was repulsive. The talk was of prayer, Jesus, and the possibility of a new life. Bill apparently spoke a few words himself, although he was not able to recall what he said (Thomsen 1975).

At home, Bill tried to taper off alcohol but was unsuccessful. His fear of brain damage and his uncontrollable drinking led him to Charles B. Towns Hospital, where he sought the help of Dr. William D. Silkworth. Silkworth was a neurologist whose dream of building his own hospital had collapsed along with his savings during the Depression. He had a compassionate interest in helping alcoholic persons and is estimated to have treated over 50,000 during his career (Thomsen 1975). Bill was admitted to Towns Hospital for what was probably the fourth time. On the second day, Ebby visited and at Bill's request explained the "formula" for sobriety: "Realize you are licked, admit it, and get willing to turn your life over to the will of God" (Kurtz 1979, p. 19).

What happened to Bill Wilson in that hospital bed was not fully described by him until two decades later (Wilson 1957). He was deeply depressed, but he fought the notion that there was a power greater than himself and reported that in his despair

> [I cried out,] If there is a God, let Him show Himself! I am ready to do anything, anything! Suddenly the room lit up with a great white light. I was caught up into an ecstasy which there are no words to describe. It seemed to me, in the mind's eye, that I was on a mountain and that wind not of air but of spirit was blowing. And then it burst upon me that I was a free man. Slowly the ecstasy subsided. I lay on the bed, but now for a time I was in another world, a new world of consciousness. All about me and through me there was a wonderful feeling of Presence, and I thought to myself, "So this is the God of the preachers!" A great peace stole over me and I thought, "No matter how wrong things seem to be, they are all right. Things are all right with God and His world." (Kurtz 1979, pp. 19–20)

Bill asked a nurse to find Dr. Silkworth. He feared and wanted to know if this experience represented brain damage. Silkworth listened to Bill's experience, asked questions, and responded that Bill was "perfectly sane, in my opinion" (Thomsen 1975, p. 224). Silkworth explained that he had read about such things and that they could produce profound changes.

He encouraged Bill to "hang on to it.... It is so much better than what you had a couple of hours ago" (p. 224).

After discharge from Towns Hospital, Bill returned to the Oxford Group—this time, he was sober. He and his wife, Lois, attended the meetings, and Bill would go after the meeting with other members to a local cafeteria. Three postconversion experiences strengthened Bill's sobriety and his determination to carry the message to other alcoholic persons: the counseling of Dr. Silkworth, the exchange of experiences with other alcoholic persons at Steward's Cafeteria, and the support of Rev. Sam Shoemaker. Silkworth provided a medical explanation for the alcoholic's plight: an "allergy." Of course, alcoholism is not an allergy, but the term was a useful analogy. Furthermore, Silkworth avoided focusing on the past and emphasized positive aspects of the individual's life and struggle with recovery. In this regard, his approach may have been a forerunner of motivational interviewing. The informal meetings of the alcoholics at the cafeteria, with their natural inclination to share experiences in a setting that was nonjudgmental, clearly convinced Bill Wilson that one alcoholic talking to another was a tool—a profound dynamic—for moving forward into a life free of alcohol. Rev. Shoemaker, the Episcopal priest, gave Bill and others a new perspective on prayer—namely, listening to or meditating on what God wants for you as an alternative or in addition to requests and petitions (Thomsen 1975).

According to Thomsen (1975), over the 6 months after leaving Towns Hospital, Bill fervently told his story to other alcoholic persons. He stayed sober, but they did not. He was frustrated that Oxford Group members were lukewarm at best with the idea of alcoholism being a disease. They were interested in moral regeneration. Discouraged, Bill spoke with Dr. Silkworth, who told him to stop preaching and to emphasize the physical destruction of alcohol (Thomsen 1975). Bill continued to struggle with whether to emphasize sin or sickness. Meanwhile, he was back working as a broker, which is what took him to Akron, Ohio, in May 1935.

Bill was involved in a proxy fight to take over a small machine tool factory. He and his colleagues lost; the colleagues left Akron shortly thereafter, and Bill was left alone on the Saturday before Mother's Day. Dejected, he began to rationalize the desire to drink. A bar was down the hall, and he walked toward it, but in near panic about what he was about to do, he went back to the lobby instead. In his telling of this incident years later, Bill said he knew he had to talk to someone, preferably another alcoholic person. He called a minister whose name was listed in the church directory located in the lobby. Rev. Walter Tunks received Bill's call and responded to his request for help, giving him 10 names. After numerous calls, Bill reached an Oxford Group member, Ms. Henrietta Seiberling.

Ms. Seiberling, the daughter-in-law of the president of Goodyear Tire and Rubber Company, understood Bill's plight and graciously asked him to her house. She was not alcoholic herself but had been trying to help a local surgeon, Dr. Bob Smith, with his alcoholism. She arranged for Dr. Bob and Bill to meet at her home the next day (Thomsen 1975).

Dr. Bob had attempted many treatments and had a strong connection with the local Oxford Group. He was considered hopeless. Bob and his wife, Anne, met Bill at Ms. Seiberling's on that Sunday. Dr. Bob was tremulous, stooped over, and haggard looking. Bill reassured him that their visit could be brief.

It is likely that Bill shifted gears as he spoke with Dr. Bob—that is, Bill did not warn the doctor about the consequences of heavy drinking, nor did he emphasize his own turnaround as experienced during detoxification at Towns Hospital. Instead, Bill opened up about his past promises, failed hopes, and drunken despair. He reviewed his hospital stays and the visits from Ebby. He did not talk down to Dr. Bob, and in turn Dr. Bob, who was apparently very taciturn and self-reliant, saw himself in Bill's story. They knew that they understood each other (Kurtz 1979). Although Bill remained sober after their meeting, Dr. Bob soon thereafter went to a medical convention in Atlantic City and returned to Akron drunk. With assistance from his wife and Bill, however, he acquired lasting sobriety on June 10, 1935.

Kurtz's (1979) definitive history of AA identifies what he has called four "founding moments" in the development and evolution of the group. These moments, mentioned previously, are highlighted again here because of their salience:

1. *The relationship between Carl Jung and Roland H.* This was a failed therapeutic experience, as acknowledged by Jung. However, Jung's discussion with Roland about the possibility of spiritual change or awakening was critical to Roland's joining the Oxford Group. Roland's successful conversion followed. Bill Wilson, in 1961, wrote to Jung: "The conversations between you [and Roland] were to become the first link in the chain of events that led to the founding of Alcoholics Anonymous" (Kurtz 1979, p. 8).

2. *Ebby T's 1934 visit with Bill Wilson in Wilson's kitchen in New York City.* Ebby had been guided by Roland to "get religion." Bill was drinking when Ebby visited. Ebby turned down Bill's offers of alcohol. Bill could not shake the image of his former co-drinker as sober and resolute. Ebby's example and his kind, patient encouragement spurred Bill to try once again—that is, to readmit himself to Towns Hospital. (Unfortunately, Ebby later relapsed and died from the consequences of alcoholism.)

3. *Bill's spiritual experience at Towns Hospital.* Either Roland or Ebby (it is not known which) directed Bill to William James's (1902/1985) famous work *The Varieties of Religious Experience.* This text enabled Bill to further understand and value the spiritual experience he had undergone in December 1934.

4. *The conversation and the subsequent interaction between Bill and Dr. Bob Smith in Akron, Ohio, in May and June 1935.* Their initial conversation captures the power of AA's eventual strategy of one alcoholic person talking to another. Kurtz (1979, p. 29) describes the conversation as follows:

> Here was someone [Wilson] who did understand, or perhaps at least could. This stranger from New York didn't ask questions and didn't preach; he offered no "you musts" or even "let's us's." He had simply told the dreary but fascinating facts about himself, about his own drinking. And now, as Wilson moved to stand up to end the conversation, he was actually thanking Dr. Smith for listening. "I called Henrietta because I needed another alcoholic. I needed you, Bob, probably a lot more than you'll ever need me. So, thanks a lot for hearing me out. I know now that I'm not going to take a drink, and I'm grateful to you." While he had been listening to Bill's story, Bob had occasionally nodded his head, muttering, "Yes, that's like me, that's just like me." Now he could bear the strain no longer. He'd listened to Bill's story, and now, by God, this "rum hound from New York" was going to listen to his. For the first time in his life, Dr. Bob Smith began to open his heart.

Growth of AA

Bill Wilson and Dr. Bob Smith spent the summer of 1935 meeting with alcoholic persons at Dr. Bob's home. When Bill returned to New York City at the end of the summer, there were four newly sober alcoholics, including Dr. Bob, in Akron.

Bill Wilson was ambitious. He tirelessly recruited alcoholics at the Oxford Group meetings in New York. He sought funding and soon faced a major temptation: in 1936, Charles Towns, the owner of Towns Hospital, wanted Bill to bring his program into that hospital. Bill would receive a portion of the profits, which would solve Bill's growing financial problems and provide an organizational structure for the growth of his group (White 1998). Fellow members (the name Alcoholics Anonymous had not yet been coined) discouraged the arrangement, however, and Bill yielded to their influence. AA since has continued to avoid affiliation with other entities.

There was no certain AA identity in the mid-1930s. The members met within the structure of the Oxford Group. Strains in this relationship soon emerged: The Oxford Group valued publicity, whereas the members preferred anonymity. The Oxford Group was Protestant; many of the alcoholics were Catholic. Oxford Group members were zealous about the strictness of their beliefs, whereas the early members of Bill's group wanted to accept any alcoholic—believer or not, Catholic, Protestant, or otherwise.

The AA identity began to take shape through the formulation of the 12 steps (originally only six), which Bill Wilson credited to three sources: the Oxford Group, Dr. William Silkworth, and William James.

The "Big Book," formally known as *Alcoholics Anonymous*, was written by Bill Wilson beginning in 1938. The book was published in 1939, and initial reviews in medical circles were derogatory, saying the book had "no scientific merit or interest" ("Book Reviews: Alcoholics Anonymous" 1940). Twenty thousand direct mail notices of the book were sent to physicians, but only two orders were made (Thomsen 1975). Later, through articles in popular magazines such as the *Saturday Evening Post*, sales of the book took off and national publicity developed.

The group now known as Alcoholics Anonymous officially adopted its name in 1939, at which time the group had an estimated 100 members. A rapid growth of the group occurred as members spread the word about AA beyond New York City and Ohio and as radio shows and newspaper articles publicized AA. Sales of the "Big Book" greatly increased, and Bill Wilson and Bob Smith were rumored to have split the royalties, although an audit dispelled this rumor. The growing pains continued: critics complained of a lack of rules, too little authority, and insufficient organizational structure. Ultimately, "AA committed itself to corporate poverty, group authority rather than personal authority and leadership, and the lowest level of organization necessary to carry AA's message of recovery" (White 1998, p. 137).

By 1946, AA's 12 traditions were formulated. The 12 traditions provide the guidelines for AA organizational behavior and provide principles to protect the group life of AA (Alcoholics Anonymous 1978). A central office was established in New York City in 1945. In 1950, Dr. Bob, the cofounder of AA, died. He had lived long enough to witness AA's explosive growth to nearly 90,000 members at the time of his death. Bill Wilson died on January 24, 1971.

AA Survey Data

Since 1968, the General Service Office of AA in New York City has conducted a membership survey about every 3 years. No formal membership lists are maintained, and some local groups do not list themselves with the General Service Office. Table 14–1 lists AA membership and group information as of January 1, 2010.

A 2007 membership survey (Alcoholics Anonymous 2007) documented increasing collaboration among physicians, other health care providers, and AA. Thirty-nine percent of current members reported being referred to AA by a health care professional; 63% of current members received treatment or some formal counseling prior to joining AA; and 74% of these stated that such treatment played an important part in their decision to go to AA. The increasing transparency between AA and medicine is reflected further by a report stating that 74% of members' physicians know they are in AA.

How Members Discover AA

As mentioned, 39% of members in the 2007 survey were referred by a health care provider. Another 31% were self-motivated, 33% were referred through an AA member, 24% by family, 11% by court order, 4% by

TABLE 14–1.   **Alcoholics Anonymous estimates of groups and members as of January 1, 2010**

	Groups	Members
United States	56,694	1,264,716
Canada	4,887	94,163
Subtotal	61,581	1,358,879
Correctional facilities, U.S. and Canada	1,589	39,731
Internationalists[a]	3	0
Lone members	0	157
Total	63,173	1,398,767
Outside United States and Canada[b]	52,600	704,266
Grand total	**115,773**	**2,103,033**

Note. The AA General Service Office does not keep membership records. The information shown here is based on reports given by groups listed with GSO and does not represent an actual count of those who consider themselves AA members.

[a][Internationalists are seagoing members in naval service or the merchant marine.]

[b]We are aware of AA activity in more than 180 countries, including 60 autonomous general service offices in other lands. Annually we attempt to contact those GSOs and groups that request to be listed in our records. Where current data is lacking we use an earlier year's figure.

Source. Reprinted from January 1, 2010, update to "Alcoholics Anonymous: Estimates of A.A. Groups and Members." Alcoholics Anonymous, personal communication, June 2010. Used with permission.

an employer or fellow employee, and 1% by clergy (Alcoholics Anonymous 2007).

Length of Sobriety

According to the latest AA survey, 31% of members report less than 1 year of sobriety, 24% report 1–5 years, 12% report 5–10 years, and 33% report more than 10 years. These data document that newcomers to AA can expect to meet alcoholic persons with long-term sobriety (Alcoholic Anonymous 2007). Occasionally, the newcomer is envious of those with long-term success in the program. Envy can be defused by the reminder that a person stays sober "one day at a time" and that the old-timer may be as close to a next drink as the newcomer.

Current Demographics

Table 14–2 presents the demographic makeup of AA as of 2007.

TABLE 14–2. Alcoholics Anonymous membership demographics (%)

Marital status		**Occupation**	
Married	35	Retired	16
Single	34	Self-employed/other	11
Divorced	23	Manager/administrator	10
Other	8	Professional/technical	10
		Skilled trade	8
Ethnicity		Unemployed	8
White	85.1	Laborer	6
Black	5.7	Health professional	5
Hispanic	4.8	Disabled (not working)	5
Native American	1.6	Sales worker	4
Asian and other	2.8	Student	4
		Service worker	3
		Educator	3
Age		Clerical worker	2
Under age 21	2.3	Homemaker	2
Ages 21–30	11.3	Transportation (equipment operator)	2
Ages 31–40	16.5	Craft worker	1
Ages 41–50	28.5		
Ages 51–60	23.8		
Ages 61–70	12.3		
Over 70	5.3		

Note. Data from U.S. and Canadian members.

Source. Reprinted from "Alcoholics Anonymous: Estimates of A.A. Groups and Members." 2007. Available at: http://www.aa.org/en_media_ resources.cfm?PageID=74. Accessed February 24, 2010. Used with permission.

The AA Program

The program of AA is considered a fellowship. A *fellowship* is a "mutual association of persons on equal and friendly terms; a mutual sharing, as of experience, activity, or interest" (*Webster's New Twentieth Century Dictionary of the English Language* 1980). The fellowship of AA is structured to sustain the primary focus of AA, which is "to stay sober and help other alcoholics to achieve sobriety" (Alcoholics Anonymous 1992). Structured features of AA include meetings, AA literature, and the 12 steps and 12 traditions.

Meetings

AA meetings may be open or closed. An open meeting welcomes guests and those attempting to recover from alcoholism. Closed meetings should be attended only by those who consider themselves AA members or are contemplating membership. There are several types of meetings:

1. *Speaker meetings.* During a speaker meeting, a member tells his or her story to the group in attendance, putting emphasis on what happened (e.g., the effect of alcohol in that person's life), what was done about it (how the person got sober), and what the person is doing now to stay sober. Experienced AA members often assess the quality of one's sobriety by how much emphasis is placed on the "drunkalogue" or the "war stories" versus how much the speaker emphasizes his or her current focus on remaining sober. (Quality is related to current recovery activities and not the gory details of drunkenness.)
2. *Step meetings.* During step meetings, one of the 12 steps is introduced by a group leader and discussed by the members. This is an effort to more fully appreciate the importance of each step and to develop a deeper understanding of the same for one's life.
3. *Discussion meetings.* Discussion meetings involve a group discussion focused on a salient aspect of recovery; for example, the group might discuss humility or resentments and learn from each other's experience of trying to apply the former or overcome the latter.

The AA Literature

Each AA meeting starts with the leader of the meeting reading the AA preamble. The preamble concisely reviews what AA is and is not:

> Alcoholics Anonymous is a fellowship of men and women who share their experience, strength, and hope with each other that they may solve their common problem and help others to recover from alcoholism. The only requirement for membership is a desire to stop drinking. There are no

dues or fees for AA membership; we are self-supporting through our own contributions. AA is not allied with any sect, denomination, politics, organization, or institution; does not wish to engage in any controversy, neither endorses nor opposes any causes. Our primary purpose is to stay sober and help other alcoholics to achieve sobriety. (Alcoholics Anonymous 1992)

The AA General Service Office (Box 459, Grand Central Station, New York, NY 10163) publishes a variety of pamphlets and books that describe what AA is, share AA wisdom, and guide recovering alcoholic persons. The AA literature is available in several different languages and can be ordered through AA by telephone (212-870-3400).

The best known of the AA literature is *Alcoholics Anonymous*, known as the "Big Book." First published in 1939, it has sold nearly 30 million copies. Bill Wilson wrote the first 164 pages, after which personal stories are presented.

The 12 Steps and 12 Traditions

The 12 steps (Table 14–3) and the 12 traditions (Table 14–4) summarize the principles of AA and are widely printed, in formats ranging from wallet cards to placards. One gains sobriety, in part, by working through the 12 steps. The 12 traditions reinforce the integrity of the AA approach. Sponsorship is another structured feature of AA.

Each new member is encouraged to have a sponsor. The sponsor is an experienced member of AA with a respectable track record of sobriety. Typically, one would be expected to be sober at least 1 year before becoming a sponsor. A sponsor is a mentor. He or she is available for phone calls and works the steps with the newcomer—especially Steps 4 and 5, in which the new member makes "a fearless moral inventory" (Step 4) of himself or herself and shares the same (Step 5) with his or her sponsor.

AA emphasizes "principles before personalities"—that is, individuals are encouraged to choose a sponsor who will best allow them to grow within the program. The sponsor does not have to be the best friend you ever had or be socioeconomically or temperamentally similar. Some sponsors are very easygoing and put few demands on the fellow member, whereas others require daily readings and daily contact.

AA is not effective simply by having established the structures outlined here. The process of AA is a powerful but not fully understood dynamic. This process includes spiritual growth, a tempering of pathological narcissism, empathy, interpersonal support, group adhesion, and variables perhaps as unique as each individual participant. (A review of possible mechanisms can be found in Nace 2005 or Tonigan and Connors 2008.)

TABLE 14–3. **The 12 steps of Alcoholics Anonymous**

1. We admitted we were powerless over alcohol—that our lives had become unmanageable.

2. Came to believe that a Power greater than ourselves could restore us to sanity.

3. Made a decision to turn our will and our lives over to the care of God as we understood Him.

4. Made a searching and fearless moral inventory of ourselves.

5. Admitted to God, to ourselves, and to another human being the exact nature of our wrongs.

6. Were entirely ready to have God remove all these defects of character.

7. Humbly asked Him to remove our shortcomings.

8. Made a list of all persons we had harmed, and became willing to make amends to them all.

9. Made direct amends to such people wherever possible, except when to do so would injure them or others.

10. Continued to take personal inventory and when we were wrong promptly admitted it.

11. Sought through prayer and meditation to improve our conscious contact with God, as we understood Him, praying only for knowledge of His will for us and the power to carry that out.

12. Having had a spiritual awakening as the result of these Steps, we tried to carry this message to alcoholics, and to practice these principles in all our affairs.

Source. Reprinted from Alcoholics Anonymous: *Twelve Steps and Twelve Traditions.* New York, Alcoholics Anonymous World Services, 1978. Used with permission.

The Experiences of Patients

Clinicians will find that patients in AA feel understood. They feel accepted. They are not judged or expected to change their personalities. They are encouraged to "keep coming back" and are not told what to do but rather are told what worked for others.

> **Sarah,** as an infant, would hold her breath when her mother left the room. This protest over separation led, at times, to loss of consciousness. Later, Sarah dreaded school and recalls daily anxiety at the start of class each day, including through graduate school. She obtained a doctorate degree in spite of escalating alcohol use. Her teaching career was checkered with unexplained absences (related to binge drinking) and eventually with episodes of rehabilitation and hospitalization. Brief periods of sobriety were punctuated with binge drinking, which often involved having 24 beers per day. By her 30s, Sarah had gained control over her lifelong severe anxiety disorder through use of a variety of medications, but the drinking continued.

TABLE 14–4. **The 12 traditions of Alcoholics Anonymous (AA)**

1. Our common welfare should come first; personal recovery depends upon AA unity.

2. For our group purpose there is but one ultimate authority—a loving God as He may express Himself in our group conscience. Our leaders are but trusted servants; they do not govern.

3. The only requirement for AA membership is a desire to stop drinking.

4. Each group should be autonomous except in matters affecting other groups or AA as a whole.

5. Each group has but one primary purpose—to carry its message to the alcoholic who still suffers.

6. An AA group ought never endorse, finance, or lend the AA name to any related facility or outside enterprise, lest problems of money, property, and prestige divert us from our primary purpose.

7. Every AA group ought to be fully self-supporting, declining outside contributions.

8. Alcoholics Anonymous should remain forever nonprofessional, but our service centers may employ special workers.

9. AA, as such, ought never be organized; but we may create special service boards or committees directly responsible to those they serve.

10. Alcoholics Anonymous has no opinion on outside issues; hence the AA name ought never be drawn into public controversy.

11. Our public relations policy is based on attraction rather than promotion; we need always maintain personal anonymity at the level of press, radio, and films.

12. Anonymity is the spiritual foundation of all our Traditions, ever reminding us to place principles before personalities.

Source. Reprinted from Alcoholics Anonymous: *Twelve Steps and Twelve Traditions.* New York, Alcoholics Anonymous World Services, 1978. Used with permission.

Sarah grew up in a middle-class home free of alcohol or drug problems. Her mother was "nervous" but not formally diagnosed. Sarah, her two siblings, and her parents had no religious affiliation. This was a home indifferent to spirituality, religion, or ultimate concerns.

Her psychiatrist continually urged her to try AA. Her discomfort with the "religiosity" kept her away. The tedious pattern of frequent (once or twice per week) heavy binge drinking, her growing social isolation, and a developing depression resulted in a return to a 30-day inpatient rehabilitation program. She found fault with much of the program, but gradually and unexpectedly felt early promptings of an inner peace. Early one morning, she saw a deer on the grounds of this rural rehabilitation center. The deer paused, fixed its gaze on Sarah, and then cantered across the field. Her delight in this natural scene was followed by an unfolding acceptance—an acceptance of who she was, her powerlessness over many things in her life, and her powerlessness over alcohol. She heard the AA message differently at this point. It was comforting; it made sense. Her natural intellectual curiosity prompted her to read widely the "Big Book," *Twelve Steps and Twelve Traditions*, and, eventually, Christian texts provided by her sponsor.

Sarah's commitment to sobriety is firm. She is pensive about the years she lived in spiritual indifference. She is seeking to know God, and her mother and sister are joining her. Periodic intense cravings occur. The cravings have reduced her to tears at times, but she has learned to reach out to others and is gaining confidence without complacency. The absence of alcohol has diminished her anxiety. She is taking less medication, and psychotherapy with her psychiatrist has shifted in depth.

Sarah's case is illustrative in several ways: the ease with which religion and ultimate concerns can be ignored in a comfortable materialistic culture; the transmission of this indifference from one generation to another; and the eventual discovery of a drug (in her case, alcohol) to relieve dysphoria and transform (however briefly) one's sense of self. Furthermore, the dependency on alcohol secondary to her anxiety disorder led to occupational and social dysfunction, loss of control, and despair. A concerned physician steered her back to an intensive recovery program. From there, a transforming spiritual reality was experienced. Sarah did not ignore this experience but embraced it, undeterred by cognitive dissonance. The AA program, the gentle mentoring of a sponsor, and the surprising support of her family opened the future for Sarah—a future where her considerable talents can be realized.

Hope, cohesiveness, acceptance, and other positive aspects of the AA experience bind many fledgling members to the fellowship. The incentive to drink remains powerful for many, even some who successfully engage in the program. Relapses are accepted—indeed, they are expected—and no one is turned away or dismissed from AA as a result of relapse. A drunken participant may be asked to leave a meeting but is encouraged to return the following day.

> **Roy,** a 48-year-old internist, returned from his third inpatient rehabilitation treatment for alcohol dependence. His response to treatment over the past 6 years had been poor. AA attendance had been sporadic. Psychotherapy had been provided by a variety of professionals. Now he faced major changes: His wife had filed for divorce while he was in residential treatment. He was not allowed to return to his home, was not permitted by his wife to accompany their 18-year-old daughter to the university she was about to attend, and had a hostile relationship with his 20-year-old son, who was also alcoholic.
>
> After 1 week of trying to reengage with his family, Roy began drinking. He called his previous psychiatrist on a Sunday night, was seen the next

morning, and started taking disulfiram and an antidepressant. The psychiatrist, who was familiar with Roy's extensive treatment history, encouraged him to try to turn things around on an outpatient basis. Roy was relieved that he could continue his work, which was largely administrative rather than clinical. After the Monday appointment, he was seen on Wednesday of the same week and scheduled for Friday morning. On Thursday night, he was sleepless. Roy, a person without a commitment to religion or spirituality, had an inchoate sense of God and was what is often referred to as a "cultural Christian," in contrast to a "believer." Yet on that Thursday night, something changed. Roy reported that he prayed to God that he would either stop craving alcohol or be allowed to drink himself to death. The constant tension between wanting/needing a drink and the obvious consequences had become intolerable.

Roy showed up at his appointment that Friday morning reporting that he had lost the desire to drink. He did not know how; there had been no "white light" experience. He knew that he had felt desperate and prayed desperately. Neither his psychiatrist nor Roy knew quite what to make of this, but at least Roy seemed safe to remain on outpatient status. A week later he stopped taking disulfiram, confident that the tension over alcohol was over. It was. Six years later, he remains sober and married. He and his son conduct an AA meeting at a halfway house for newly released prisoners. He still has not become "religious," but he remains grateful for a transformation that reversed his downward spiral.

In addition to the craving or incentive to return to alcohol, many people encountering AA have personal reactions that deter their participation. The clinician should be alert to the following common responses and motivate the patient to overcome them.

- *"I wasn't as bad as that."* Patients often find differences between themselves and the people they meet at AA. The patient may never have been in jail or lost a job. Regardless of specific experiences, the AA wisdom is to look for similarities, not differences.
- *"I can't identify with that group."* Perhaps the participants seem too young, too old, or not up to one's social standards. Such responses often serve a defensive function. The clinician can encourage the patient to visit other groups or help the patient gain a deeper understanding of his or her resistances.
- *"They're too religious"* or *"It's a cult."* Further exposure is always necessary. These invalid responses typically serve as a defense against relinquishing the dependency on alcohol. Repeated exposure to AA, including visiting different meetings, is likely to vitiate these initial problematic reactions.
- *"Someone tried to hit on me."* It is possible, but not very common, that an AA member will use the group as a potential source for sexual com-

panionship. Other meetings may be chosen. Furthermore, the newcomer may use such an experience to learn how to set boundaries and to develop his or her priorities.

Clinicians' exhortations to patients to attend meetings as part of their recovery will tap into some patients' pathology beyond the expected denial and defensive efforts listed here. Two categories stand out: those with anxiety disorders and those with paranoid or schizoid features. Examples are provided in the following cases:

> **Phil,** a college student, was taken home from his university after a near-suicide attempt—Phil had been drunk while making preparations to overdose. His fraternity brothers called his parents. This was his third suicide attempt (all of which had occurred while drunk) in 12 months. Phil knew he was alcoholic, feared drinking because of the subsequent severe depression, and wanted help. He wanted to try AA again. The anxiety that built up as he thought of attending meetings was more than he wanted to endure. He would probably have to drink just to get there. Phil had a severe pervasive social phobia. Sertraline gradually began to dampen his symptoms, and injectable naltrexone lessened his alcohol cravings. With encouragement as well as pressure from his parents, he reluctantly agreed to try AA again. Emphasis was placed on not letting his symptoms control his life and on moving out into a venue that would assist him in his goal of sobriety. Phil built on his earlier success in attending classes, because he knew that as he became familiar with group members, attendance would be easier.

> **George** had tried several rehabilitation programs over the previous 10 years. Now in his mid-50s, he was living alone, alienated from his siblings, and trying to maintain a family apartment rental business. He called his doctor to get chlordiazepoxide (Librium). George did not trust people. There was a woman he thought he might marry. Although she was a "chronic liar," he figured that she could help take care of him. George was experiencing alcohol withdrawal seizures more frequently. He ranted against AA, rehabilitation, and so on. He was inclined to give his views on God, religion, and the evils he saw in these concepts, rather than focus on his increasingly acute alcohol-related complications. He was haughty and always disdainful of what his doctor and others advised. George's mixed personality disorder included schizoid, paranoid, and narcissistic traits. He remained noncompliant except during the most acute crisis, which typically took place during his efforts to taper his drinking. There have been no indications of a change in attitude for George, and his prognosis would seem poor.

Physicians who treat alcoholic persons encounter resistance in most patients. Persistence on the physician's part can lead patients to either grateful improvement and acceptance of their alcoholism or, less common, a transferring awareness of their condition and a willingness to follow the program of AA and other treatment recommendations. Some circumstances involve comorbid conditions, as the previous two cases illustrate. Specific attention to comorbidity in synchrony with addressing the substance use disorder is essential.

The Reach of Alcoholics Anonymous

Since AA's founding in 1935, its reach to alcoholic individuals has been monumental, extending to more than 2 million members in more than 100,000 groups across at least 150 countries. These numbers, however, portray only one facet of AA's reach. AA's influence is found in many facets of today's efforts to address substance use disorders.

- Marty Mann, a woman who recovered from alcoholism in the early 1940s (with the help of AA) had a vision of educating the public about alcoholism. She shared her vision with Bill Wilson, but Bill, in accord with AA tradition, did not want to directly affiliate AA with a public educational campaign. Ms. Mann sought advice from Dr. E. M. Jellinek, who was affiliated with the Yale Center for Alcohol Studies. Jellinek, a scientist, found funding for Mann, whose primary "credentials" were her personal recovery and her zeal to educate the public. Mann founded the National Committee for Education on Alcoholism in 1944. In 1954, the group became known as the National Council on Alcoholism, and Mann served as director of this committee from 1954 to 1968. She lectured across the country for 35 years and influenced legislation to formulate a public health response to alcoholism (White 1998).
- A second sphere of influence has been the infusion of AA tenets in professionally based treatment programs. The Minnesota Model exemplifies the changed attitudes toward alcoholic persons that were emerging in the mid-twentieth century. This model has dominated the alcoholism treatment industry and still survives to some extent in the era of managed care. The model asserts that 1) alcoholism is involuntary and a primary disease, 2) alcoholism is chronic and progressive, 3) a multidisciplinary team with recovery counselors is the optimal approach, and 4) AA step work and follow-up are critical (Anderson 1981).
- The Minnesota Model integrated professionally managed treatment with the grassroots model of AA. Spirituality became a component of professional treatment, and the model has been extended to the treatment of drug abuse.

- Most self-help groups today borrow, with modifications, the 12-step approach of AA. Narcotics Anonymous, Cocaine Anonymous, Gamblers Anonymous, and Overeaters Anonymous are examples. Al-Anon is an additional example that provides a 12-step formulation for family members of an alcoholic person.

Conclusion

AA was preceded by temperance societies, fraternal organizations, and religious groups that had an interest in arresting the destruction wrought by alcoholism. The commitment of two recovered alcoholic men led to the founding of the most successful approach to alcoholism to date—Alcoholics Anonymous. AA has skillfully avoided extending its reach beyond helping alcoholic persons. It has a clear structure to follow for the individual desiring not to drink. The success of the AA program is reflected in the number of participants and its spread across the world. Furthermore, the AA approach has influenced modern rehabilitation efforts and most self-help groups.

Key Clinical Concepts

- The founding of AA was the culmination of decades of effort to help alcoholic persons by religious organizations, secular groups, and physicians.
- The integrity of the AA organization has been sustained by avoiding any affiliation with outside entities and by remaining faithful to its mission to help alcoholic individuals.
- The fellowship of AA provides a structure for daily living through appreciation of the 12 steps and 12 traditions that foster sobriety and personal maturity.
- The efficacy of AA is reflected by its growth, its influence on substance abuse treatment programs, and the increasing referral to AA by health care providers.

Suggested Reading

Alcoholics Anonymous: Twelve Steps and Twelve Traditions. New York, Alcoholics Anonymous World Services, 1978

Alcoholics Anonymous: Alcoholics Anonymous, 4th Edition. New York, Alcoholics Anonymous World Services, 2001

Kurtz E: Not-God: A History of Alcoholics Anonymous. Center City, MN, Hazelden, 1979

Thomsen R: Bill W. New York, Harper & Row, 1975

White WL: Slaying the Dragon: The History of Addiction Treatment and Recovery in America. Bloomington, IL, Chestnut Health Systems/Lighthouse Institute, 1998

References

Alcoholics Anonymous: Twelve Steps and Twelve Traditions. New York, Alcoholics Anonymous World Services, 1978

Alcoholics Anonymous: Grapevine. New York, The AA Grapevine, 1992

Alcoholics Anonymous: Estimates of AA Groups and Members. 2007. Available at: http://www.aa.org/en_media_ resources.cfm?PageID=74. Accessed February 24, 2010.

Anderson D: Perspectives on Treatment: The Minnesota Experience. Center City, MN, Hazelden Educational Materials, 1981

Book Reviews: Alcoholics Anonymous. J Nerv Ment Dis 92:399, 1940

Fahey DM: Temperance and Racism: John Bull, Johnny Reb, and the Good Templars. Lexington, KY, Lexington University Press, 1996

Forcehimes AA, Feldstein SW, Miller WR: Glatt's curve revisited: a study investigating the progression of recovery in Alcoholics Anonymous. Alcohol Treat Q 26:241–258, 2008

James W: The Varieties of Religious Experience (1902). Cambridge, MA, Harvard University Press, 1985

Kurtz E: Not-God: A History of Alcoholics Anonymous. Center City, MN, Hazelden, 1979

Maxwell M: The Washingtonian movement. Q J Stud Alcohol 2:410–451, 1950

Miller WR, C'de Baca J: Quantum Change: When Epiphanies and Sudden Insights Transform Ordinary Lives. New York, Guilford, 2001

Nace EP: Alcoholics Anonymous, in Substance Abuse: A Comprehensive Textbook, 4th Edition. Edited by Lowinson JH, Ruiz P, Millman RB, et al. Philadelphia, PA, Lippincott Williams & Wilkins, 2005, pp 587–599

Prochaska J, DiClemente C: The Transtheoretical Approach: Crossing Traditional Boundaries of Theory. Chicago, IL, Dow Jones Irwin, 1984

Thomsen R: Bill W. New York, Harper & Row, 1975

Tonigan JS, Connors GJ: Psychological mechanisms in Alcoholics Anonymous, in The American Psychiatric Publishing Textbook of Substance Abuse Treatment, 4th Edition. Edited by Galanter M, Kleber HD. Washington, DC, American Psychiatric Publishing, 2008, pp 491–498

Tyrell I: Sobering Up. Westport, CT, Greenwood Press, 1979

Webster's New Twentieth Century Dictionary of the English Language, Unabridged, 2nd Edition. New York, William Collins, 1980

White WL: Slaying the Dragon: The History of Addiction Treatment and Recovery in America. Bloomington, IL, Chestnut Health Systems/Lighthouse Institute, 1998

Wilson WG: Alcoholics Anonymous Comes of Age. New York, Alcoholics Anonymous Publishing, 1957

Index

Page numbers printed in **boldface** type refer to tables or figures.